ACCESS YOUR ONLINE RESOURCES

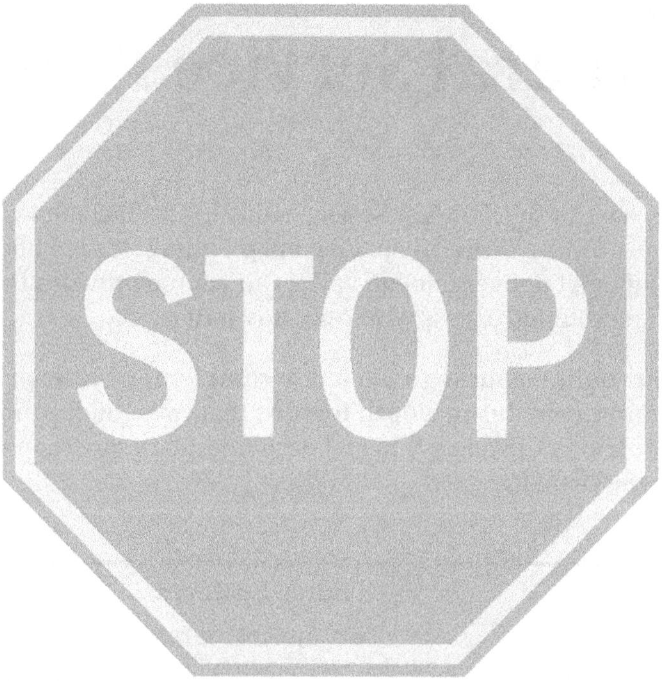

DON'T MISS OUT ON THE ONLINE RESOURCES INCLUDED WITH YOUR PURCHASE!

Your purchase of this product unlocks access to our Online Resources page. Elevate your study experience with our **interactive practice test interface**, along with all of the additional resources that we couldn't include in this book.

Flip to the Online Resources section at the end of this book to find the link and a QR code to get started!

Mometrix
TEST PREPARATION

Mometrix TEST PREPARATION

Funeral Service Exam Secrets Study Guide

Written and edited by the Mometrix Funeral Director Certification Test Team

Mometrix offers volume discount pricing to institutions. For more information or a price quote, please contact our sales department at sales@mometrix.com or 888-248-1219.

Paperback
ISBN 13: 978-1-60971-768-1
ISBN 10: 1-60971-768-6

Ebook
ISBN 13: 978-1-62120-568-5
ISBN 10: 1-62120-568-1

Hardback
ISBN 13: 978-1-5167-0572-6
ISBN 10: 1-5167-0572-6

DEAR FUTURE EXAM SUCCESS STORY

First of all, **THANK YOU** for purchasing Mometrix study materials!

Second, congratulations! You are one of the few determined test-takers who are committed to doing whatever it takes to excel on your exam. **You have come to the right place.** We developed these study materials with one goal in mind: to deliver you the information you need in a format that's concise and easy to use.

In addition to optimizing your guide for the content of the test, we've outlined our recommended steps for breaking down the preparation process into small, attainable goals so you can make sure you stay on track.

We've also analyzed the entire test-taking process, identifying the most common pitfalls and showing how you can overcome them and be ready for any curveball the test throws you.

Standardized testing is one of the biggest obstacles on your road to success, which only increases the importance of doing well in the high-pressure, high-stakes environment of test day. Your results on this test could have a significant impact on your future, and this guide provides the information and practical advice to help you achieve your full potential on test day.

Your success is our success

We would love to hear from you! If you would like to share the story of your exam success or if you have any questions or comments in regard to our products, please contact us at **800-673-8175** or **support@mometrix.com**.

Thanks again for your business and we wish you continued success!

Sincerely,
The Mometrix Test Preparation Team

TABLE OF CONTENTS

Introduction

Thank you for purchasing this resource! You have made the choice to prepare yourself for a test that could have a huge impact on your future, and this guide is designed to help you be fully ready for test day. Obviously, it's important to have a solid understanding of the test material, but you also need to be prepared for the unique environment and stressors of the test, so that you can perform to the best of your abilities.

For this purpose, the first section that appears in this guide is the **Secret Keys**. We've devoted countless hours to meticulously researching what works and what doesn't, and we've boiled down our findings to the five most impactful steps you can take to improve your performance on the test. We start at the beginning with study planning and move through the preparation process, all the way to the testing strategies that will help you get the most out of what you know when you're finally sitting in front of the test.

We recommend that you start preparing for your test as far in advance as possible. However, if you've bought this guide as a last-minute study resource and only have a few days before your test, we recommend that you skip over the first two Secret Keys since they address a long-term study plan.

If you struggle with **test anxiety**, we strongly encourage you to check out our recommendations for how you can overcome it. Test anxiety is a formidable foe, but it can be beaten, and we want to make sure you have the tools you need to defeat it.

Secret Key #1 – Plan Big, Study Small

There's a lot riding on your performance. If you want to ace this test, you're going to need to keep your skills sharp and the material fresh in your mind. You need a plan that lets you review everything you need to know while still fitting in your schedule. We'll break this strategy down into three categories.

Information Organization

Start with the information you already have: the official test outline. From this, you can make a complete list of all the concepts you need to cover before the test. Organize these concepts into groups that can be studied together, and create a list of any related vocabulary you need to learn so you can brush up on any difficult terms. You'll want to keep this vocabulary list handy once you actually start studying since you may need to add to it along the way.

Time Management

Once you have your set of study concepts, decide how to spread them out over the time you have left before the test. Break your study plan into small, clear goals so you have a manageable task for each day and know exactly what you're doing. Then just focus on one small step at a time. When you manage your time this way, you don't need to spend hours at a time studying. Studying a small block of content for a short period each day helps you retain information better and avoid stressing over how much you have left to do. You can relax knowing that you have a plan to cover everything in time. In order for this strategy to be effective though, you have to start studying early and stick to your schedule. Avoid the exhaustion and futility that comes from last-minute cramming!

Study Environment

The environment you study in has a big impact on your learning. Studying in a coffee shop, while probably more enjoyable, is not likely to be as fruitful as studying in a quiet room. It's important to keep distractions to a minimum. You're only planning to study for a short block of time, so make the most of it. Don't pause to check your phone or get up to find a snack. It's also important to **avoid multitasking**. Research has consistently shown that multitasking will make your studying dramatically less effective. Your study area should also be comfortable and well-lit so you don't have the distraction of straining your eyes or sitting on an uncomfortable chair.

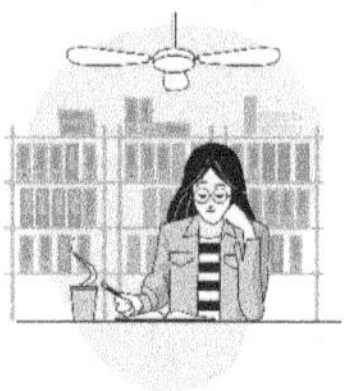

The time of day you study is also important. You want to be rested and alert. Don't wait until just before bedtime. Study when you'll be most likely to comprehend and remember. Even better, if you know what time of day your test will be, set that time aside for study. That way your brain will be used to working on that subject at that specific time and you'll have a better chance of recalling information.

Finally, it can be helpful to team up with others who are studying for the same test. Your actual studying should be done in as isolated an environment as possible, but the work of organizing the information and setting up the study plan can be divided up. In between study sessions, you can discuss with your teammates the concepts that you're all studying and quiz each other on the details. Just be sure that your teammates are as serious about the test as you are. If you find that your study time is being replaced with social time, you might need to find a new team.

Secret Key #2 – Make Your Studying Count

You're devoting a lot of time and effort to preparing for this test, so you want to be absolutely certain it will pay off. This means doing more than just reading the content and hoping you can remember it on test day. It's important to make every minute of study count. There are two main areas you can focus on to make your studying count.

Retention

It doesn't matter how much time you study if you can't remember the material. You need to make sure you are retaining the concepts. To check your retention of the information you're learning, try recalling it at later times with minimal prompting. Try carrying around flashcards and glance at one or two from time to time or ask a friend who's also studying for the test to quiz you.

To enhance your retention, look for ways to put the information into practice so that you can apply it rather than simply recalling it. If you're using the information in practical ways, it will be much easier to remember. Similarly, it helps to solidify a concept in your mind if you're not only reading it to yourself but also explaining it to someone else. Ask a friend to let you teach them about a concept you're a little shaky on (or speak aloud to an imaginary audience if necessary). As you try to summarize, define, give examples, and answer your friend's questions, you'll understand the concepts better and they will stay with you longer. Finally, step back for a big picture view and ask yourself how each piece of information fits with the whole subject. When you link the different concepts together and see them working together as a whole, it's easier to remember the individual components.

Finally, practice showing your work on any multi-step problems, even if you're just studying. Writing out each step you take to solve a problem will help solidify the process in your mind, and you'll be more likely to remember it during the test.

Modality

Modality simply refers to the means or method by which you study. Choosing a study modality that fits your own individual learning style is crucial. No two people learn best in exactly the same way, so it's important to know your strengths and use them to your advantage.

For example, if you learn best by visualization, focus on visualizing a concept in your mind and draw an image or a diagram. Try color-coding your notes, illustrating them, or creating symbols that will trigger your mind to recall a learned concept. If you learn best by hearing or discussing information, find a study partner who learns the same way or read aloud to yourself. Think about how to put the information in your own words. Imagine that you are giving a lecture on the topic and record yourself so you can listen to it later.

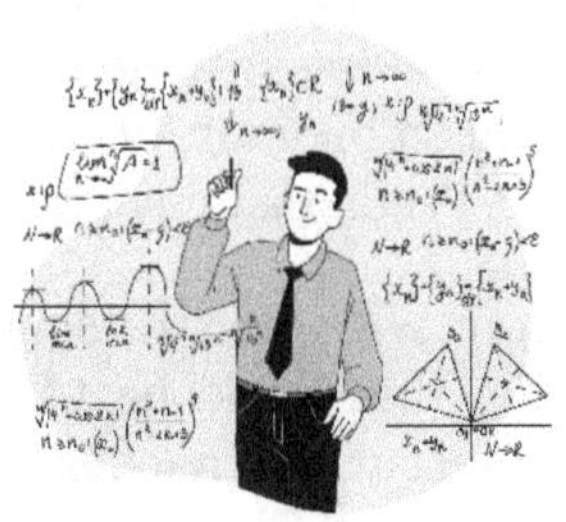

For any learning style, flashcards can be helpful. Organize the information so you can take advantage of spare moments to review. Underline key words or phrases. Use different colors for different categories. Mnemonic devices (such as creating a short list in which every item starts with the same letter) can also help with retention. Find what works best for you and use it to store the information in your mind most effectively and easily.

Secret Key #3 – Practice the Right Way

Your success on test day depends not only on how many hours you put into preparing, but also on whether you prepared the right way. It's good to check along the way to see if your studying is paying off. One of the most effective ways to do this is by taking practice tests to evaluate your progress. Practice tests are useful because they show exactly where you need to improve. Every time you take a practice test, pay special attention to these three groups of questions:

- The questions you got wrong
- The questions you had to guess on, even if you guessed right
- The questions you found difficult or slow to work through

This will show you exactly what your weak areas are, and where you need to devote more study time. Ask yourself why each of these questions gave you trouble. Was it because you didn't understand the material? Was it because you didn't remember the vocabulary? Do you need more repetitions on this type of question to build speed and confidence? Dig into those questions and figure out how you can strengthen your weak areas as you go back to review the material.

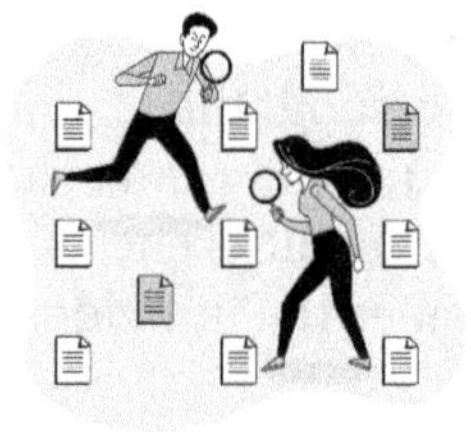

Additionally, many practice tests have a section explaining the answer choices. It can be tempting to read the explanation and think that you now have a good understanding of the concept. However, an explanation likely only covers part of the question's broader context. Even if the explanation makes perfect sense, **go back and investigate** every concept related to the question until you're positive you have a thorough understanding.

As you go along, keep in mind that the practice test is just that: practice. Memorizing these questions and answers will not be very helpful on the actual test because it is unlikely to have any of the same exact questions. If you only know the right answers to the sample questions, you won't be prepared for the real thing. **Study the concepts** until you understand them fully, and then you'll be able to answer any question that shows up on the test.

It's important to wait on the practice tests until you're ready. If you take a test on your first day of study, you may be overwhelmed by the amount of material covered and how much you need to learn. Work up to it gradually.

On test day, you'll need to be prepared for answering questions, managing your time, and using the test-taking strategies you've learned. It's a lot to balance, like a mental marathon that will have a big impact on your future. Like training for a marathon, you'll need to start slowly and work your way up. When test day arrives, you'll be ready.

Start with the strategies you've read in the first two Secret Keys—plan your course and study in the way that works best for you. If you have time, consider using multiple study resources to get different approaches to the same concepts. It can be helpful to see difficult concepts from more than one angle. Then find a good source for practice tests. Many times, the test website will suggest potential study resources or provide sample tests.

Practice Test Strategy

If you're able to find at least three practice tests, we recommend this strategy:

UNTIMED AND OPEN-BOOK PRACTICE

Take the first test with no time constraints and with your notes and study guide handy. Take your time and focus on applying the strategies you've learned.

TIMED AND OPEN-BOOK PRACTICE

Take the second practice test open-book as well, but set a timer and practice pacing yourself to finish in time.

TIMED AND CLOSED-BOOK PRACTICE

Take any other practice tests as if it were test day. Set a timer and put away your study materials. Sit at a table or desk in a quiet room, imagine yourself at the testing center, and answer questions as quickly and accurately as possible.

Keep repeating timed and closed-book tests on a regular basis until you run out of practice tests or it's time for the actual test. Your mind will be ready for the schedule and stress of test day, and you'll be able to focus on recalling the material you've learned.

Secret Key #4 – Pace Yourself

Once you're fully prepared for the material on the test, your biggest challenge on test day will be managing your time. Just knowing that the clock is ticking can make you panic even if you have plenty of time left. Work on pacing yourself so you can build confidence against the time constraints of the exam. Pacing is a difficult skill to master, especially in a high-pressure environment, so **practice is vital**.

Set time expectations for your pace based on how much time is available. For example, if a section has 60 questions and the time limit is 30 minutes, you know you have to average 30 seconds or less per question in order to answer them all. Although 30 seconds is the hard limit, set 25 seconds per question as your goal, so you reserve extra time to spend on harder questions. When you budget extra time for the harder questions, you no longer have any reason to stress when those questions take longer to answer.

Don't let this time expectation distract you from working through the test at a calm, steady pace, but keep it in mind so you don't spend too much time on any one question. Recognize that taking extra time on one question you don't understand may keep you from answering two that you do understand later in the test. If your time limit for a question is up and you're still not sure of the answer, mark it and move on, and come back to it later if the time and the test format allow. If the testing format doesn't allow you to return to earlier questions, just make an educated guess; then put it out of your mind and move on.

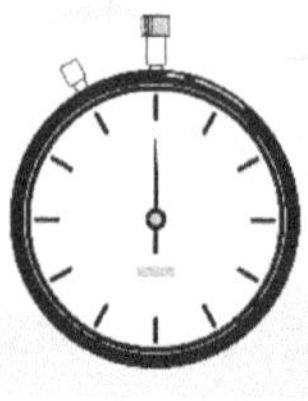

On the easier questions, be careful not to rush. It may seem wise to hurry through them so you have more time for the challenging ones, but it's not worth missing one if you know the concept and just didn't take the time to read the question fully. Work efficiently but make sure you understand the question and have looked at all of the answer choices, since more than one may seem right at first.

Even if you're paying attention to the time, you may find yourself a little behind at some point. You should speed up to get back on track, but do so wisely. Don't panic; just take a few seconds less on each question until you're caught up. Don't guess without thinking, but do look through the answer choices and eliminate any you know are wrong. If you can get down to two choices, it is often worthwhile to guess from those. Once you've chosen an answer, move on and don't dwell on any that you skipped or had to hurry through. If a question was taking too long, chances are it was one of the harder ones, so you weren't as likely to get it right anyway.

On the other hand, if you find yourself getting ahead of schedule, it may be beneficial to slow down a little. The more quickly you work, the more likely you are to make a careless mistake that will affect your score. You've budgeted time for each question, so don't be afraid to spend that time. Practice an efficient but careful pace to get the most out of the time you have.

Secret Key #5 – Have a Plan for Guessing

When you're taking the test, you may find yourself stuck on a question. Some of the answer choices seem better than others, but you don't see the one answer choice that is obviously correct. What do you do?

The scenario described above is very common, yet most test takers have not effectively prepared for it. Developing and practicing a plan for guessing may be one of the single most effective uses of your time as you get ready for the exam.

In developing your plan for guessing, there are three questions to address:

- When should you start the guessing process?
- How should you narrow down the choices?
- Which answer should you choose?

When to Start the Guessing Process

Unless your plan for guessing is to select C every time (which, despite its merits, is not what we recommend), you need to leave yourself enough time to apply your answer elimination strategies. Since you have a limited amount of time for each question, that means that if you're going to give yourself the best shot at guessing correctly, you have to decide quickly whether or not you will guess.

Of course, the best-case scenario is that you don't have to guess at all, so first, see if you can answer the question based on your knowledge of the subject and basic reasoning skills. Focus on the key words in the question and try to jog your memory of related topics. Give yourself a chance to bring the knowledge to mind, but once you realize that you don't have (or you can't access) the knowledge you need to answer the question, it's time to start the guessing process.

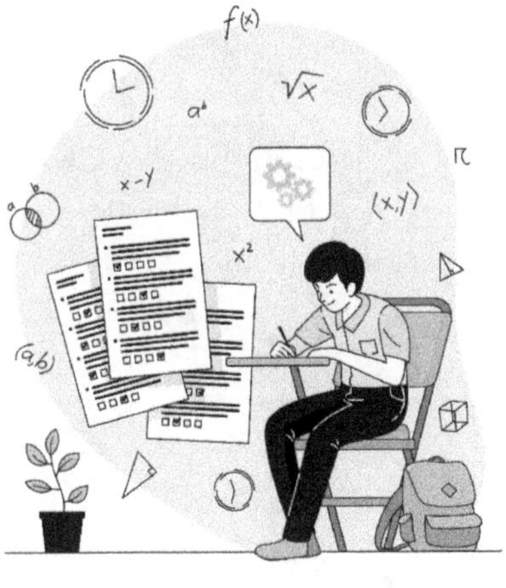

It's almost always better to start the guessing process too early than too late. It only takes a few seconds to remember something and answer the question from knowledge. Carefully eliminating wrong answer choices takes longer. Plus, going through the process of eliminating answer choices can actually help jog your memory.

Summary: Start the guessing process as soon as you decide that you can't answer the question based on your knowledge.

How to Narrow Down the Choices

The next chapter in this book (**Test-Taking Strategies**) includes a wide range of strategies for how to approach questions and how to look for answer choices to eliminate. You will definitely want to read those carefully, practice them, and figure out which ones work best for you. Here though, we're going to address a mindset rather than a particular strategy.

Your odds of guessing an answer correctly depend on how many options you are choosing from.

Number of options left	5	4	3	2	1
Odds of guessing correctly	20%	25%	33%	50%	100%

You can see from this chart just how valuable it is to be able to eliminate incorrect answers and make an educated guess, but there are two things that many test takers do that cause them to miss out on the benefits of guessing:

- Accidentally eliminating the correct answer
- Selecting an answer based on an impression

We'll look at the first one here, and the second one in the next section.

To avoid accidentally eliminating the correct answer, we recommend a thought exercise called **the $5 challenge**. In this challenge, you only eliminate an answer choice from contention if you are willing to bet $5 on it being wrong. Why $5? Five dollars is a small but not insignificant amount of money. It's an amount you could afford to lose but wouldn't want to throw away. And while losing $5 once might not hurt too much, doing it twenty times will set you back $100. In the same way, each small decision you make—eliminating a choice here, guessing on a question there—won't by itself impact your score very much, but when you put them all together, they can make a big difference. By holding each answer choice elimination decision to a higher standard, you can reduce the risk of accidentally eliminating the correct answer.

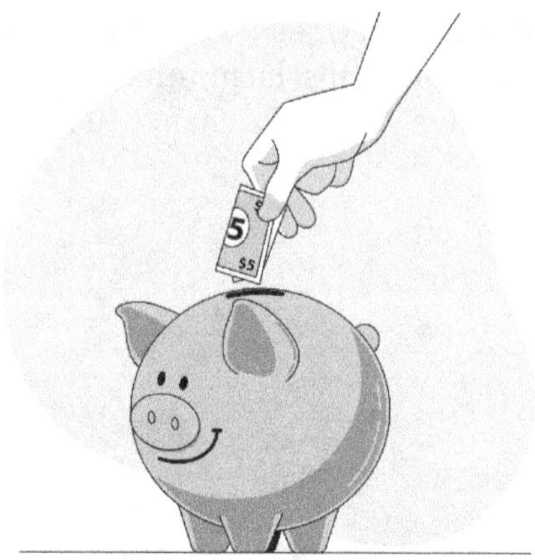

The $5 challenge can also be applied in a positive sense: If you are willing to bet $5 that an answer choice *is* correct, go ahead and mark it as correct.

Summary: Only eliminate an answer choice if you are willing to bet $5 that it is wrong.

Which Answer to Choose

You're taking the test. You've run into a hard question and decided you'll have to guess. You've eliminated all the answer choices you're willing to bet $5 on. Now you have to pick an answer. Why do we even need to talk about this? Why can't you just pick whichever one you feel like when the time comes?

The answer to these questions is that if you don't come into the test with a plan, you'll rely on your impression to select an answer choice, and if you do that, you risk falling into a trap. The test writers know that everyone who takes their test will be guessing on some of the questions, so they intentionally write wrong answer choices to seem plausible. You still have to pick an answer though, and if the wrong answer choices are designed to look right, how can you ever be sure that you're not falling for their trap? The best solution we've found to this dilemma is to take the decision out of your hands entirely. Here is the process we recommend:

Once you've eliminated any choices that you are confident (willing to bet $5) are wrong, select the first remaining choice as your answer.

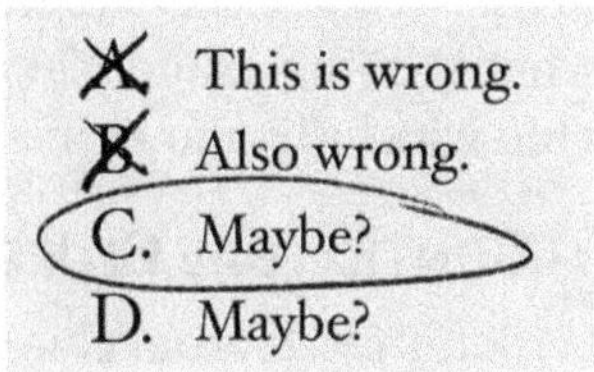

Whether you choose to select the first remaining choice, the second, or the last, the important thing is that you use some preselected standard. Using this approach guarantees that you will not be enticed into selecting an answer choice that looks right, because you are not basing your decision on how the answer choices look.

This is not meant to make you question your knowledge. Instead, it is to help you recognize the difference between your knowledge and your impressions. There's a huge difference between thinking an answer is right because of what you know, and thinking an answer is right because it looks or sounds like it should be right.

Summary: To ensure that your selection is appropriately random, make a predetermined selection from among all answer choices you have not eliminated.

Test-Taking Strategies

This section contains a list of test-taking strategies that you may find helpful as you work through the test. By taking what you know and applying logical thought, you can maximize your chances of answering any question correctly!

It is very important to realize that every question is different and every person is different: no single strategy will work on every question, and no single strategy will work for every person. That's why we've included all of them here, so you can try them out and determine which ones work best for different types of questions and which ones work best for you.

Question Strategies

✓ Read Carefully

Read the question and the answer choices carefully. Don't miss the question because you misread the terms. You have plenty of time to read each question thoroughly and make sure you understand what is being asked. Yet a happy medium must be attained, so don't waste too much time. You must read carefully and efficiently.

✓ Contextual Clues

Look for contextual clues. If the question includes a word you are not familiar with, look at the immediate context for some indication of what the word might mean. Contextual clues can often give you all the information you need to decipher the meaning of an unfamiliar word. Even if you can't determine the meaning, you may be able to narrow down the possibilities enough to make a solid guess at the answer to the question.

✓ Prefixes

If you're having trouble with a word in the question or answer choices, try dissecting it. Take advantage of every clue that the word might include. Prefixes can be a huge help. Usually, they allow you to determine a basic meaning. *Pre-* means before, *post-* means after, *pro-* is positive, *de-* is negative. From prefixes, you can get an idea of the general meaning of the word and try to put it into context.

✓ Hedge Words

Watch out for critical hedge words, such as *likely, may, can, often, almost, mostly, usually, generally, rarely,* and *sometimes.* Question writers insert these hedge phrases to cover every possibility. Often an answer choice will be wrong simply because it leaves no room for exception. Be on guard for answer choices that have definitive words such as *exactly* and *always.*

✓ Switchback Words

Stay alert for *switchbacks*. These are the words and phrases frequently used to alert you to shifts in thought. The most common switchback words are *but, although,* and *however*. Others include *nevertheless, on the other hand, even though, while, in spite of, despite,* and *regardless of.* Switchback words are important to catch because they can change the direction of the question or an answer choice.

⊘ Face Value

When in doubt, use common sense. Accept the situation in the problem at face value. Don't read too much into it. These problems will not require you to make wild assumptions. If you have to go beyond creativity and warp time or space in order to have an answer choice fit the question, then you should move on and consider the other answer choices. These are normal problems rooted in reality. The applicable relationship or explanation may not be readily apparent, but it is there for you to figure out. Use your common sense to interpret anything that isn't clear.

Answer Choice Strategies

⊘ Answer Selection

The most thorough way to pick an answer choice is to identify and eliminate wrong answers until only one is left, then confirm it is the correct answer. Sometimes an answer choice may immediately seem right, but be careful. The test writers will usually put more than one reasonable answer choice on each question, so take a second to read all of them and make sure that the other choices are not equally obvious. As long as you have time left, it is better to read every answer choice than to pick the first one that looks right without checking the others.

⊘ Answer Choice Families

An answer choice family consists of two (in rare cases, three) answer choices that are very similar in construction and cannot all be true at the same time. If you see two answer choices that are direct opposites or parallels, one of them is usually the correct answer. For instance, if one answer choice says that quantity x increases and another either says that quantity x decreases (opposite) or says that quantity y increases (parallel), then those answer choices would fall into the same family. An answer choice that doesn't match the construction of the answer choice family is more likely to be incorrect. Most questions will not have answer choice families, but when they do appear, you should be prepared to recognize them.

⊘ Eliminate Answers

Eliminate answer choices as soon as you realize they are wrong, but make sure you consider all possibilities. If you are eliminating answer choices and realize that the last one you are left with is also wrong, don't panic. Start over and consider each choice again. There may be something you missed the first time that you will realize on the second pass.

⊘ Avoid Fact Traps

Don't be distracted by an answer choice that is factually true but doesn't answer the question. You are looking for the choice that answers the question. Stay focused on what the question is asking for so you don't accidentally pick an answer that is true but incorrect. Always go back to the question and make sure the answer choice you've selected actually answers the question and is not merely a true statement.

⊘ Extreme Statements

In general, you should avoid answers that put forth extreme actions as standard practice or proclaim controversial ideas as established fact. An answer choice that states the "process should be used in certain situations, if..." is much more likely to be correct than one that states the "process should be discontinued completely." The first is a calm rational statement and doesn't even make a definitive, uncompromising stance, using a hedge word *if* to provide wiggle room, whereas the second choice is far more extreme.

⊘ Benchmark

As you read through the answer choices and you come across one that seems to answer the question well, mentally select that answer choice. This is not your final answer, but it's the one that will help you evaluate the other answer choices. The one that you selected is your benchmark or standard for judging each of the other answer choices. Every other answer choice must be compared to your benchmark. That choice is correct until proven otherwise by another answer choice beating it. If you find a better answer, then that one becomes your new benchmark. Once you've decided that no other choice answers the question as well as your benchmark, you have your final answer.

⊘ Predict the Answer

Before you even start looking at the answer choices, it is often best to try to predict the answer. When you come up with the answer on your own, it is easier to avoid distractions and traps because you will know exactly what to look for. The right answer choice is unlikely to be word-for-word what you came up with, but it should be a close match. Even if you are confident that you have the right answer, you should still take the time to read each option before moving on.

General Strategies

⊘ Tough Questions

If you are stumped on a problem or it appears too hard or too difficult, don't waste time. Move on! Remember though, if you can quickly check for obviously incorrect answer choices, your chances of guessing correctly are greatly improved. Before you completely give up, at least try to knock out a couple of possible answers. Eliminate what you can and then guess at the remaining answer choices before moving on.

⊘ Check Your Work

Since you will probably not know every term listed and the answer to every question, it is important that you get credit for the ones that you do know. Don't miss any questions through careless mistakes. If at all possible, try to take a second to look back over your answer selection and make sure you've selected the correct answer choice and haven't made a costly careless mistake (such as marking an answer choice that you didn't mean to mark). This quick double check should more than pay for itself in caught mistakes for the time it costs.

⊘ Pace Yourself

It's easy to be overwhelmed when you're looking at a page full of questions; your mind is confused and full of random thoughts, and the clock is ticking down faster than you would like. Calm down and maintain the pace that you have set for yourself. Especially as you get down to the last few minutes of the test, don't let the small numbers on the clock make you panic. As long as you are on track by monitoring your pace, you are guaranteed to have time for each question.

⊘ Don't Rush

It is very easy to make errors when you are in a hurry. Maintaining a fast pace in answering questions is pointless if it makes you miss questions that you would have gotten right otherwise. Test writers like to include distracting information and wrong answers that seem right. Taking a little extra time to avoid careless mistakes can make all the difference in your test score. Find a pace that allows you to be confident in the answers that you select.

⊘ Keep Moving

Panicking will not help you pass the test, so do your best to stay calm and keep moving. Taking deep breaths and going through the answer elimination steps you practiced can help to break through a stress barrier and keep your pace.

Final Notes

The combination of a solid foundation of content knowledge and the confidence that comes from practicing your plan for applying that knowledge is the key to maximizing your performance on test day. As your foundation of content knowledge is built up and strengthened, you'll find that the strategies included in this chapter become more and more effective in helping you quickly sift through the distractions and traps of the test to isolate the correct answer.

Now that you're preparing to move forward into the test content chapters of this book, be sure to keep your goal in mind. As you read, think about how you will be able to apply this information on the test. If you've already seen sample questions for the test and you have an idea of the question format and style, try to come up with questions of your own that you can answer based on what you're reading. This will give you valuable practice applying your knowledge in the same ways you can expect to on test day.

Good luck and good studying!

NBE Arts

Funeral Arranging and Directing

Notification of Death

The notification of death, or the **first call** to the funeral home, is made by the family, hospice nurse, nursing facility, or hospital to request the removal and transfer of the deceased to the funeral home. This notification is done almost exclusively (98% of the time) by telephone. It is important to obtain the address for removal. In some cases, the call may start as a simple inquiry, and the funeral director can guide the caller through various options. The Funeral Rule requires **telephone price disclosure**, so the director must be prepared with pricing information. Throughout the call, the funeral director must communicate with compassion and clarity to assist clients with difficult decisions.

Telephone Etiquette

The funeral director should answer the phone by identifying the **name of the firm** rather than using a greeting such as "good morning." The tone should be formal, with clear diction and pronunciation. While gathering the required information, the funeral director should be patient and calm, but neither cheerful nor monotone. After receiving the information, he or she should summarize the call for accuracy and should assure the client that his or her desires will be met. In closing, the director should provide an estimated time of arrival but avoid saying, "We will be right there" or "Thank you." Lastly, the funeral director should explain that the next step is the **arrangement conference** and make an appointment if possible. When the call is completed, the funeral director should wait for the client to hang up first.

First Call Form

The **first call form** (or first call sheet) is one of the most important forms in the funeral home business—it guides the funeral director in asking the necessary questions and provides a written record of the obtained information. The caller may or may not be the person who will be responsible for making the arrangements. If the caller is not the responsible person, the funeral director should obtain contact information for the responsible person. If there is a question about the cause of death, a **coroner** or **medical examiner** may request an autopsy, which is performed by the medical examiner, a pathologist, or a forensic pathologist (a medical doctor who is specifically trained to determine a cause of death). The cause of death is added to the **death certificate**, which must be signed by the physician, coroner, or medical examiner in accordance with state law. In the case of an unnatural death (accidental, suicide, homicide, undetermined, or pending determination), the death certificate must be signed by the coroner or medical examiner.

First Call Information

The following is a list of the information to be obtained and recorded during the first call:

- Full name of deceased
- Location of deceased
- Name, phone number, and relationship of caller to the deceased
- Name, phone number, and address of next of kin (if not the caller) and whether he or she has been notified
- Name of attending physician and whether he or she has been notified
- Date of birth and date and time of death

- Whether pre-need services have been arranged (guaranteed/non-guaranteed contract)
- Whether disposition decisions have been made that necessitate permission to embalm (if the caller is the next of kin)
- Person in charge of making the arrangement decisions (if not the caller)
- Whether the decedent is ready for transfer, waiting on family to arrive, or waiting on a coroner's or organ donation release
- Any special circumstances or considerations (e.g., weight of the decedent, stairs or other obstacles, extremely emotional family members, special requests, or religious needs)

DEATH AT A HOSPITAL OR INSTITUTION

In the case of a death call from a hospital or other institution, the call may not be from the next of kin or surviving spouse. In this case, it is critical to obtain the name, address, and phone number that the institution has on record for the **family contact**. The following is a list of information to be obtained during the first call for removal from a hospital or institution:

- Has the family release form been signed?
- Has the attending physician been notified?
- Will an autopsy be required (and has the medical examiner been notified)?
- Has permission been given to embalm?

TRANSFER OF REMAINS

The removal and relocation of the deceased from the place of death to the funeral home is called the **transfer of remains**. The information obtained during the first call should be only what is necessary to transfer the deceased to the funeral home, and the details should be documented on a **first call form** in order of importance. The funeral director should establish whether the caller is the **next of kin** (nearest relative) or the **surviving spouse** (the term **survivor** refers to one who outlives someone else). **Kin** refers to blood relatives, so legally the surviving spouse is not kin. The funeral director should identify the **informant** to ascertain whether decisions regarding **disposition** have been made. The informant signs release documents, disclosure forms, and contractual agreements. Hospitals and nursing facilities may have forms to be signed by the family and/or funeral home representative to confirm the transfer of custody and any personal possessions that accompany the body.

GENERAL TRANSFER PROCEDURES

The following is a list of procedures for transferring the deceased from a home or institution:

- Confirm identity.
- Confirm legal authority to transfer with coroner or medical examiner, if necessary.
- Use protective equipment (universal precautions).
- Wrap body in sheet or body bag.
- Immediately take deceased to transfer vehicle.
- Provide the family with information about the funeral home and its services if there is one.
- Obtain permission to embalm if applicable.

In the case of a home removal, the family should be given the choice whether to stay in the room or step out while the deceased is placed in the body bag. The family must also be asked for permission to cover the face and zip the bag; if the family declines, this can be completed after the decedent is in the vehicle for transfer. In addition, the family should be given the opportunity to discuss method of disposition, schedule an arrangement conference, and receive a copy of the funeral home's General Price List at this time.

Transfer Vehicle and Personnel

The vehicle used to transport the deceased from the place of death to the funeral home is called a **transfer vehicle**. It should be maintained in good condition at all times. Some funeral homes use a **hearse** to perform this function. In other cases, a van or other vehicle of sufficient size may be used. During a home removal, it is advisable to use two personnel for the removal. Always replace any furniture that was moved during the removal. Sometimes a **livery service** or **private carrier** contracts with the funeral home to make removals.

Transfer Equipment

The following is a list of transfer equipment items that should be kept in the transfer vehicle at all times:

- Mortuary/ambulance cot
- Collapsible stretcher
- Straps
- Cot cover
- Sheets
- Rubber or plastic sheets
- Towels
- Moist hand wipes
- Disaster pouches
- Pillow or head block
- Personal protective equipment (PPE)

Arrangement Conference

The arrangement conference is the meeting between the funeral director and the decedent's family to discuss service details, financial details, and legal documents. Service details to be discussed include legal and religious requirements, cultural and religious customs, and event planning to be coordinated by the funeral home. The family should be given a variety of options to meet their needs and desires. The funeral director requests several items from the family, including a recent picture of the deceased. This picture can be used as a reference for embalming preparation as well as for preparing an online or newspaper **obituary**. The obituary serves as the public death notice and may contain funeral service information and a short biography of the deceased along with the picture. Merchandise and sundry items are also selected during the arrangement conference. A **memorial folder** is a printed pamphlet for attendees and usually includes the birth and death dates, a photograph, service information, and typically a poem, verse, or song lyric that holds meaning for the decedent and/or the family.

Legal Document Preparation

During the **funeral arrangement conference**, the funeral director gathers specific information regarding the deceased as well as the family's wishes for the funeral service and the financial details of the contract. The informant provides the **vital statistics**, including the personal information of the deceased regarding birth, marriage, divorce, and death. These statistics are used to complete the **death certificate** and **burial/disposition transit permit**. The death certificate describes final disposition and final medical information, including the **cause of death**. It is also used to settle the estate and file insurance benefits. The burial/disposition transit permit is issued by a governmental agency after the death certificate has been filed. This permit authorizes the funeral director to transport and/or make the final disposition of the deceased. It includes the signatures of the funeral director, the issuing governmental agency, and the sexton.

Arrangement Conference Items

The following is a list of items the family should bring to the **arrangement conference** to aid in preparing for the funeral and ensuring that all available death benefits are received:

- A recent picture of the deceased for reference in preparation or the obituary
- Social Security number of the deceased (required for death certificate and Social Security benefits)
- Military discharge papers if the deceased was a veteran
- Guaranteed/non-guaranteed contract information if applicable
- Life insurance papers
- Information about the desired presentation of the deceased, including clothing and jewelry to be worn

In addition, the funeral director should talk with the family to gather information about the deceased that would help to plan a service that will have personal meaning. This information should include the desired service or ritual, presentation, clothing, and personal items.

Arrangement Conference Responsibilities of Funeral Director

The funeral director should go over the following items with the family:

- General Price List (GPL), urn price list, casket price list, and outer burial container price list as applicable
- Authorizations for disposition
- Time and place of service and final disposition
- Use of clergy or officiant
- Merchandise and personalization selections
- Funeral service type
- Vehicle use
- Applicable government benefits or programs (Social Security, military, employer death benefits, etc.)
- Financial responsibility and payment for the contract

Arrangement Conference Authorizations Completed by the Next of Kin

During the arrangement conference, the funeral director must secure proper authorizations specific to the service requested by the next of kin (NOK). Permission to transfer the decedent into the care of the funeral home is typically given orally during the initial phone call with the family; however, a document confirming this permission should be signed during the arrangement conference. Embalming authorization can also be secured orally, but this needs to be explicitly stated and not implied; written authorization is good practice. The funeral director must clearly explain when embalming is necessary and when it is not. For cremation, the NOK signs an authorization form giving permission to cremate. The form also should contain basic information about the decedent, the authorizing person(s), any medical devices, removal and disposition of personal effects, and final disposition of cremated remains, along with an indemnification. If the NOK selects minimum care services, a form should be signed confirming this. The Federal Trade Commission requires that the NOK be given a **Statement of Funeral Goods and Services Selected** breaking down the prices of selected services, merchandise, and cash advances. Payment options are discussed, and the financially responsible person should sign a funeral contract agreeing to purchase the chosen services and merchandise.

Pre-Planned/Pre-Funded Funeral Arrangements and the Impact of Alterations

Individuals may arrange their own funerals in advance of their deaths in a pre-need arrangement conference, which covers many of the same details as an at-need conference, including the location, service type, and merchandise. These arrangements are subject to the same state and federal regulations, including the FTC Funeral Rule, as at-need arrangements. **Pre-funded funeral arrangements** are made and funded, or paid for, in advance of the need, while **pre-planned funeral arrangements** are made in advance but not funded. Pre-funded contracts can be either **guaranteed** or **non-guaranteed**, and they may be **revocable** (breakable) or **irrevocable**. Contract details should include information on what changes are or are not possible, how to make changes, and what will happen in the event that the funeral home cannot fulfill the contract (e.g., selected merchandise is not available). Any alterations to items previously guaranteed in terms of cost could result in additional expenses, with the money in the trust applied toward the current cost of the new goods and services selected. The next of kin will usually honor the requests made in a pre-funded/pre-planned contract; however, legally, the next of kin can make changes to the service style and merchandise. Disagreements between family members on whether to honor the requests of the deceased can be settled in court.

Pre-Planned Funeral Financial Arrangements

Funeral arrangements made in advance of death are considered **pre-planned funeral arrangements** since the funeral arrangement decisions are made before death. The reasons for pre-planning funeral arrangements include securing personal wishes, making informed decisions, relieving survivors, and reducing assets for Medicaid eligibility. If the pre-arrangements are paid for in advance, they are considered **pre-funded funeral arrangements**. In some cases, the pre-funded arrangements come from a **life insurance policy** that has been assigned to go toward funeral expenses upon death. Another form of pre-funding is establishing a **trust account**, which establishes a legal fiduciary responsibility for the funeral home as a trustee. An **individual trust account** is held by an individual. A **master trust account** is a pooled trust account; the funeral home may participate in an established master trust program. The price of **cash advance items** (flowers, cemetery or crematory service charges, obituary notices, etc.) cannot be guaranteed to stay the same.

Professional Liability Related to Documentation and Funeral Plans

Funeral directors face liabilities related to not only decedent care but also legal and contractual terms determined during the funeral planning stages. In the event of a violation, the funeral director incurs liability to the state and/or family. To minimize liability, the funeral director should document all communication with the family, religious leaders, or other individuals or businesses involved in planning or performing services.

Statutory duties include securing and filing paperwork (death certificates, burial permits, transportation permits, cremation documentation, etc.). State law dictates the amount of time allotted to complete and file legal documentation. Failure to do so can result in sanctions; extensions may be applied for and granted for extenuating circumstances.

Contractual obligations include both oral and written agreements in which the director promises to execute services. A breach of contract results in liability for damages for emotional distress.

Implied duties are those that are assumed, while **expressed duties** are clearly defined. The most common breaches are:

- **Negligent embalming:** the embalming outcome is below the standard of care
- **Negligent funeral directing:** failure to perform services involved in funeral directing or failure to honor requests
- **Safeguarding the body:** keeping the body safe from harm
- **Privacy**: confidentiality of decedent and family
- **Defective merchandise**: the director is responsible for merchandise liability unless clearly disclaimed
- **Transportation:** safely transport decedent and mourners
- **Aftercare:** malpractice for unqualified counseling services

Funeral Service Codes of Ethics and Informal Professional Norms

Various organizations have published professional **codes of conduct** or **codes of ethics** for funeral directors. Although details differ, they echo similar principles for maintaining an elevated standard of care throughout the industry while suggesting goals and ideals for funeral directors and funeral homes.

Funeral directors are ethically obligated to meet the needs of the families they serve by providing quality, nonjudgmental, confidential, respectful, dignified, and professional care to both the families and the deceased while following all national and state legislation. Funeral directors have a professional responsibility to be fair and honest as they serve the public. They must comply with all governmental and health and safety regulations set forth for the profession to keep themselves and the public safe.

Informal professional norms for funeral directors include professional attire. Services are usually conducted in formal business attire such as suits; when transferring decedents into the care of the funeral home or between locations, semi-formal business attire is worn. Attire is conservative and should not feature bright colors or wild patterns. While stylish clothing is acceptable, funeral directors should blend in and not draw attention away from the family or deceased. Clothing gives a first impression and reflects professionalism.

Modifications to Plans Following the Arrangement Conference

The next of kin has the right to alter requested services following the arrangements. Occasionally, families completely change disposition, such as changing a traditional burial to cremation or adding services prior to a burial or cremation. A planned closed casket may end up staying open following the private family viewing. Difficulty arises when service times/dates are changed after publication of an announcement of services. In this case, a notice of **change of services** can be published, but some of the public may miss this change.

It is crucial for the funeral director to ensure that the family is aware of when cremation will take place. Because cremation is irreversible, there must be a hard cutoff time for requesting disposition changes or a final viewing. Clear and concise information, along with repetition, can gently help families understand the finality. Funeral directors can often sense when families are wavering in their decisions, and they should prepare for the possibility that a family member will call asking for a final viewing a few minutes before the cremation is scheduled to begin.

Directors should accommodate modifications when they are able; however, it is not always possible.

Government Social Services Benefit Programs

A variety of government benefits and programs are available to families, including those administered by the **Social Security Administration** and the **Department of Veterans Affairs.** The Social Security Administration provides benefits for survivors upon completion of the **SSA-721** (statement of death) and the **SSA-8** (application for the lump sum benefit payment of $255). The Department of Veterans Affairs can determine if the survivors are entitled to veterans' benefits. In both cases, the funeral director can assist the family in understanding and obtaining any benefits to which they are entitled. The time limit for filing the Social Security lump sum burial claim is two years after death. In some cases, Medicare or Medicaid may pay part of the cost of custodial care, which is a fee for the period in which a body is held at the funeral home.

Veteran Burial Eligibility

The status of a **deceased veteran** can impact both the funeral service and the disposition. A veteran is an individual who is no longer active-duty military personnel but has served in a branch of the US Armed Forces for a certain amount of time and has received discharge papers (the type of discharge —honorable, dishonorable, or medical—is identified on **Form DD-214**). A veteran may be eligible for burial in a **national cemetery** established by the government for the exclusive use of veterans and eligible family members. These cemeteries may be nationally operated or state operated. The Department of Veterans Affairs operates national veteran cemeteries in some states, while other states operate state veteran cemeteries.

Elements of a Veteran's Burial Service

If a family requests a military service, the funeral director is responsible for communicating directly with the deceased's branch of service to determine eligibility. Usually, a **chaplain** is selected by the military to conduct the religious aspects of a funeral service for a variety of denominations. In addition, a **color guard**, **firing squad**, **bugler**, and **military escort** may be assigned to attend the funeral in case of active-duty death, and **honorary pallbearers** may serve as an honor guard for the deceased. An eligible veteran can receive an inscribed **memorial**.

Veteran's Burial Service

During a military funeral service, the American flag is draped on the casket before it is loaded into the hearse, typically once the casket is closed or following the service in a church. A 21-gun salute is performed. Following the committal, the military personnel fold the flag and present it to the next of kin. Finally, taps is played. The following is a list of individuals who are typically present at the **military service**:

- Chaplain
- Bugler
- Color bearers
- Color guards
- Commander of the Post
- Firing squad
- Commander of the firing squad
- Casket bearers

If the veteran is buried at a non-military cemetery, the funeral director coordinates with the local Department of Veterans Affairs or active-duty military personnel to have military honors (the folding of the flag, taps, and usually a gun salute) accorded.

PRIORITY OF SURVIVORS FOR VETERAN BENEFITS

A veteran is eligible for a variety of **burial expense reimbursements** and benefits for all legal disposition methods based on the status of his or her discharge. The benefits are paid to the survivor in order of highest priority, beginning with the veteran's **surviving spouse** or **survivor of a legal union**. Next in line are the veteran's children, regardless of age. If there are no children, the veteran's parents are eligible. Finally, if there are no surviving parents, spouses, or children, the executor or administrator of the deceased veteran's estate receives the benefits. Benefit amounts are different for **service-related deaths** than for deaths in a VA hospital.

VETERANS ALLOWANCES AND BURIAL BENEFITS

The family should request the **burial expense reimbursement** from the Veterans Benefits Administration. This is for the following benefits:

- A **burial plot** located in one of the VA cemeteries, including an additional space for the veteran's spouse if reserved. These are often double-depth burial vaults and cannot be selected in advance or at the time of loss. They are assigned at the time of loss by the cemetery official.
- A **burial expense allowance** of $300 toward burial expenses or up to $2,000 (plus transportation of the deceased) if the death is service-related **(Form 21P-530)**.
- A **plot allowance** if not using a VA cemetery. If the veteran died on or after October 1, 2015, the VA will pay $747 for a plot **(Form 21P-530)**.

VETERAN'S MEMORIAL AND MISCELLANEOUS BENEFITS

A veteran is eligible for a variety of memorial benefits and miscellaneous recognitions based on his or her discharge status.

A **veteran's memorial** is available for eligible veterans **(Form 40-1330)**. The inscription layout is standardized with service rank, date of birth, and date of death, as well as three to four words selected by the family. In a non-VA cemetery, the fees for cemetery installation are not included. The following styles are available:

- Memorial headstone (flat or upright granite or marble)
- Flat bronze 24" × 12" (does not include granite base)
- Niche-size bronze

Miscellaneous benefits include:

- A **United States flag**, under certain conditions. Most funeral homes provide this regardless **(Form 27-2008)**.
- A **Presidential Memorial Certificate** for veterans who were not dishonorably discharged **(Form 40-0247)**.

PRE-SERVICE DETAILS THAT NEED TO BE COMPLETED FOLLOWING THE ARRANGEMENT CONFERENCE

Before the service, the funeral director should:

- Transfer the decedent into the care of the funeral home.
- Prepare the body for identification viewing or embalm.
- Verify availability of service space, officiant, musicians, and veterans/fraternal organizations for the day and time the family requested (before publishing anything).

- Submit the death notice to selected newspapers.
- Secure (electronic or physical) custody of the death certificate. Using vital statistics, complete and file the death certificate and burial/transportation permits.
- Compose the obituary and send it to family for approval, then submit the obituary to selected newspapers and applicable websites.
- Order the casket (or urn) and keepsakes with specific delivery needs.
- Order the vault or outer burial container with order and setup needs, cemetery information, service times, and estimated arrival at the cemetery.
- Contact the cemetery sexton to mark out the grave and the gravedigger to open.
- Order flowers.
- Dress, casket, and cosmeticize the decedent in preparation for services and schedule a hairdresser or, following the identification viewing, proceed with cremation after the legal holding period, coroner authorization, and family authorizations are complete.
- Schedule staff and vehicles for services.
- Design and create sundry items, memorial folders/prayer cards, the register book, service programs, and video tributes.
- Create a temporary marker or order final engraving on the memorial stone.

Tasks to Be Done Immediately Prior to a Visitation or Service

Just before a visitation or service, the funeral director should:

- Move the casket or urn (or in lieu of an urn, the selected photograph/centerpiece) into the visitation or service space.
- Arrange flowers around the casket/urn with nearest and dearest closest, typically displayed as follows: spray from the spouse on or above the casket or behind or around the urn; children on the left; siblings on the right; and grandchildren inside the casket or in front of the urn. Families may order shared flower pieces, so always check the cards and ribbons. Pay attention to aesthetics while arranging the remaining flowers, factoring in size and colors. Make the flower book.
- Set out the register book, pen, and memorial folders/prayer cards along with any family-specific accessories (prie-dieu/kneeler, candles, Mass tray, crucifix, American flag, etc.).
- If using a signboard, display it prominently and verify all information for accuracy.
- Start background music and tribute videos.
- Arrange photographs and memory displays on easels and tables.
- Attend to housekeeping including checking lighting, vacuuming, emptying garbage cans, stocking bathrooms, and arranging chairs and furniture as needed.
- Check the entire space in a final walk-through prior to the family arriving. If the casket is open, do a final check of the decedent to ensure that no adjustments are needed.

Transitioning from the Visitation to the Service and Graveside Service

Before transitioning between funeral elements or locations, the funeral director should discuss the following with the family:

- What will remain in the casket with the deceased and what will be returned to the family (e.g., jewelry; personal items like hats, medals, rosaries; and interior display items)?
- Which flowers are going to the church and the cemetery, which will be taken home, and which will be donated to a church or nursing facility?
- What order do they want to process in? At a minimum, record each driver's name; the color and model of the car and the names of passengers can also be helpful information.

The funeral director should also instruct the pallbearers where and what time to meet. They might be used only to carry the casket from the hearse to the graveside. Other times they will be needed to go from the funeral home to the hearse, the hearse into the church, the church to the hearse, and the hearse to graveside. Sometimes they ceremonially escort the casket during the processional and recessional during the service.

When services are spread out over multiple days, speak with the next of kin once guests have left after the visitation. When services are held in a single day, details can be discussed with the family before the guests arrive.

Tasks That Need to Be Performed by Funeral Directors and Assistants During the Services

At any funeral service, the family should be greeted at the door by the funeral director. Once coats are hung and everyone has arrived, the family can be escorted into the service space for their first viewing of the deceased or the urn. Any alterations requested by the family should be made by the funeral director with help from support staff. During a visitation, a staff member should greet guests; hang coats; and direct people to sign the guestbook, pick up a memorial folder/prayer card, and join the receiving line. The funeral director should periodically check in with the family and discreetly monitor the deceased if the casket is open.

In preparation for the service, make sure musical selections are ready and livestream video equipment is set up, connected, and tested. A few minutes prior to starting a service, the funeral director should seat the family and encourage guests to find a seat. Make sure the podium and microphone are set up. Pass out service folders and assist the clergy with any last-minute needs.

In concluding the service, the funeral director should thank attendants for coming on behalf of the family and give any necessary instructions for the procession if applicable.

Types of Funeral Service

A **traditional service** is conducted with the body of the deceased present and follows a prescribed, orderly ritual dictated by religious belief or social custom. It may also include a **wake**, or watch over the deceased, usually an evening visitation time. A **contemporary funeral rite** includes more modern elements that add to or replace traditional rites. These can include religious aspects and customization/personalization such as music, readings, poems, and video tributes. An **adaptive funeral rite** is modified in some way by the family members and is typically more modern or is arranged to fulfill a desired need of the family. A **memorial service** does not have the body present and is often conducted for cremation disposition, with or without the presence of the **cremated remains**. A **humanistic service** has no religious aspects whatsoever.

Visitation

A visitation is a public or private viewing of the deceased in the casket (open or closed) either the day before or directly before the **funeral service**. During the viewing, attendees typically sign a **register** or **memorial book**. The **guest book**, or **register book,** is a record for the deceased including information on date of birth and date of death, location of the service (church or chapel), family and pallbearers, and signature lines for attendees. **Prayer cards** are small cards with a prayer on one side and information about the deceased on the other. These are often used in Catholic funeral services.

Ceremony

During the arrangement conference, the funeral director and the family decide on the type of ceremony. A **ceremony** is a formally organized event to celebrate or pay homage to the deceased. A **funeral service** is a ceremony conducted by an officiant immediately before burial or cremation. The officiant in most cases receives an **honorarium** or **gratuity** as a modest payment for conducting the service. **Funeral rites** are broadly defined as any form of funeral ceremony. A ceremony can be less formal than a funeral service, such as a **memorial gathering**. This is a ceremony coordinated by a professional third party or a family member who may have been trained as a celebrant. A **memorial service** is a style of service, religious or otherwise, in which the physical body is not present. It can be formal or informal and officiated by a religious leader, celebrant, or family member.

Funeral Directing Inside a Facility

Funeral coordination is a critical role of the funeral director. The family seating arrangements are reserved in advance. Family flower arrangements should be closest to the casket and should have symmetry and balance, with the casket in the center. A **pallbearer** or **casket bearer** is an attendee who assists in carrying the casket during the funeral and committal service. The funeral director provides instructions to the pallbearers and directs their role during the ceremony. During the **eulogy**, one or more persons gives a short speech commemorating the deceased. An **elegy** is a song or poem that expresses sadness for the loss of a loved one. Some services involve **genuflection**, or reverently kneeling on the right knee. The service ends with a **dismissal** as the funeral director facilitates the movement of all parties out of the building.

Funeral Procession

Following the funeral director's dismissal, the pallbearers load the casket into the funeral coach, and the **cortege** or **funeral procession** prepares to leave for the cemetery. At this time the flowers that were around the casket are loaded into the flower van, which travels to the cemetery ahead of the procession. At the cemetery, for a ground burial, the flowers are arranged on and around artificial grass. Although one or more elements may not be present, the general **order of the vehicles** departing to the cemetery is:

- Lead cars:
    - Police escort
    - Lead car
    - Clergy
    - Pallbearers
- Hearse
- Family:
    - Close family limousine
    - Family cars
- Attendees

Importance of Religious Funeral Rites

Many religious groups have specific **funeral rites** and customs. A funeral director should be familiar with the religious groups in his or her area and their typical rites, rituals, and customs surrounding the preparation and disposition of the deceased. The exact form of these rites can vary based on the sect, congregation, location, individuals, and circumstances. For example, while some religions generally prohibit autopsies, many sects and individuals are willing to make an exception if the cause of death is unknown or there is reason to suspect foul play. In addition, while some religions traditionally complete disposition (burial or cremation) within 24 hours of death, local laws may not permit this. In this case, followers of these religions will generally seek disposition as soon as it is legal and feasible. Local clergy (or other leaders if a group does not have clergy) should be consulted when planning any religious funeral, and their recommendations should be followed.

Roman Catholic Funeral Rites

Funeral Elements

A **rosary service** is a special vigil service visitation ceremony, usually held at a funeral home the night before the funeral Mass. It includes special prayers that are recited with a crucifix and rosary beads. A **vigil light** is placed at each end of the casket during the visitation.

In the Roman Catholic faith, a funeral service is called a **funeral Mass** or **funeral liturgy**. A **Mass card** is purchased and given to the family to communicate that the giver is praying for the deceased at Mass. The officiant in charge of a Roman Catholic Mass is called a **celebrant**. **Prayer cards** are individual cards for funeral attendees that contain the name of the deceased and a verse or prayer. The casket is placed at right angles to the raised platform (the **altar**). Deceased laypersons and nuns are placed with their feet toward the altar. The casket of the priest is placed with the head toward the altar. The **prayer rail** or **prie-dieu** is placed in front of the casket so that individuals can approach the casket and kneel.

Funeral Mass

Catholic funerals often start with a viewing, or wake, a day or two before the funeral Mass. During the funeral ceremony, the casket is sprinkled with holy water; then the emblematic cloth of the church, the **pall**, is draped over the closed casket. Atop the pall is placed the cross and Bible as a symbol of faith and baptism. A **Paschal candle**, which denotes the everlasting light of Christ, is placed near the casket during the funeral Mass. The Mass includes readings from the Bible, a homily delivered by the priest, a Communion ceremony, and hymns and church music with singing led by the **cantor**. The **final commendation** signifies the end of the funeral Mass. The funeral then moves to the cemetery, where the priest performs the **Rite of Committal** before the casket is lowered into the grave.

Eastern Orthodox Church (Orthodox Church) Funeral Rites

Priest is the title given to a member of the clergy ordained to lead religious ceremonial rites. The term **deacon** refers to a clerical position, one who serves in the church in various capacities. A **cantor** participates in services by chanting, accompanying the priest. The **Divine Liturgy** is a ceremony that includes readings and hymns celebrating the Eucharist. The **Parastas** is the nighttime funeral service of a vigil. The **Trisagion** service is a group of three short memorial services or blessings containing hymns sung the night before, the day of, and at the end of the funeral. The **solea** is the open area located in front of the altar. An **icon** is a picture or painting symbolizing a holy person, usually made in mosaic or on wood. The **iconostasis** is a panel hung with icons and located at the front of the church, dividing the solea from the sanctuary.

Protestant Funeral Rites

Protestants are Christians who believe in God, the Trinity, and salvation with the promise of eternal life through the death and resurrection of Jesus. Common denominations classified as Protestant are Methodist, Lutheran, Anglican, Presbyterian, Baptist, Reformed, and some nondenominational Christian churches. The **pastor** or **minister** leads the funeral service in the church or at the funeral home. At church, some denominations use a **pall** on the casket or urn and often process into the sanctuary at the beginning of the service. Historically, Protestant funeral services focused on passing into everlasting life and could be broken down into the ritual of reading scriptures and prayers, music, the sermon, and the **committal service**. Today, services can additionally include contemporary or traditional music along with eulogies and references to the decedent's life. Following the funeral service, a recession out of the church is led by the pastor, followed by the casket or urn, family members, and then attendees. At a graveside service, Protestant ministers have a committal service. Ceremonies for some denominations will include casting dirt or soil upon the casket or urn. A funeral gathering is often held following the completion of the services, often at the church, the family home, or a public gathering space.

Jewish Rite

Once the body is casketed, family members or congregants **(shomers)** sit watch, or **shmira,** with the body, reciting psalms until the funeral. The service is held at the **synagogue** or funeral home. Typically, the casket is closed; however, some families have a private viewing. Prior to the service, the **mourners** gather in a private room. The rabbi places a black ribbon on each of the mourners and then cuts the ribbon while they recite a prayer; this ceremony is called **keriah** (tearing of a garment or black ribbon). The funeral service contains prayers, music, readings, and a **hesped**, or eulogy. Following the procession to the cemetery, pallbearers carry the casket to the graveside, pausing seven times on the way. Psalm 91 and the **Mourner's Kaddish** are recited at the graveside. The rabbi may place dirt from Israel atop the casket before it is lowered into the grave. Family and attendees shovel dirt into the grave as an "ultimate" **mitzvah,** a kindness done knowing it won't be repaid. Following the services, the family **sits shiva** for seven days, during which family and friends pay respects. In the Reform tradition, shiva is held for three days. Sending flowers is not appropriate, but sending food is.

Islamic Rite

The Islamic funeral prayer service can take place at the mosque (outside the mosque or in a designated prayer room) or a funeral home. During the funeral service, the deceased and attendees face **Mecca,** the holy center of Islam. The service and prayers are led by the **imam**, a holy leader. Traditionally, only men attended services, but today some sects allow women to participate. Attendees may be separated by gender within the service space. Loud expressions of grief or extreme emotions are not permitted. The procession to the gravesite is silent. Within some Muslim communities, only men attend the graveside service. The body is lowered into the ground and positioned to face Mecca; the funeral director must coordinate with the cemetery because not all cemetery plots are laid out with this consideration. At the graveside, all attendees throw three handfuls of dirt into the grave. Grave liners are required by most cemeteries, so to meet Islamic religious requirements, they are placed upside-down over the body or casket. After a death, a forty-day mourning period is traditional, though most modern-day Muslims follow a three-day mourning period.

Buddhist Funeral Rites

Buddhist funerals do not have many requirements. Buddhism prohibits the use of the terms "death" or "deceased" and instead uses "passed on." Buddhists hope to achieve a state of **Nirvana** after death, or perfect freedom and peace. The **bonze** is the name of the Buddhist priest. The **makura-gyo** is the bedside prayer said by the bonze. The **service of encasketing** is a traditional ceremony performed in conjunction with the placement of the deceased into the casket. A hymn called the **Gatha** may be sung as part of the funeral ceremony. The funeral itself may include chanting, prayers, and funeral readings. Food offerings may be brought into the funeral home. Incense is burned. The **words of appreciation** are the portion of the religious ceremony when the funeral attendees are thanked for coming to the ceremony. The family typically wears white, while guests wear dark colors; bright colors and jewelry are avoided. Buddhists are typically cremated, but burial or other forms of disposition are permitted.

Mormon Funeral Rite

Mormons are members of the Church of Jesus Christ of Latter-Day Saints. The church was founded by the prophet Joseph Smith, who translated the writings of the prophets that were originally compiled by the prophet Mormon. This translation is called the **Book of Mormon**. Within the religion, cremation is not encouraged, embalming is allowed, caskets can be open or closed, and services may be at the church, funeral home, or graveside. Most of the funeral details are left for the next of kin to decide. The funeral should be held within a week of death. If a decedent has **temple clothing**, a family member or church member of the same gender may dress him or her in this all-white attire. The funeral consists of music, scriptures, and prayers. The officiant is a **bishop** from the deceased's church. A cross or crucifix is not permitted during the services. A **committal service** is held at the graveside following the service. The church often hosts the family and attendees for a meal afterwards.

Hindu Funeral Rite

Hindu funerals take place as soon after death as possible, and Hindus are usually cremated immediately following the funeral. The cremation ceremony traditionally takes place within 24 hours of death but may be delayed based on state laws regarding waiting periods before cremation or other circumstances. The decedent's body is washed by family members and friends, then displayed in an open casket during the **mukhagni**, or cremation ceremony. Funeral attendees wear white. After the cremation, the decedent's ashes are scattered at a location of the family's choosing. While non-Hindus may attend the funeral, only Hindus participate in funeral **mantras**, or chants.

Other Religious Funeral Rites

The **Christian Science** church (the Church of Christ, Scientist) does not have clergy or specific funeral rites. The funeral service of a Christian Scientist may be held anywhere except at the Christian Science church; it is led by a fellow practitioner. **Jehovah's Witnesses** hold funeral services at their place of worship, known as the **Kingdom Hall**. The choices of embalming and disposition are up to the family.

Role of Fraternal and Social Organizations in Funeral Services

Many fraternal and social organizations offer a ceremony conducted at the visitation, before or after the service, or at the graveside to commemorate the decedent's membership and dedication to the organization. Many churches do not allow these ceremonies to take place in the church, so they are conducted at the funeral home or graveside. This does not mean the church condemns the organization or ceremony; they may just have stipulations for their sanctuaries and worship places to be used for ceremonies of their beliefs only.

The type of ceremony offered by any given organization can vary by location. When gathering information from the family, ask about organizations the decedent was involved with because the family may want to have the organization involved if they offer a special service.

Organizations that offer ceremonies include:

- Freemasons
- Elks
- Grange
- Independent Order of Odd Fellows
- Order of the Eastern Star
- International Association of Rebekah Assembly
- Knights of Columbus

- Moose
- Firefighters
- Police
- Military and veteran's organizations

Shipping Human Remains Domestically

Ship-outs involve sending a body to another funeral home; **ship-ins** involve receiving a body from another funeral home. Notification of death or request for service can come from the family or another funeral home. The family may know what funeral home will send or receive the body, or they may ask for recommendations. When services are prior to transportation, the decedent is shipped in a casket; when services are at the receiving location, a casket is typically not used for shipping. Services may take place in both locations. **Trade calls** are when one funeral home contacts another for transportation, documentation, embalming, and/or coordinating air transportation. **Interstate** shipping may require embalming, depending on the laws of the recipient state. Flights can be booked with airlines directly or with private shipping companies. Embalming is required for air transportation unless religious beliefs prevent it. Unembalmed bodies are transported with dry ice or ice packs. In cases with leaking, decomposition, or extended shipping timelines for unembalmed decedents, a **Ziegler case** (a zinc-lined container with a one-piece zinc top screwed to the base portion that holds the body) is used. Cremated remains can only be shipped through the US Postal Service's Priority Mail Express. FedEx and UPS will not ship cremated remains.

Shipping Both Casketed and Non-Casketed Human Remains

These are the steps for shipping casketed remains:

1. Lower the bed of the casket.
2. Cover the face and hands so cosmetics do not transfer onto interior fabrics.
3. Place a box between the bottom of the feet and foot end of the casket to prevent sliding.
4. Lock metal caskets, but place the cap in a shipping envelope to prevent damage to the casket due to changing air pressure in flight (wooden caskets have no risk of compression damage because they aren't airtight).
5. Secure the casket in an **air tray** shipping unit with a wooden bottom and cardboard top (see final steps below).

These are the steps for shipping non-casketed remains:

1. Dress the decedent in plastic garments (pants, at minimum) and a hospital gown.
2. Wrap the body in a sheet (not plastic because plastic accumulates moisture/mold).
3. Place the decedent in a **combination case**, a particleboard box with a cardboard tray and cover that meets shipping regulations.
4. Place clothing and personal possessions in a garment bag at the decedent's feet.
5. Secure the body with straps on the interior of the combination case, and secure the cardboard lid with exterior straps.

For both air trays and combination cases, tape a shipping envelope with the decedent's name, receiving funeral home, and flight information to the box. The envelope should contain the burial/transportation permit along with any other necessary documentation (death certificate, affidavits, embalming report, apostilles, etc.).

International Shipping of Human Remains

An **apostille** is an officially accepted certification that can be used internationally. The apostille and all other documents must be translated into the language of the receiving country. When a funeral home must forward remains to another country, the first step is to notify the **consulate** of the receiving country to coordinate the transfer. It is important to maintain compliance with both customs at the entry point and the laws of the receiving country. In some cases, an affidavit of "no contagious disease" may be required along with an embalming certificate. When remains are transported to the US from a foreign country (such as when a US citizen dies abroad), the consular officer from the nearest US embassy or consulate notifies the **State Department**, which contacts the family or representative. An embalmed body may be shipped in a casket. Required documentation varies among countries and airlines and may be extensive. Cremated remains may be shipped internationally through the US Postal Service.

Final Disposition Services

Final disposition is the physical act of placing the decedent in his or her final resting place. **Direct disposition** does not include any formal viewing, service, or ceremony with the body of the deceased. A **committal service** is the segment of the actual funeral service that is held at the site of final disposition. A **graveside service** refers to any ceremony, with or without religious elements, held at the site of final disposition. A **grave** is a designated site excavated for the **burial** of the deceased. **Entombment** is the process by which the casket containing the deceased is placed into a crypt.

Methods of Final Disposition

Cremation accelerates the decomposition of a body by heat (1,400–1,800 °F) from gas burners in a **retort**, which is a specially designed brick chamber in a crematory. Upon completion of cremation, the remaining bone fragments are raked from the chamber and allowed to cool until they can be pulverized and placed in an **urn** or other receptacle. The cremated remains are then returned to the family. **Anatomical donation** is the donation of the body for research or medical use of the organs. If the body is not cremated or donated, an embalmer may prepare the body for viewing prior to burial. Some funeral homes charge an additional fee for this preparation.

Alternative Disposition

Disposition at sea refers to either the burial at sea of a casket or the scattering at sea of cremated remains. This must occur at open sea, a minimum of three nautical miles from shore, and is reported to the EPA. **Green burial** is the act of interring a body that has not been embalmed in a biodegradable casket or bag in a section of the cemetery specifically designated for natural burials. Green burial has minimal environmental impact. **Cryonics** is a procedure that preserves the tissue of the deceased in extreme low temperatures with the intent of restoring it to life at a future date with advances in medical science. The process of **resomation**, or alkaline hydrolysis, is the process of reducing the body tissues to bone fragments with heat (360 °F), pressure, and an alkaline solution of potassium hydroxide.

Cemetery Disposition Options

A **cemetery** is land that is legally designated for the burial of human remains and includes a variety of final disposition options. In some cases, the deceased is interred in an adult-size casket within an outer burial container or, in the case of a cremated body, interred in an urn. A cemetery **lot** is a portion of a cemetery that is subdivided into one or more interment spaces for burial. A **crypt** is a compartmentalized space in a building such as a mausoleum for the placement of human remains in a casket or an urn. A **niche** is a compartmentalized space in a building such as a columbarium for the placement of cremated remains. A **scattering garden** is a section of a cemetery where cremated remains are placed in a non-retrievable space and commingled with other cremated remains. A **receiving vault** is a cemetery building designed for the temporary storage and placement of the deceased before the final burial or entombment.

Considerations for Cremation

Because the act of **cremation** is irreversible, proper identification and legal authorization are the most important responsibilities of the funeral director. **Identification viewing** involves one or more members of the immediate family confirming the identity of the deceased before cremation can take place. The authorizing party who instructed the funeral home to cremate the body is required to sign a legal form specific to the state in which the death occurred. The container used for cremation may be the same one used for the funeral service if it is wooden. A **rental casket** is a specially designed casket with a cardboard interior that later encases the body for the cremation process. **Alternative containers** are designed for direct cremation or use in ceremonial cremation services. They are constructed of lightweight fiberboard or corrugated cardboard and are relatively inexpensive.

Services with Cremation

In **traditional cremation**, the body is present at the funeral ceremony, and cremation takes place afterward. Traditional cremation is a common choice and often includes embalming for the visitation or viewing. With **direct cremation**, no funeral service is held prior to cremation. In this case there is no viewing of the deceased except as required for identification. A **memorial service** is a funeral tribute to the life of the deceased without the body present. It can be held in a variety of locations and can take place days, weeks, or months after death. This service may or may not include an **urn** receptacle with the cremated body. A **memorial gathering** is an informal service to remember the life of a deceased loved one.

Disposition of Cremated Remains

The final disposition of cremated remains can be in a variety of places, including the ground (**earth burial**). Cremated remains may also be placed in a **mausoleum**. This is common when a person chooses a full-casket burial but a spouse or family member chooses an urn, and they are entombed in a single crypt. A **columbarium** is a structure dedicated for the inurnment of strictly cremated remains. The **scattering** of cremated remains is the dispersion of the bone fragments over the ground or at sea according to legal requirements.

Anatomical Donation Programs

Written to promote organ donation and whole-body donation, the **Uniform Anatomical Gift Act (UAGA)** was adopted by all states. The act states that people can designate their body for donation upon death if they are over 18 years old and of sound mind. This designation can be stated in a will, legal donation form, or valid driver's license. Surviving spouses or legal **next of kin (NOK)** can also authorize donation if no one within the same or a higher-level kinship contests it. The act specifies donees, hospitals, medical and dental schools, and medical storage banks, and donors can be used for research, education, or advancement of science. **Whole-body donation** is typically to medical schools for education and research. Bodies can remain intact for cadaver labs, or they can be sectioned for specific research. **Organ donation** occurs following death or brain death in a medical facility. Additionally, some people donate one or more organs to a specific research organization. Often this is researched and arranged for by the decedent or family; however, NOK sometimes have funeral homes coordinate this. These facilities will provide families or the funeral director with requirements, decedent care, transportation, and procurement procedures to facilitate donation.

Full Body Donation and Organ Donation

Full body donation: Upon death and the family's request, the funeral home contacts the donation facility to start the approval process. To establish medical history and evaluate candidacy, donation facility staff ask the funeral director, family, or medical care providers questions. Once approved, the director secures donation authorizations from the NOK, obtains the death certificate and permit, and coordinates the transportation to the medical facility. When the facility is finished with the body, it is cremated; NOK can request that the cremated remains be returned. When not returned to the family, the remains are buried in a cemetery contracted with the facility and marked with a number to maintain anonymity. The family can plan a memorial service at their convenience.

Organ donation: Upon death or brain death, medical facilities are required to make referrals to donation organizations; a liaison contacts NOK to attain authorizations. Bone, ligaments, tendons, integument (skin), corneas, and heart valves can be donated post-mortem, while viable organs are donated upon brain death. Procurement teams may come to the medical facility or have the decedent transferred to a procurement center. Afterwards, the funeral home is contacted to take custody. The family can select services and disposition of their choice, with or without the body present.

Funeral Service Marketing/Merchandising

Casket Terminology

A **casket** is an inflexible, decorative container made of wood, metal, or similar material with an interior lining. A **coffin** is an inflexible container and is usually made of wood, constructed to be wide at the shoulders and narrow at the feet. **Alternative containers** are designed for direct disposition and are constructed of lightweight fiberboard or corrugated cardboard; these are inexpensive, non-decorative containers. An **air tray** is constructed with a solid wood base and a corrugated cardboard covering to protect a casket during transportation. A **combination case** is constructed of particleboard or wood with a cardboard tray for transportation by air. A **Ziegler case** is designed for advanced decomposition and includes a gasket seal. This case is inserted into a casket or used as a separate shipping container.

Wood Casket Materials

The exterior dimensions of a standard wood casket are 81"× 28"× 24". **Softwood caskets** originate from conifers and are less expensive. The grain is wide, and the wood is light and soft. **Hardwood caskets** originate from deciduous trees and are more expensive. The compact grain is tighter, and the wood is heavier and firmer than softwood. Examples of hardwood trees used in caskets include oak, birch, poplar, walnut, mahogany, and cherry. **Select hardwood caskets** are constructed from several different kinds of wood. A **laminate casket** is constructed of sheets of finer wood material glued onto a less expensive base. **Wood veneer** is a type of laminate with an outer layer of better-quality wood over an inner layer of less expensive wood. Wood caskets can be unfinished or have a natural finish and may be stained or unstained.

Metal Casket Materials

The exterior dimensions of a standard metal casket are 83" × 28" × 24". The term **gauge** is a measurement of metal thickness equivalent to the number of metal sheets that could be layered to equal an inch, so a higher number indicates a thinner sheet. Most caskets are between 16 and 20 gauge. An **alloy** is a blend of two or more metals. **Ferrous** metal caskets are constructed from iron, including steel or stainless steel. **Steel** is a metal alloy composed of iron and carbon. **Stainless steel caskets** are constructed of steel with at least 11% chromium and occasionally nickel, and they are noted to be rust-resistant. A **galvanized metal** has been covered with zinc for improved resistance to rust. Any metal alloy that is not made with iron is considered to be a **nonferrous** metal. The term **wrought** refers to the process of rolling the metal into sheets. A **copper casket** is formed from sheets of pliable copper. A **copper deposit casket** is constructed with an electrolytic process that deposits copper molecules on the casket. A **bronze casket** is an alloy of 90% copper and 10% tin and zinc. Bronze is more durable than copper or steel.

Exterior Casket Finishes

A **brushed finish** is first painted, then scratched, completed with a sealer, and finally buffed to high gloss. This is usually done for stainless steel, copper, and bronze caskets. A **plated finish** is achieved by coating the base metal of a casket or part with a different metal through an electrolytic process. A **sprayed finish** is painted on a metal surface. A **hammertone finish** is a paint finish that is sprayed on to give the appearance of minor indentations in the metal. A **crinkled finish** is a coating process that wrinkles upon drying. A **matte finish** is flat and dull without gloss. A **satin finish** is semi-gloss with a low luster.

Casket Parts

The **body** is the part of the casket that includes the molding along the uppermost edge of the body panels, the body panel base molding, and the casket bottom. The **cap** or lid is the uppermost portion. The **shell** refers to the cap and body pieces of the casket. The **fishtails** (pies) are two wedge-shaped portions of the lid at each end of the crown. The **body panels** are both the sides and ends of the casket shell, and the **foot panels** are inside the cap interior at the foot of the casket, opposite the **head panel**. The **rim** (ogee) is a molding component of the cap in an S-shape. The **crown** is the uppermost portion of the cap, on top of the rim. **Base molding** is the molding along the lowest rim of the body panels.

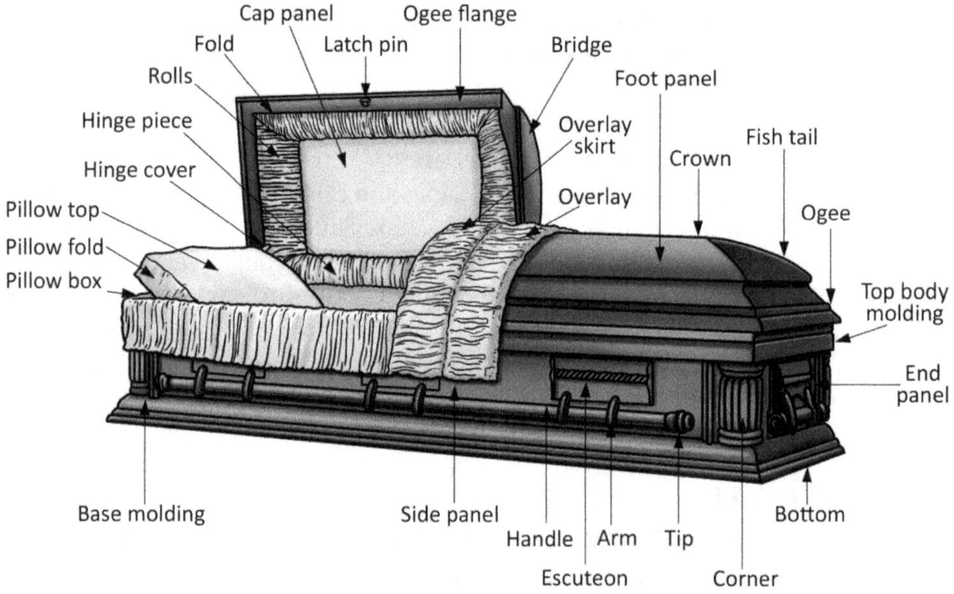

Casket Closures

The two closure methods for caskets are **gasketed** and **non-gasketed**. There are four non-gasketed closure methods. The **latch** method secures the cap to the body after the lid is closed. The **threaded fastener** utilizes a threaded screw that fastens on the hinged cap. **Chemical compounds** to close a casket include an epoxy or butyl tape. A **hermetically sealed** casket is closed by fusion or soldering and creates an airtight seal. A gasketed casket has a rubber lining between the base and lid. The gasket closure method of a casket has several component parts. The **gasket** itself is made of rubber. The **gasket channel** holds the transverse gasket to seal the space between the head and foot caps. The **hinge cover** (hinge skirt) connects the cap to the casket body. The **locking mechanism** locks the cap to the body.

Casket Shapes and Hardware

A **perfection full-couch casket** is one in which the top rim frame (ogee), crown, fish tail and pies are crafted in a single piece which can be raised together. A **perfection half-couch casket** is one in which the top rim frame (ogee), crown, and pies are formed in two separate pieces. An **elliptic** casket has ends shaped in half circles. A **round corner** casket has welded round corner pieces. A **flaring square** is a side body panel of the shell that is narrow at the bottom of the casket and flares out toward the top. The **hardware** of a casket refers to the decorative handles, ornamental fixtures, and custom décor attached to the casket shell. **Cast hardware** is the most expensive type of metal hardware and uses molten metal poured into a mold. **Stamped hardware** is produced by pressing out shapes with hydraulics and is less expensive.

Casket Handles and Components

The **bar** is the handle attached to the lug or arm that the pallbearer grasps to hold the casket. The bar is either fixed or swinging. The **swing bar** casket handle is attached on a hinged arm and is moveable. The **stationary bar** is set on a motionless arm and is unmovable. There are several components to the casket handles. The **arm** is the piece of the handle that connects the bar to the lug. The **bail handle** is the solitary grip in which the lug, arm, and bar are combined. The **lug** (ear) is the part of the handle that attaches to the body of the casket. The **tip** is the ornamental piece attached to the end of the bar. The **corner** is the hardware attached at each of the four corners of the casket body.

Casket Textile Materials

Interior fabric choices include linen, crepe, broadcloth, doeskin, plush, satin, and velvet. A **crushed interior** is created with a lining material on a metal form, pressed on with weight, and steamed into place. A **shirred interior** is lined with material that is gathered and sewn in place. A **tufted interior** incorporates a padded material sewn between the lining and backing material to create a raised, cushioned look. A **tailored interior** has a tightly drawn lining. The **overlay** (throw) is the cloth that covers the foot panel. The **apron** is the portion of the overlay that drapes into the body of the casket and attaches to the foot panel in a half-couch casket. In a full-couch casket, the throw covers the decedent from the waist down; full-couch caskets do not have aprons. The **cove** (roll-puffing) is a lining inside the casket of the rim, adjacent to the cap panel. The **masselin** is an upholstery material made of pressed paper in a sheet form. **Head panels** are specialty items inserted over the inner panel. These include emblems, symbols, or custom-drawn impressions.

Infant and Oversized Caskets

Infant caskets are often casket/vault combinations. Some suppliers construct infant/child caskets with the same materials as standard caskets. While available sizes vary between suppliers, some start as small as 12" in exterior length. The interior dimensions are most important in choosing a casket to fit the decedent. Standard wood caskets measure 75" × 22" × 16–22", while metals are 78" × 23" × 16–24". **Oversized casket** interiors are wider than 24"; most are 29–36" wide and 82–84" long. Sizes increase in increments of 2". Oversized caskets can have crank beds or loose cellulose/foam batting, allowing for positioning flexibility. These caskets are manufactured with or without gaskets, with polycarbonate or steel hardware, and with stationary or swing bars (which are narrower than stationary bars when in the down position). Oversized caskets require additional hardware lugs and bottom braces. Handling considerations for oversized decedents include measuring the body at the widest part (from elbow to elbow); removing the lid for casketing ease; determining whether the casket requires two church trucks; checking the width of all hallways and doors at the funeral home, church, and vehicle; and determining whether oversized caskets need oversized vaults and oversized graves.

Outer Burial Containers

Outer burial containers (OBC) are often required by cemeteries. Their purpose is to prevent the ground from settling, withstand the weight and pressure of the surrounding soil, and accommodate the weight of passing cemetery equipment. **Grave liners** are composed of concrete, wood, polymers, or fiberglass. They withstand the weight of the earth but do not seal or have protective measures. The grave liner can be a grave box (a base box and a lid) or sectional (untreated concrete slabs that are lowered around and atop the casket); grave boxes are the most common form. **Burial vaults** can be sealed to protect against environmental elements. They can be composed of treated and enhanced concrete, metals, polypropylene, or fiberglass. OBCs typically have an interior dimension of 86" long × 30" wide × 25" high and an exterior dimension of 90" long × 34" wide × 33" high. Exact measurements vary between companies. Oversized OBCs are available for oversized caskets. For these cases, the grave openings need to be dug wider than standard. Some cemeteries have extra space factored into the grave spaces to accommodate larger OBCs, while others may require the family to purchase two spaces.

Cremation and Alternative Containers

Alternative cremation containers are simple nonmetal receptacles for human remains, often composed of cardboard, particleboard, polyethylene, or other combustible materials. They contain the body prior to cremation and are used for the cremation process. **Cremation caskets** are made of combustible materials with minimal metal components and range from simple to ornate. Many have finished interiors and can be used for services prior to cremation. Families may select a cremation casket for services with the body present, a ceremonial cremation, or even a direct cremation. **Ceremonial rental caskets** are used for services with the body present, prior to cremation. A cardboard container with interior fabrics is fitted inside the interior of the casket for services. For the cremation process, the cardboard container is rolled out of the foot end of the casket. The casket shell is then reused with a new liner and fabrics.

Cremated remains are placed in an **urn**. When an urn is not selected, the remains are placed in a plastic bag inside a **temporary container** (an industry-standard plastic box) inside a cardboard box. Urns are available in many sizes and materials to serve different functions; they can be biodegradable and can be used for burial, decoration, scattering, or keepsakes.

Sales of Merchandise and Services and Selection Room Approaches

The funeral home should establish a plan for sales of merchandise and services. This plan should include a profile of the funeral home's clients and techniques for increasing sales to them. It should also include specific sales objectives, such as increasing profit by 10% in one year.

In presenting merchandise, funeral directors must know their products, prices, and delivery/turn-around timelines and clearly answer questions from families. In the **direct selection room approach**, the director remains in the selection room throughout the entire process, giving support and answering questions. In contrast, in the **indirect selection room approach**, the director gives the family an overview of the room and then leaves them to discuss options in private.

Selecting Suppliers and Vendors

There are many considerations for selecting merchandise suppliers, including the type and quality of items they offer. Large companies have **sales representatives (reps)** who facilitate orders and sales. Reps meet with funeral directors to showcase the array and quality of products offered. They provide information on changes, discontinued items, upcoming sales, and new products, and they offer insight into what is currently selling well. Reps will help design selection rooms to feature their products. Consider whether vendors have informational brochures, sales magazines, or web portals available for funeral directors to directly show clients without the need for alterations. These aids are extremely helpful because selection rooms are limited in space. Select companies with merchandise in-stock at nearby warehouses or that have expedited shipping available. Look into discounts and incentives. Quality customer service and representative availability from vendors is important. Funeral directors need a point of contact for product issues to ensure timely resolution. Reps routinely check in with funeral directors to ensure satisfaction with products and services.

Ordering Merchandise

A **cash discount** is a reduced sale price and is valid for immediate sales only. A **quantity discount** is a reduced sale price for buying multiple items. A **rebate** returns monies to the purchaser at a later date. A **consignment** is an agreement between a wholesaler and retailer for units to be on loan or display, to be paid as they are sold. **Inventory** refers to goods for future sale. **Inventory turnover** refers to the amount of stock that sells over a year or period. **Economic order quantity (EOQ)** is the quantity of units to be purchased for the greatest savings. **Casket handling fees** may be imposed on the consumer by a funeral home if a casket is purchased from a third-party seller. According to the Federal Trade Commission, funeral providers must accept merchandise from a third-party seller and cannot charge a fee for the use of such merchandise, and so, while they are fairly common, casket handling fees are illegal.

Selection Room

A **selection room** should be located near or adjacent to the arrangement room. Selection rooms should be decorated with neutral colors. Casket display equipment includes a **casket stand** for single unit support or a **casket rack** that can display or store two caskets, one above the other. A **church truck** is an accordion unit with wheels for casket transport, capable of being transported in a hearse; older units may be solid or simply fold rather than accordion. A **demonstration group** is a display of select casket units that show the customer the various materials used in construction. A **fractional display** is a casket selection room with partial casket panels or ends and corners rather than full caskets. Selection rooms can display products from one company or feature multiple suppliers.

Pre-Need Sales Plans and Presentation Styles

Funeral homes have three options for establishing a pre-need program: establish it themselves, hire dedicated pre-need staff, or outsource to a specialized pre-need company. **Passive pre-need programs** are when the funeral director waits for people to request pre-need appointments. These programs are usually minimal, consisting of brochures displayed in the funeral home or newspaper advertisements to provide some information about pre-planning. **Active pre-need programs** are when funeral homes actively encourage and recruit people to make pre-arrangements. This approach uses multiple sources of **direct marketing** (such as mail, television, or radio advertisements) and community events to educate and secure future clientele. Many funeral homes use funeral directors to make pre-need appointments; however, some states do not require pre-need staff to be licensed funeral directors. To implement a successful pre-need program, a funeral home must establish program goals, advertise, designate staff or hire someone to dedicate time for pre-need arrangements, and evaluate components to expand those that are successful and adjust those that are not.

Determining Pricing of Merchandise and Services

The Federal Trade Commission (FTC) requires itemized pricing, but packages are allowed if families are given a **General Price List (GPL)** that lists everything separately. Types of pricing systems include:

- **Itemized:** Services and merchandise are priced individually.
- **Unit pricing:** Services and merchandise are combined into one total.
- **Bi-Unit pricing:** Services and merchandise are separately grouped in price.
- **Functional pricing:** Services and merchandise are listed by category.
- **Package pricing:** Specific service styles and merchandise are grouped together.

After merchandise is selected, the funeral director needs to remove the selected items from inventory and/or order products. When ordering, provide necessary details to the supplier, including customization, add-ons, and delivery schedule, to ensure that items arrive in time for the services.

Pricing Philosophies and Pricing Packages for Funerals

Methods used to determine prices for merchandise include:

- **Fixed multiple** or **times factor**: The wholesale price is marked up by a fixed amount—this makes things easy but does not factor in the **Consumer Value Index (CVI)**, which is the wholesale cost divided by the retail price.
- **Gradual recovery**: This is characterized by varied markup, which increases for higher-cost items. Less markup on the low-end puts the best value on lower-priced products.
- **Declining price structure:** As wholesale costs increase, the markup decreases, which improves CVI, encouraging higher-end purchases.
- **Modified declining price:** This is characterized by declining price structures with a lower markup on the lowest-end casket.

Gross profit margins (retail cost minus wholesale cost) are calculated to track profitability. Tracking inventory is important for re-ordering and evaluating what sells well and what doesn't. Using **inventory turnover**, or how much of a product is sold within a given timeframe, funeral directors can calculate their **economic order quality (EOQ)**, or the quantity ordered that will minimize total costs. Tracking **sales frequency**, the number of sales in a price category over a specific timeframe, is helpful in evaluating sales. Computer programs can accurately track and analyze sales of services and merchandise. Knowing what items sell well will guide future inventory purchases, ultimately leading to more sales and higher profits.

Retail Pricing Analysis

The **average (mean)** price is calculated by adding several prices and dividing the sum by the number of units. The **median (midpoint)** is the middle price: half the units are priced above this number and the other half below. The **mode** is the most common price. The **range** is the difference between the highest and lowest prices. A **quartile** is one of four equal divisions of data when the numbers are listed in order from smallest to largest; for example, the 25% quartile of prices is the lowest 25% of prices. **Income** is defined as business revenue received for the sale of goods and services. A **break-even analysis** studies a business position to determine the minimum volume of sales required to equal its expenses, resulting in neither profit nor loss.

Price List Documents and Itemization

The **statement of funeral goods and services selected** is a written document itemizing all goods and services chosen by the customer, including cost. A **non-declinable basic service fee** is the funeral home's charge for basic professional use of the facility and staff and is a minimum required charge when the customer selects the funeral home. **Sundry items** include register books, acknowledgement cards, thank you cards, and other small items. The **cash advance** is a portion of the funeral home contract that lists items purchased by the funeral home on behalf of the family, on their request, from a third-party seller, such as flowers, a newspaper obituary, cemetery fees, or an honorarium for an officiant. There is no markup or margin on these pass-through purchases, but the consumer may be required to pay in advance so the funeral home can order them.

Marketing

Marketing is the business planning and strategy methodology for the advertising and sale of goods and services to the consumer. **Demographics** are statistical population studies that measure size, composition, and socioeconomic conditions. A **market** is a group of people with purchasing power and unsatisfied needs and wants. **Market research** is the analysis of demographics and psychographics in a target market. An **economic base** is a local population of wealth produced in an area, including community employment. The **market value approach** determines a business's value by comparing the revenues of other businesses offering similar goods and services in similar market segments. **Public relations** is the process of promoting a business in a positive, community-oriented manner. **Advertising** is the process of creating public awareness of a service or commodity for sale through various mediums. **Sales promotions** are how a business represents certain products or services as a special value by offering incentives to purchase during a certain period.

Accounting

Accounting is the communication and interpretation of financial information according to standardized business practice. **Bookkeeping** is the process of entering accounting details into a **journal** to record all financial transactions. **Assets** are the various forms of property owned by the business. **Accounts receivable** are a form of business asset representing payment due to the business. **Inventory** is a form of business asset that includes goods and materials intended for resale and distribution. **Liabilities** are the debts owed by the business. **Accounts payable** are a form of business liability representing monies due from the business to another party. A **debit** is a business journal entry that increases an asset account. A **credit** is a business journal entry that decreases an asset account.

Considerations of Customer Service

A main consideration of **customer service** within funeral homes is pricing. Funeral homes need to be profitable while remaining both fair to clients and competitive with other area funeral homes. In providing service options to families, directors need to be aware and respectful of budgets. Present options and let the family select what they are comfortable with. If they disclose a price cap for services and merchandise, guide them to options that are realistic for their needs and budget. Successful funeral directors have exceptional customer service. It is essential that customers find value in both the services and merchandise the funeral home provides. People have exceedingly high expectations, and meeting them can be challenging. By actively listening, paying attention to detail, flexibly meeting (reasonable and legal) requests without judgement, and providing compassionate yet proficient service, funeral directors can serve families well. Tools such as follow-up aftercare and customer service surveys are available to help provide insight into how the director and staff performed. Feedback from families gives insight into how the funeral home and staff are operating and gives an opportunity for both compliments and constructive criticism.

Business Plans

Creating a **business plan** is one of the first steps of starting a business. It describes the business, including its organization, marketing strategies, management structure, services and/or products and how they surpass competition, and funding needs. A business plan can be used to gain investors and secure loans. **Primary objectives** are the essential goals required for a business to be successful. These relate to profitability, productivity, growth, and efficiency. A funeral home's primary objectives include profiting by caring for the dead while fulfilling family requests. **Secondary objectives** are how the business will meet primary objectives. Providing quality services can lead to referrals, which contribute to profit and business growth. **Short-term goals**

and objectives are what a business plans to attain in less than a year, often within a period of weeks or months. They are smaller goals, laid out in steps, to keep moving toward long-term goals. **Long-term goals** take longer to achieve and are bigger-picture goals. A short-term goal is starting a pre-need program with educational events and programs. This takes steps toward long-term growth goals of serving more families in years to come. Short-term goals can help maintain employee morale and motivation while working toward long-term goals.

FUNERAL HOME MANAGEMENT

Funeral home management includes motivating people and resources to accomplish objectives and goals throughout the funeral home. Managers oversee various aspects of the funeral home, including employees, maintenance, compliance with regulations, and customer satisfaction. There are four functions of management:

- **Planning**: Crucial to the success of a business, a manager must plan and strategize, in great detail, projects and tasks that need to be accomplished by staff members to meet the goals and objectives of the business.
- **Organization**: Managers coordinate staff members, divide workloads, and allocate resources to meet both day-to-day and long-term goals. Nurturing teamwork and unity within the workplace sets the groundwork for a productive and positive work environment.
- **Directing/Actuating**: By listening to problems and facilitating healthy solutions while removing workplace toxicity, successful managers encourage, support, and motivate employees to reach objectives.
- **Evaluating/Controlling**: Managers are responsible for attaining the goals set out by the business. Evaluations measure the success or shortcomings of staff, services, and/or merchandise. When goals are not met or performances are inadequate, the manager must take control to redirect, reevaluate, and revise to a successful course.

AREAS OF MANAGEMENT WITHIN THE FUNERAL HOME

A **funeral service manager** must have a broad knowledge base to be successful. Some funeral homes have one manager, while others may have several. The following is a list of management categories that need to be overseen and directed:

- **Finances**: accounting, budgeting, asset and liability management (cash flow, inventory, and receivables), price structure and evaluation, and billing
- **Marketing**: promoting products, advertising, customer and public relations, and pre-need programming and events
- **Human resources**: employee staffing, including hiring, firing, evaluations, compensation, promotions, and training
- **Facilities**: physical building care, construction, and maintenance; groundskeeping; fleet management; meeting governmental regulations (OSHA, ADA, EPA)
- **Funeral service management**: funeral services and dispositions, religious rites, product and merchandise knowledge, decedent care, securing and filing legal documentation, and aftercare programs
- **Office**: computers and equipment maintenance, recordkeeping, phone calls and correspondence, pre-need and at-need documentation, scheduling, and banking

Successful management within these departments and collaboration between managers will lead to a successful and thriving business.

Psychology in Funeral Service

Psychological Needs of the Bereaved and the Role of Funeral Rites and Services

Throughout the grieving process, the surviving family and friends must progress through various stages of grief to successfully restructure their lives without their loved one. This **grief work** can be broken down into stages, although everyone grieves and reacts differently as they process their emotions. The bereaved must come to terms with their loss, accept the pain that comes with this acknowledgement, transition from a living to memorialized relationship, reestablish and redefine their life without this person, and redirect emotional energy. The relationship between the decedent and the bereaved, the manner of death, and the bereaved's prior loss experience all factor into the complexity of grief work.

Funeral rites can address some of the psychological and psychosocial needs of the bereaved. They allow family to focus on accomplishing specific, time-sensitive tasks; share memories and talk about their loved one; outwardly mourn their loss within a socially acceptable platform where they won't be judged or feel embarrassed; participate in comforting religious or spiritual ceremonies and traditions; view the decedent; receive community and social support; and receive information about grief therapy and available bereavement support.

Bereavement, Grief, and Mourning

The death of a person is a form of loss also known as **bereavement**. A bereaved person is assaulted by a range of emotions, which are categorized as **grief**. J. William Worden categorizes grief into four classes: masked, exaggerated, chronic, and delayed. Exaggerated is the most extreme form. **Mourning** is an emotional expression of loss by a person who experiences grief and is undergoing the process of incorporating the loss into his or her daily reality. A person with grief syndrome, according to Worden, displays psychological and somatic symptoms. A person exhibiting a masked grief may not recognize that his or her actions or behaviors are a result of grief.

Types of Grief

Anomic grief is difficult for the survivor because he or she has not established an acceptable method to deal with the grief. One example of this type of grief can be found when a parent loses a child. The parent had expected the child to outlive him or her and did not establish a method to deal with the mourning process. The parent is likely to be disoriented for some time.

Anticipatory grief occurs when death is imminent, usually after a long illness. Death may come as a relief since the survivor has likely watched the loved one suffer and has had time to grasp the fact that life is limited.

Delayed grief occurs when feelings of loss are put off until the person can cope with those feelings at a future time.

Exaggerated grief is an extreme form of grief that can cause a person to become motionless and unable to keep functioning.

Masked grief is exhibited by a person in an unaware state who does not recognize that his/her actions or behaviors are a result of grief.

Complicated grief is a chronic grief that remains unresolved for a seemingly endless period of time.

Acute Grief

Acute grief can be linked to emotional, physical, behavioral, and cognitive factors. People can experience grief from not just losing a loved one but also from ending a relationship or losing a job, pet, or possession. The level of grief suffered may depend on the individual's personality. Many factors can trigger **grief responses**. For example, family upbringing can have a direct impact on how a person deals with grief. A person's culture or religious beliefs may also influence the grieving process. Bereavement is a natural part of life, and everyone can expect to lose loved ones at some point. Extended family relationships, children, marriage, and mental health can be negatively impacted during the mourning process. Thus, it is important for a person in mourning to seek **emotional support**.

Psychological, Sociological, and Physiological Influences on Grief

Grief affects everyone differently. An individual's grief journey can be separated into **psychological** (internal), **sociological** (external), and **physiological** (biological) influences. Psychological factors that influence grief include:

- **The relationship between the deceased and survivor**: The level of love, attachment, and dependency influence mourning.
- **Nature of death**: Natural and expected deaths (extended illness or deterioration with advanced age) allow families to say goodbye, find closure, and mentally prepare. Unexpected, sudden deaths cause complicated grief journeys. This complexity compounds when the death involves violence or suicide.
- **Prior experience with grief and loss**: Reactions and resolution to previous losses predict an individual's response to their current loss and how they will progress through new grief.

Sociological influences involve the mourner's community, family structure, religion, and economic status. Funeral rites factor into the grief journey, providing an environment to outwardly express emotions and receive social support. Physiological influences include sleep, nutrition, exercise, and sometimes alcohol and drug use, whether prescription or self-selected. Understanding these influences will help funeral directors successfully and nonjudgmentally work with people navigating grief journeys.

Theories of Grief

Lindemann's Grief Syndrome

Studies have shown that similar **physical symptoms of grief** appear among those who suffer from grief. Erich Lindemann reported these commonalities in 1944, his findings based on a study of young survivors of a traumatic fire. **Somatic distress** may come in waves or be intermittent, each episode lasting from 20 minutes to an hour. These symptoms may include tightness in the throat, a choking sensation or shortness of breath, sighing heavily or often, a feeling of emptiness in the stomach region, a lack of muscular power and vitality, and intense pain or tension. These physical conditions are a real and valid complaint among those who suffer from **grief syndrome**. The grieving individual may not even be aware or only vaguely aware that he or she is exhibiting signs of somatic distress associated with grief syndrome.

Attachment Theory

John Bowlby observed a mother's instinct to protect her young and hypothesized that an infant's desire to explore and develop is strengthened by the attachment with his or her mother. This was contrary to Sigmund Freud's views on the breaking of this attachment. Chris Fraley and Philip Shaver went on to say that romantic relationships have similarities to the infant and mother relationships or attachments. This theory holds that a person's desire to experience safety and security is made evident whenever he or she is near someone to whom he or she is attached. The positive side of this attachment is found in the way that a romantic partnership is shared throughout a person's lifetime. However, when the spouse dies, the sense of loss is amplified by this same attachment.

Tasks of Mourning and Grief Therapy

J. William Worden described the **four tasks of mourning** that a counselor can help a grieving person through in **grief therapy**. The first task is **acceptance** of the death. The bereaved may have difficulty accepting the finality of death and the loss of that person. The second task involves **processing** emotions. Physical and emotional pain is now a part of everyday existence. Then, the person must **adjust** to a new environment without the deceased person, including performing tasks previously accomplished by the deceased. This can create anxiety over the new responsibilities as well as frustration and anger that the deceased person is no longer there to do the work. In the fourth and final task, the survivor must **emotionally break ties** with the deceased. This break allows the survivor to continue with life and form new relationships, which can be difficult because the survivor may feel as if he or she is betraying or dishonoring the deceased by moving on.

Stages of Dying

Elisabeth Kübler-Ross described the **stages of death and dying** based on her studies surrounding the dying process.

- The first stage involves **denial and isolation**. For example, an individual may stay away from the deathbed of a loved one in an attempt to avoid the situation. Many people avoid situations in which they are unsure how to react or to respond.
- The second stage is **anger**. A person may be angry with God for letting a situation occur or angry at the environment, doctors, nurses, or friends and family members. The person may feel that no one else is going through the situation with quite the same intensity.
- The third stage involves **bargaining**. This may involve an internal argument with God as the person tries to negotiate over the impending death.
- The fourth stage involves **depression**. A person in this stage expresses regrets over past losses. Reactive depression is expressed in response to lost jobs, lost hobbies, or a loss of mobility. Preparatory depression is expressed in relation to expected future losses, such as a loss of independence due to age.
- The fifth stage is **acceptance**, when the person comes to terms with the inevitability of his or her own death.

Stages of Grief

Previously it was believed that grief, like dying, could be categorized into five stages: **denial**, **anger**, **bargaining**, **depression**, and **acceptance**. However, there are now other models of grief that are based on processes and dynamics rather than simple stages. One such model involves phases of processing the death. The first phase comes from a need for self-preservation. Shock, numbness, or a sense of unreality may appear as strength. The next phase includes a yearning and searching for the person that has been lost. It is not unusual for a person to search crowds for the face of a lost loved one. This yearning may be called "pining away" for the loved one. Another phase in the process of grief is disorganization and despair. This is recognized as depression and can last for years. The culmination of this process ends with acceptance. Acceptance involves a reorganization and rebuilding of the survivor's life without the presence of the deceased.

Denial and Acceptance

Denial is a normal reaction when someone dies suddenly or violently. **Denial**, often the first step in the grieving process, begins as a coping system for the grieving person. The mind shies away from the loss and begins to deny the reality of the loved one's death. The person in denial is experiencing a type of **shock** and may even appear calm and controlled. This period of denial can be short or may last a long time. Religious and cultural groups can be of enormous comfort to the person experiencing loss. Viewing the body may also reduce the length of denial. During the grieving process, loved ones must reach a point of **emotional release**. Writing the death announcement can provide a significant psychological benefit to the grieving party. Funeral rites can allow those who are grieving to express sorrow over the departure of a loved one. The idea that the deceased is resting peacefully can provide comfort, and this idea may be enhanced by viewing the body if circumstances permit. Making the funeral arrangements can also help the person to accept the death, accelerating the grieving process. By accepting the death of the loved one, a person can finally reach **closure**.

Reactions to Grief

A grieving person may feel anger, frustration, abandonment, or resentment. Anger may be directed at the loved one who has died or sometimes at other family members. The grieving person may feel that others are not grieving enough or may even blame the death of a loved one on an attending physician or other party. **Guilt** is also often experienced during loss. Guilt is the result of unresolved issues with the deceased person and may be the result of a misperception by the survivor that the death could have been averted by some action on his or her part. Many people experience **powerlessness** and **hopelessness** over the death of a loved one. Some exhibit signs of sleeplessness, disrupted sleep patterns, or an overpowering sense of loss. Others can become extremely violent, moody, or sensitive and may withdraw socially and become deeply depressed. Lethargy and troubling doubts are common; many even question their faith and belief systems. Some become incapable of expressing emotion during this time. The funeral director must take all these factors into consideration when dealing with family members who exhibit these reactions to grief. The director should remain **diplomatic** and **sympathetic** during encounters with grieving family members.

Grief Process Risks

The grief process can make a person extremely **vulnerable**. Some people experience nightmares or sleep disorders during this time. Others experience loss or increase in appetite, and still others develop a habit of making repetitive motions in an attempt to avoid the pain of loss. A person may experience events, such as hearing the deceased's favorite song or going to a place that the bereaved and the deceased visited together, that trigger a fresh emotional response to the loss. In some cases, a person deeply affected by grief may experience **hallucinations**. These hallucinations usually involve seeing or hearing the loved one come into a room or stand at the doorway in a familiar way. The experiences can be auditory, visual, olfactory, positional, or gustatory in nature, and these sensations may still be evident a year or two after the loss. If these sensations continue or worsen after a lengthy period of time, the bereaved should seek professional help.

Death of a Child or a Spouse

Children can die as a result of stillbirth, sudden infant death syndrome (SIDS), illness, or accidents. Many parents are unable to accept the child's death and experience extreme guilt. The intensity of grief often leads to marital problems, depression, and occasionally attempted suicide. Another form of intense bereavement is caused by the death of a spouse. The surviving spouse often expresses a sense of loss of self and may have difficulty adjusting to the added obligations of carrying on the deceased's duties. Many find that social occasions are difficult and so may isolate themselves from social events. Still others are left out of social activities involving couples. The separation of the dyad (a group of two people) can be one of life's most traumatic events.

Children and Grief

Children can express grief in a variety of ways, depending on personality and age. In children up to age 2, there is a sense of loss that may be transferred from the caregiver to the self. The child's eating, toilet, or sleeping habits may be affected. Children from 2 to 6 years of age may still not understand the concepts of death or time. A child may fail to mourn, may personify the death, or may have other nonverbal communication disturbances. Some young children may believe that the deceased person should eat, drink, and perform other natural functions. Some think that the parent can come back if the child just wishes hard enough. Children ages 6 to 9 may view death as a monster that has taken the parent away. The child may question the causes of death. From ages 9 to 12, the child may believe that death is a punishment, perhaps for previous arguments with the parent. The child may feel apprehension over the funeral and burial and may have concerns about who will take over as caregiver.

Impact of Natural Deaths on the Grieving Process

Extended illness, degrading health, pre-existing conditions, and advanced age all help prepare family and friends for death, giving them time to process mortality and their inevitable loss and begin mentally preparing for their grief journey. This also gives them time to consider or begin preliminary plans for disposition, easing the post-death burden of funeral decisions. Family and friends have time to express their love, make peace with their dying loved one, or create a few final memories. These opportunities support later grief work. However, the surprise of a loved one dying suddenly (e.g., from myocardial infarction, stroke, or aneurysm) complicates grief work. If the survivor was present for the medical event, this can add traumatic memories and emotional distress. The age of the decedent influences the survivor's grief journey and how they may rationalize the death, feel anger for premature loss, experience sadness for missed life events of the survivors, and have difficulty restructuring life without the decedent. Miscarriages and stillbirths can bring up feelings of guilt and anger; trauma from the expulsion, removal, or birth of the fetus/baby; loneliness, isolation, and lack of support; feeling minimized by others in their grief; and crushed dreams and anticipation of the future. An unknown cause of fetal or infant death complicates grief further.

Role of Hospice in Preparing the Family for Death

Hospice provides medical care and support to people who are terminally ill and/or declining in health. Care can be provided in homes, nursing facilities, hospice centers, or hospice units within hospitals. Hospice programs and companies abide by state and federal regulations. Patients must meet specific criteria to be eligible for **hospice care** (prognosis of six months or less to live; terminally ill or in a state of decline; not on life-extending medications; difficulty with self-care, mobility, and communication; and typically a need for pain management). In addition to physical care, hospice provides emotional care; medical, dietary, and spiritual counseling; and access to resources. It prepares both the patient and the patient's family for the death. They have a schedule of care but are on call to provide additional support to the patient and family as needed.

Following death, hospice helps with many immediate tasks such as contacting the funeral home, removing medical equipment and devices from the home/facility, and cleaning or tidying up the death space after the person is transferred out of the home. Over the next few weeks, hospice personnel stay in touch with the family, checking in with them, providing resources, and inviting them to bereavement events and support groups.

Impact of Deaths from Neurodegenerative Diseases

Alzheimer's disease slowly degrades mental function and physical health until death. This extended **neurodegenerative disease** is difficult for families. Often, a family member assumes the demanding role of caregiver. As the demands increase, the caregiver feels isolated from the community and often is left unsupported. The family mourns the loss of their loved one prior to death because Alzheimer's affects temperament, disposition, and characteristics as the disease progresses. As the brain deteriorates, patients may lose the ability to recognize family, which causes additional stress as the family watches their loved one forget who they are. Following death, caregivers can feel relief, experience guilt for feeling that relief, and have continued trauma from the memories of their loved one's deterioration. The caregiver can remain isolated after the death because it can be difficult or overwhelming to restart activities and social interactions after not having the time or energy for them for years prior. They also may have lost many societal connections and friends as their caregiving role increased. Other neurodegenerative diseases requiring immense family support and intensive caregiving (e.g., multiple sclerosis, amyotrophic lateral sclerosis, Parkinson's disease, and muscular dystrophy) are similarly emotionally and physically taxing to the caregiver and produce similar grief responses.

Impact of Deaths from SIDS on the Grieving Process

Sudden infant death syndrome (SIDS): The unexpected, sudden loss of an infant creates complicated grief work. The unknown cause of death causes parents and caregivers to feel guilt for not providing sufficient care to the baby. The community can also leave the family feeling judged and isolated by implying that the family was neglectful or harmed the baby. Siblings are significantly impacted by SIDS. They grieve the loss, fight guilt, deal with their parents' reaction to grief, and can direct anger towards their parents or the baby. SIDS deaths are typically investigated by the coroner/medical examiner and police, which causes additional duress to families in the days immediately following the death.

Impact of Deaths from AIDS on the Grieving Process

Acquired immune deficiency syndrome (AIDS): Some illnesses, like AIDS, have a stigma attached to them which impacts the survivors' grief work. In addition to grieving, these survivors can feel shame and experience isolation from their community. The fear of contracting the disease from their loved one can cause guilt as they distance themselves from their dying loved one.

Some survivors become advocates by creating a platform to educate the public, raise awareness, propose protective guidelines, provide resources to others affected by the disease, and memorialize their loved one.

Impact of Unnatural Deaths on the Grieving Process

Families suffering a loss from **suicide** deal with guilt, anger, desertion, isolation, depression, and community stigmas (e.g., blame, lack of support and empathy, and negative views of the deceased). The term "commit suicide" reflects the negative perceptions associated with the act of suicide. Religious organizations usually provide extensive support following a loss, but some condemn this act, leaving survivors feeling isolated without the comfort of their religion, judged, hurt, and ashamed. The bereaved have an intense desire to know why the person chose to die by suicide.

Death by **homicide** results in extremely complicated grief work. Survivors must come to terms with the death, the manner and violence of the death, the untimeliness of the death, emotions such as anger and fear, resulting trauma (if the death was witnessed), and the investigative and trial procedures.

Unexpected, sudden deaths from an **accident** leave the bereaved in shock; overwhelmed; struggling with denial, anger, and acceptance; feeling lonely and abandoned from the sudden detachment; and traumatized from witnessing or being involved in the accident. Accidental deaths rob survivors of the farewells and goodbyes that accompany anticipated deaths.

In the case of a missing person presumed or legally declared dead, the bereaved struggle with acceptance of the death, the unknown, and the inability to lay their loved one to rest.

Value of Participation in Funeral Rites

Funeral ceremonies and rites play an important role in the grief process. Planning services, making decisions and selections, writing obituaries, and attending memorial services are all part of participating in honoring the life of a loved one. These tasks and gatherings provide structure and guidance for the family while helping to distract from grief and allow them to refocus. Participation in the preparation of the body (as seen in some religions) and in funeral/memorial services can be cathartic. Funeral directors should encourage reasonable participation wherever the family members are comfortable. Funeral rites encourage the community to unite around grieving families, providing them with love and support as they restructure their lives without the decedent. Participation can consist of simply receiving friends and family at a visitation or gathering, or it can be involvement in services such as readings, eulogies, lighting candles, pallbearing, laying flowers on the grave, and more. Within some belief systems, **grave goods**—items given to the dead prior to disposition—can be important in the grief process; sending decedents off with important or meaningful items, sentimental or religious, is a way to ensure that they have what they need for the afterlife.

Funeral Service Counseling

Counseling and Therapy

Funeral directors should be aware of the types of counseling that grieving families and friends may receive from therapists. **Grief counseling** is therapy for the persons involved in the grief process. This therapy allows people to gain a healthy perspective on the circumstances of their loss and to accept that loss in a natural grieving process. It is reserved for **uncomplicated** forms of grief. **Grief therapy** is appropriate for those who are experiencing forms of **abnormal grief**, such as delayed grief, inhibited grief, and prolonged grief. The aim is to help a person overcome the defenses that are impeding and blocking the natural process of mourning. **Crisis counseling** addresses short-lived or temporary needs of a person who is unable to function because of the intensity of grief. This grief may manifest as confusion, pain, or other strong emotions.

The Role Funeral Directors Play in Counseling Families

From the first call to aftercare, funeral directors act as advisors and support systems for families beginning their grief journey; in this role, they are **funeral service counselors**. Funeral service counselors are not therapists or grief counselors, but they do use many of the same skills. Reading body language, facial expressions, and posture allows the director to surmise how people are feeling, determine how open they are, and understand their emotional state. Active listening, asking questions, commenting on observations, acknowledging and validating feelings, and encouraging participation help establish a relationship with the family to guide them through their loss. Facilitating disposition decisions and walking families through service and memorialization options helps them feel supported, which reduces angst, stress, and overwhelm. Following services, funeral directors can refer families to aftercare programs facilitated by the funeral home or other community organizations that can continue to support them.

While funeral service counselors can validate emotions, guide families in funeral-related decision-making, and make industry-specific suggestions to ease the burden of their grief, they should not act as therapists. Grief-therapy resources should be provided to families to ensure that they get the support and help they need to process their grief in a healthy way.

The Funeral Director as Facilitator

The funeral director works closely with the bereaved to help them **feel at ease** during the process of funeral planning. The director may offer alternatives or suggestions to help the survivors plan a meaningful service that reflects the life of the deceased while being healing for friends and family who attend. This is not a therapy session. Instead, a funeral service director offers detailed examples and choices for the bereaved family. A good funeral service director illustrates with ease, clearly outlining and explaining the products and services offered. The director does not take an active part in the decision-making process. Instead, he or she should have a smooth, professional demeanor that makes him or her **unobtrusive** to the survivors as they work through decisions. The clients must be allowed to make their own decisions given the information that the funeral service director expertly provides.

Interpersonal Skills Necessary for Funeral Directors

Funeral directors use verbal and nonverbal interpersonal skills to communicate effectively with families. Facial expressions, eye contact, body language, and posture are all forms of **nonverbal communication**. It is important for funeral directors to be mindful of their own nonverbal communication and how it may impact the families. Additionally, directors can use their familiarity with nonverbal communication to read how family members are feeling throughout their funeral experience. These cues can reveal if someone is stressed, overwhelmed, uncomfortable, confused, or open to guidance or suggestions. Observations can be extremely helpful in navigating the best way to communicate and approach people. **Verbal communication** is oral, including discussions, questions, reflections, and comments. **Listening skills** are imperative for funeral directors to effectively communicate with grieving families. Factors that decrease how well someone listens include biases, emotional strain, distractions, overwhelming amounts of information, and fatigue. Active listening, conveying understanding and empathy, eliminating distractions, reading nonverbal cues, and sharing commonalities can establish trust and comfortable rapport. Responding appropriately is part of listening and understanding. Validating emotions can aid in comforting and providing support to people on a long grief journey.

Counseling Aspects Seen Through Pre-Need, at-Need, and Aftercare Services

There are many ways funeral directors can support families and communities through grief journeys. While directors are not therapists or counselors, they do provide grief facilitation. Never refer to support programs as therapy. Through **pre-need** programs, funeral directors educate and guide individuals who often have a clear mind and are not under emotional duress in planning their own services. These appointments can have counseling or emotional-support aspects as clients are reflecting on their own mortality. There can be many emotions at play when pre-planning with a family whose loved one just received a terminal diagnosis or entered hospice care. Funeral directors provide significant **at-need** emotional support and counseling during arrangements with families at a time of loss. They guide a family through funeral planning and help them begin to process the loss through talking, sharing stories, and validating emotions. **Aftercare** programs vary in complexity. They can consist of a phone call to check in with the family, brochures or resources on grief and loss, emails or newsletters with helpful information and encouragement, or community programs where families can connect with others suffering a loss. Referrals to therapists and trained grief counselors can be provided.

Legal and Regulatory Compliance

The American Legal System

The American legal system is divided into federal law governing the nation, state law governing individual states, and local law governing municipalities within states. The **federal court** system is divided into US District Courts (which conduct trials), US Courts of Appeals (which conduct appeals of trial verdicts), and the US Supreme Court (which makes final interpretations and decisions). **State court** systems vary but typically follow the same hierarchy. Courts are further divided into **criminal courts**, which preside over charges filed by authorities to determine whether crimes and violations of law have been committed, and **civil courts**, which preside over property settlements, family disputes, and allegations of loss or suffering between private parties.

Types of Law

Case law is enacted by the court as they determine the extent of and intent behind written laws as it applies to a specific case. Case law sets precedent that lower courts are expected to follow. **Constitutional law** has been developed from the interpretation of a state or federal written constitution containing the fundamental principles of government among its executive, legislative, and judiciary branches. **Common law** is used by federal or state courts when an issue is not addressed in statutes or constitutional law. Precedents, outcomes of previous cases, and universal principles are the foundation of common law rather than laws, statutes, or codes. **Civil law**, sometimes referred to as civilian law, refers to a body of laws addressing individual rights such as property rights, family matters, and contracts. **Criminal law** determines the punishment for someone convicted of breaking a law. **Statutory law** refers to a legally enforceable written statute enacted by a legislative body, such as Congress or a state legislature. An **ordinance** is a law enacted by a municipality that may address specific safety, building, or zoning requirements.

Case Law

One of the important principles of common law is that as particular areas of the law are applied in actual cases, insight is gained for future cases. When a court resolves a relatively new issue, the decision establishes a **precedent** that may affect future court decisions as similar cases arise. The term **stare decisis** refers to the practice of the courts to uphold a ruling of precedent in other cases with similar facts and is often referred to as **case law**. The **statutes of limitations** are laws that set time restrictions to the legal enforcement in a court of law regarding a particular criminal event.

Criminal Law

A **crime** is an act that violates a law based on the constitution, a statute, or an ordinance. A crime is punishable based on the legal classification of the offense. A **felony** is a severe criminal act that is punishable by prison time or, in some states, capital punishment. A **misdemeanor** is a moderate non-felony criminal act that is punishable by a lesser form of punishment such as jail time, a fine, or community service.

Civil Law

Civil law is a set of rules governing non-criminal disputes between persons in such areas as contract, property, tort, and family law. A funeral director should be aware of civil laws relating to licensure and the legal requirements of professional conduct while doing business. A **plaintiff** is an individual who proceeds in attesting a civil action against another in the form of a **petition**. A **defendant** is the party to whom the civil action is addressed through the petition of the court. A **summons** is a legally binding complaint served to a defendant, describing a violation that requires a filed response. **Liability** is legal responsibility. **Liquidated damages** define the exact remedy of a breach of contract between two parties. **Malpractice** is an improper or negligent act by a professional. **Negligence** is the failure to exercise ordinary care or the omission of something a reasonably prudent person would do under ordinary circumstances. Lack of due care could be a violation of civil law. **Mental anguish** refers to damages to a person that may or may not be accompanied by physical injury and includes distress, sorrow, or humiliation caused by an outrageous, intentional, or grossly negligent act.

Administrative Law

Administrative law refers to the body of law created to provide guidelines for federal and state administrative agencies, including state boards and health departments. The government creates an administrative agency with appointed individuals who are responsible for enforcing the legislation. The administrative agency enacts the rules and regulations that provide the details of the agency's jurisdictional authority. **Police power** is the authority of state and federal government to make and enforce laws to guard public safety and maintain order. For funeral directors, this branch of law outlines legal obligations for licensure requirements, required health standards and practices, and business operational procedures.

Tort Law

Tort law is applied to a criminal act that is determined to be the result of a civil wrongdoing or of negligence against a person or property. It includes a compilation of obligatory duties, rights, and remedies applied in civil law proceedings for victims. An unauthorized photograph of a deceased person could be considered a violation of a right to privacy and therefore fall under tort law. **Tortious interference** is the deliberate obstruction of contractual dealings. **Moral turpitude** is an act that shows inherent baseness, vileness of principle, or depravity. A **breach of contract** occurs when one of the parties to a contract does not fulfill his or her contractual obligation. **Replevin** is an action taken to recover control of personal property. Examples of torts of cremation include the commingling of cremated remains, the failure to return all remains when urn size is insufficient, and the removal of jewelry or medical devices without obtaining permission. Torts may be intentional or unintentional. A **strict liability** tort is one in which intentionality does not matter. **Defamation** is a false statement (slander when spoken, libel when written) about a person that causes harm to their reputation. Defamation laws generally do not apply to the deceased.

Damages and Awards

A **judgment** is a legally binding decision of a court of law in a given jurisdiction. Tort violations resulting in **mental anguish** are divided into categories of physical impact, intentional infliction of mental distress, contractual breaches, and negligent infliction of mental distress. The **physical impact rule** is the principle that purely emotional harm from negligence is not sufficient to levy financial damages except in limited cases of intentional acts. **Compensatory damages** are compensation for actual monetary losses. **Punitive damages** are fines paid to plaintiffs as a punishment rather than merely compensation in cases of intentionally outrageous acts, and they are not covered by liability insurance. An **outrageous act** is a behavior that defies generally accepted social conduct. **Nominal damages** are minimal awards given to the plaintiff in recognition that the defendant wronged him or her.

Mortuary Law and the Right of Custody

Mortuary law, also known as **funeral law** or **mortuary jurisprudence**, is the branch of law that relates to the rules and principles that have been established for the handling and disposition of the deceased. Following the death of an individual, the **right of custody** refers to the legal guidelines as to who can have the body in their possession and make decisions as to its disposition. **Constructive custody** refers to the individual with authority to determine disposition. When the funeral director removes the body from the place of death and transfers it to the funeral home or moves it to another location such as a cemetery or crematory, he or she has **actual custody**, or physical possession, but not constructive custody. From the time of removal until final disposition, the funeral director is the legal guardian of the decedent and is considered to be the **custodian**.

Quasi-Property

Courts have classified decedents as **quasi-property**. Owners of property are entitled to specific rights relating to ownership such as controlling possession, use, profits, and disposition. Classifying decedents as quasi-property gives next of kin (NOK) a limited version of these specific rights. They are legally allowed to possess and transport the body, designate parties to possess and transport the body on their behalf, exclude parties from possessing the decedent, deny or designate anatomical gift donation or full-body donation within the legal scope, and determine final disposition of the body by legal means. The rights to a decedent as quasi-property can be revoked and control surpassed by authorities or court of law if disposition is not completed within the legal timeframe and by legal means (e.g., NOK cannot dispose of a body in a car trunk; they would be criminally charged, and their rights to disposition would be revoked).

Paramount Right of Disposition

The **paramount right of disposition** is the legal right to possess and determine disposition of the decedent. This right is given to the next of kin according to the following hierarchy, barring extenuating circumstances:

- Surviving spouse
- Children over the age of 18
- Parents
- Siblings
- Extended relatives

Factors that may influence or alter this hierarchy include wishes of the decedent, parties waiving rights, state statutes, and relationships requiring special consideration (e.g., unmarried domestic partners). In cases where the decedent does not have family, the right of disposition may fall to a friend or caretaker.

Regulations Surrounding Disinterments

Disinterment is the exhumation of a human corpse or cremated remains from its resting place. Disinterments are ordered under the pretense of public or private interest. Disinterment permits are issued by the registrar or applicable governing body. Authorizations are required from the cemetery and everyone within the highest level of kinship (NOK) or court of law, depending on the kind of disinterment. **Public interest disinterments** are court ordered, typically to gather evidence for criminal or civil lawsuits in the pursuit of justice. The body is exhumed, examined, and usually returned to the same cemetery. This category includes disinterments ordered by eminent domain or public health and safety when remains are reinterred elsewhere. **Private purpose disinterments** are requested by NOK to relocate remains elsewhere or within the same cemetery in cases of misinterment. Directors secure authorizations from NOK and cemeteries and complete disinterment/reinterment permits. If the validity of a request is questioned, a court of law intervenes. If the outer burial container (OBC) is compromised following disinterment, the remains are removed and placed into another prior to reinterment. An OBC should not be opened unless a court order or damage necessitates it. If the casket must be removed, it should not be opened unless a court order or damage necessitates a replacement.

LIABILITY TYPES INVOLVED IN FUNERAL EXPENSE CONTRACTS

Funeral directors need to establish who is responsible for paying the funeral expenses. Liability types include:

- **Estate Liability**: Funeral expenses take precedence over debt reconciliation. States designate limits on the amount an estate can pay towards funeral expenses; however, the value of the estate and social position are factored into expense justification. An estate administrator may be held personally liable for expenses if they neglect to sign as an administrator.
- **Dependent Liability**: Common law dictates that husbands and fathers are responsible for paying funeral expenses for their spouse and dependent children. This law supersedes estate liability, unless the will clearly states that the estate will pay funeral expenses. This applies despite estrangement, separation, or lack of contract. There is no reciprocation—wives are not held responsible. Some states have updated statutes for this antiquated law; directors need to be aware of their specific state laws.
- **Contract Liability**: Any party who authorizes the funeral contract is legally liable. This person may be responsible for all expenses or for the remaining balance following estate or insurance payment.
- **State Liability**: State or government branches can be liable when ordering services on behalf of a decedent. Verify funding prior to accepting a case.

TORT LIABILITY FOR FUNERAL DIRECTORS

Funeral directors must not interfere with the **right of disposition** and must take reasonable care to ensure that funeral homes or other locations are safe. They may be liable if they fail in these duties. Common torts applicable to funeral directors include:

- **Wrongfully withholding a body:** The next of kin (NOK) has the right to custody of the decedent in the condition left by death and to select disposition without interference.
- **Loss of the body:** Misidentification resulting in wrongful interment can result in liability.
- **Mutilation of the body**: NOK has the right to receive the body in death condition without unsanctioned alterations, including unauthorized embalming and autopsy.
- **Injury to invitees:** Attendees invited onto the property must experience reasonably safe environments, indoor and outdoor.
- **Injury to pallbearers:** Injury from carrying caskets or injury to clergy at the graveside faults the director.

CONSIDERATIONS WHEN ENTERING INTO CONTRACTS WITH CLIENTS

Contract law applies to funeral homes as they enter oral or written contracts with clients to provide services and merchandise upon request. The following parties are legally able enter into contracts to handle disposition:

- **Paramount next of kin**: spouse or family member(s) within the same level of kinship, such as children, parents, and siblings
- **Estate**: has an **implied contract** as they typically finance the funeral expenses
- **Third party**: unrelated responsible party, such as state or government agency representatives, employers, or military organizations

All persons engaging in contracts must be of sound mind and legal age. It is possible for funeral homes to establish contracts with the wrong agent mistakenly or under false pretenses; upon realization, the contract needs to be voided or re-approved by the person or agent with paramount rights of disposition. Contract **delegations** occur when the funeral home accepts responsibility to order services from other parties on behalf of clients. Submitting obituaries, ordering flowers, scheduling grave openings, and purchasing merchandise are all contracted on behalf of clients as cash advances. Contract delegations also include using another funeral home or director to complete services for a client, such as coordinating a ship-in/out or utilizing a trade service.

Contractual Forms and Delivery

A **contract** is a legally binding written document in which two or more individuals agree to perform the stated elements. A **valid contract** requires four fundamentals: mutual agreement, competent parties, legal objectives, and consideration (price). Without all of these elements, it is an **unenforceable contract**. A **contract to sell** includes a promise to transfer ownership of goods from the seller to the buyer. **Contractual capacity** means that the parties who entered into the contract must be legally capable of doing so. **Future goods** are contractual obligations that cannot be delivered upon acceptance by both parties because they are not yet in existence but will be delivered in the future.

Contractual Parties and Responsibility

A **general agent** is legally authorized to conduct all or a portion of business activity on behalf of a principal. An **offer** occurs when one person, the **offeror**, expresses readiness to enter into a contractual agreement with another person, the **offeree**. Contract **acceptance** is when both parties agree to the terms of the contract. A **contract defense** is a reason that a contract cannot be enforced, such as a lack of standing (one or both parties cannot legally enter into the contract), impossibility (the contract includes clauses that simply cannot happen), or illegality (the contract includes terms that are illegal). If an agreement is made under **duress**, with one party coercing the other, it is unenforceable. **Novation** is the substitution of one of the parties with a different person in a legally binding contract. **Fraud** occurs when an individual makes an intentionally false statement that convinces the other party to enter into a contract, causing them harm.

Types of Contracts

An **express contract** is a written or oral contractual agreement in which the specifics are clearly defined. An **implied contract** is an indirect contractual agreement in which the terms and conditions are understood between the parties but neither written nor formally stated verbally. A **quasi contract** is a contractual obligation without a formal agreement between the parties, created and enforced by the courts to stop an unjust loss when no legally enforceable agreement exists. A **unilateral contract** occurs when only one of the two parties makes a promise in return for a condition to be performed by the offeree. An **executed contract** is one that has been completely fulfilled in its terms and conditions.

Assignment and Termination of Funeral Contracts and Breach of Contract

Funeral contracts can be **assigned**, or transferred, to another funeral home if services have not already been rendered. If a decedent has been transferred into the care of a funeral home, the family can request another funeral home to take custody of the body and proceed with disposition. The first funeral home is legally obligated to release the body. The family is responsible for paying the first funeral home for any services or merchandise ordered on their behalf prior to the exchange of custody. A contract may be **terminated**, or canceled, by one or both parties, subject to conditions stated in the contract. Contractual **breaches** resulting from the funeral director's actions or lack thereof can cause mental anguish and distress to clients due to the sensitive nature of the contract, and thus funeral directors are held responsible, an exception to the physical impact rule. Client breach of contract involves neglecting to remit payment for services rendered. As long as the funeral contract was executed correctly, follows state regulations and disclosures, and is signed, it is legally binding and enforceable by a court of law. **Remedies** for breaches of contract include financial damages, legal enforcement of the contract, and cancellation of the contract.

Negotiable Instruments

A **negotiable instrument** is an unrestricted guarantee by the writer to pay a specific amount of money to another party at a specified time or upon delivery of goods or services. They can be in the form of **notes,** which are promises to pay, or **drafts,** which are orders. Checks are a type of drafted negotiable instrument; they are often used by families to pay funeral expenses and by funeral homes to pay honorariums and cemetery fees. A loan to purchase or build a funeral home is a type of negotiable instrument called a promissory note. The **liabilities** of a negotiable instrument fall on the writer and all prior possessors until the instrument is fulfilled. Whoever signs the instrument assumes liability under contract with the person they give the instrument to; the signer of the check is responsible for ensuring that it does not bounce. This is called contract liability. The person who writes the negotiable instrument has primary liability to pay the bearer. Anyone else who signs the paper assumes a secondary liability in which they are only responsible to pay the bearer if the primary party fails to make payment; this person is a co-signer.

Requirements of a Negotiable Instrument

Article 3 of the **Uniform Commercial Code (UCC)** lays out the model format for states to adopt laws on negotiable instruments. There are specific requirements for a negotiable instrument: it must be written and endorsed; have an order to pay; and be unconditional, for a specific amount of money, payable in money upon demand, and made out to the person in possession of it. Any missing information deems the instrument incomplete; however, sometimes missing information is implied. For example, if there is no date, it is implied for immediate payment.

In cases of fraudulent contracts or an agreement between parties, negotiable instruments can be **discharged**, meaning they are canceled, revoked, or the payment responsibility is passed from a primary obligator to a secondary one. The reason for the discharge is referred to as a **defense**. The **holder in due course** is the person in possession of the negotiable instrument with the stipulation that they are in honest custody of an authentic instrument payable for the stated amount. If services are partially rendered, the holder is technically only entitled to a portion of the stated amount until services are rendered in full.

Commercial Paper

The **maker** is the individual responsible for the execution of the promissory note. The **payee** is the individual to whom the negotiable instrument is made payable. An **indorsement** is the signature placed on **commercial paper** (negotiable instrument) in order to transfer ownership rights instead of money. A **promissory note** is a type of commercial paper commitment by one party to pay another party at a given time in the future. **Bearer paper** is a negotiable instrument payable to the individual who is cited on the instrument and in possession of it. A **secured claim** is a debt with collateral providing a guarantee to repay the debt.

Types of Pre-Need Contracts and Regulations

Pre-need contracts can be executed as **guaranteed** or **non-guaranteed.** Financed contracts can be established as **irrevocable** (unbreakable) or **revocable** (can be terminated by the client and refunded). All contracts are transferrable to another funeral home. Pre-need funeral contracts are regulated by **state trust laws.** Funds must be deposited into a trust, escrow, or account with a financial banking institution. State law determines the percentage of funds that must be deposited and how quickly accounts must be opened upon receipt of money. An irrevocable trust is not counted as an asset for Medicaid requirements, so this is a way to fund a funeral without affecting

Medicaid eligibility. Third-party contracts are legal in some states, while others require funeral licensing. Accounts may be established individually or within a master account, depending on state regulations. **Funeral insurance** is a type of whole life insurance designated for funeral and final expenses. The funeral home can be named beneficiary of the policy, or an assignment can be completed by the beneficiary. The Federal Trade Commission (FTC) regulates pre-need funeral contracts enacted outside of the funeral home; contracts negotiated elsewhere are considered "door to door sales" of "consumer goods and services." The FTC stipulates adherence to a three-day cancellation policy with disclosures on the receipt and contract.

Estates and Probate

An **estate** is the property of a deceased person, including real and personal property. **Probate** is the filing and subsequent proving of the legality of the **will** and administration of the will after the death of the person who left it. A person who has died **testate** had a valid will. Probate proceedings generally follow the model law of the **Uniform Probate Code (UPC)**, which has been fully or partially adopted in most states. An authorized agent, acknowledged in writing, has **express authority**. **Implied authority**, which grants an agent the ability to make decisions to fulfill a contract such as a will, is not expressly written, but it is legally binding by its reasonable nature.

Legal Representatives in Probate

Following a death, the **personal representative** of the estate is responsible for distributing the assets according to the will of the deceased. A **trustee** holds the title to property until it is transferred to the recipient. The **executor** is an individual appointed by the will of the deceased to carry out its provisions. The **administrator** is responsible for this when no executor is appointed; the administrator is appointed by the **probate court** with the jurisdiction to settle the estate. A **donee beneficiary** is not mentioned in the will as a legal beneficiary but receives a gift from the estate.

Types of Wills

A **will** is a written document guiding the disposition of property, real or personal, following the death of an individual under common law. A **nuncupative will**, or deathbed will, is an oral will that is declared or dictated by a testator, in the presence of a witness, when the testator is near death from illness or injury. This form of will is only legal for the bequest of personal property and upon completion it is converted to writing. Not all states recognize nuncupative wills, and those that do may have strict limitations on the circumstances and content of these wills. This type of will is sometimes called a **soldiers' and sailors' will** because they often can only be made by a soldier in the field or sailor at sea who may dispose of personal property only. A **holographic will** is handwritten entirely by the testator. Holographic wills are not legally recognized in some states.

Required Elements of a Legal Will

There are several elements required to make a will legally binding. Details vary by state, but typical requirements are:

- The testator (person who makes the will) is at least 18 years old.
- The testator is of sound mind and has testamentary capacity.
- The will includes a declaration of intent.
- The will is in writing (with some exceptions).
- The testator signs and dates the will voluntarily, without undue influence; in some cases, a representative may sign the will instead of the testator.
- There must be disinterested witnesses (generally two) to the above who also sign the will. Only Louisiana requires that the will be notarized.

The contents of a will generally include a description of the testator's assets, beneficiary names, a description of what each beneficiary will receive, the name of the chosen executor who will ensure that the will's stipulations are fulfilled, and any special considerations such as naming a guardian for minor children or pets.

Financial Parties to a Will

A person who leaves a valid will is a **testator**. When a person dies without a will, he or she is said to die **intestate,** and a state of intestacy exists. The order of **intestate succession** is the legal succession of an heir to a property and estate when the owner has died without a will. A **fiduciary** is a trusted individual who manages money or property on behalf of another. A **beneficiary** is an individual or entity that is awarded property in a will, including life insurance from the deceased. A **codicil** is a legally binding supplement or amendment to a will that contains an additional component or directive, more details or clarification, or an alteration to the original will. The death of a **legatee**, a person who was to inherit personal property as prescribed under a will, eliminates that distribution. Sometimes the spouse or another relative of the deceased elects to challenge the will and the prescribed disposition of assets. **Abatement** is a specific reduction in a legacy bequest under a will due to insufficient assets. **Ademption** is the removal of an inheritance because the decedent no longer owned the property at the time of death.

Power of Attorney

Power of attorney is a written authorization completed by a **grantor** or **principal** who authorizes another person to act as his or her **agent** or as an "attorney in fact" to conduct certain prescribed business activities. **General power of attorney** grants one person full power of attorney, with few or no limitations, for another person. Power of attorney is automatically revoked upon death of the principal. **Durable power of attorney** exists when a person executes a power of attorney that will become or remain effective in the event he or she should become disabled. **Springing power of attorney** "springs" into legal effect upon a specific conditional occurrence as written by the authorizing party and allows another person to act as an agent only upon that occurrence. **Financial power of attorney** grants the power to make financial decisions on behalf of the principal. **Medical power of attorney** grants permission to make medical decisions on behalf of the principal.

Distribution of Estate

A **solvent estate** is one in which the assets exceed the liabilities. An **insolvent estate** is one that is unable to pay the debts of the decedent and/or the estate. In this case, the state statute controls the priority of claims. The list of claim priority falls under formal court administration and informal distribution by agreement. A **legacy** or **bequest** is a gift of personal property by will. An **inheritance** is composed of real and personal property of the deceased's estate. It transfers after death to the **heir**, who is permitted to receive it legally by a will or the laws of intestacy. A **legatee** is one who inherits **personal property** under a will. **Intangible personal property** (stocks, bonds, copyrights, etc.) has intrinsic value but no physical properties. A **devisee** is an individual who inherits **real property** (a **devise**) through a will. In funeral arrangements, the person who has the right to make decisions does so on behalf of all survivors. Generally, while the funeral may initially be paid for by anyone, the estate and next of kin are ultimately responsible for reimbursing these funeral expenses, provided that the expenses are **reasonable** under applicable legal tests.

Regulations Enacted by the Federal Trade Commission Under the Funeral Rule

The Federal Trade Commission (FTC) regulates the funeral industry through the Funeral Industry Practices Rule, or the **Funeral Rule,** which ensures consumers have access to price lists and information to make informed decisions and select funeral goods and services they desire without false representation, biased influence, or persuasion. The Rule is enforced upon any business that sells both goods and services relating to funerals. When a cemetery sells only products and merchandise, they aren't subject to this regulation. The format and contents of the General Price List, Casket Price List, Outer Burial Container Price List, and Statement of Funeral Goods and Services Selected are all dictated by the FTC under the Funeral Rule.

The rule prohibits **tying arrangements**, which require purchases to receive a service (e.g., must buy an urn to be cremated). Exemptions include:

- A non-declinable basic service fee is charged.
- State or federal law requires a purchase.
- Consumers request a combination of goods and/or services that are impractical, unsafe, or extremely cumbersome to meet—in these instances, selecting one service may require another for safety and practicality (e.g., public visitation requires embalming).
- Merchandise from another party must be accepted, but facilitation (shipping, storage, and receiving) is not required.

Mandated Disclosures and Requirements Under the Funeral Rule

The mandated disclosures and requirements under the Funeral Rule prevent manipulated or misguided decisions by family while under the distress of grief and the stress of making quick decisions. The following subjects must be addressed:

- **Embalming**: This is not required by law except in specific situations and not required for direct cremations or direct burials. Refrigeration (in most states) is an alternative option for cremation or closed casket services.
- **Direct cremations**: Caskets are not required by law; alternative containers must be available for purchase.
- **Outer burial containers (OBC)**: These are not required by law but usually required by the cemetery. Current information regarding local cemeteries should be kept up-to-date to prevent any misrepresentations regarding OBC.
- **Crematory, cemetery, and legal requirements**: The Statement of Funeral Goods and Services Selected provides space to disclose and explain specific regulations.
- **Cash advances**: Markups, discounts, and commissions applied to third-party charges paid by the funeral home on behalf of the family must be acknowledged for each applicable item.
- **Guarantees for protection and preservation**: Funeral directors should not warrant or claim goods or services will provide lasting protection or prevent decay. It is not necessary to explain that embalming only delays decomposition, but infinite preservation cannot be suggested.

Statement of Funeral Goods and Services Selected

The Statement of Funeral Goods and Services Selected functions as a detailed invoice, listing each service and good selected by the family. Prices are taken directly off the General Price List (GPL). Applicable cash advance items, even if they need to be estimated, are included to give the family a realistic total of expenses. Prices must be listed individually. If a package was selected, that price is listed as one item but with a description of the services and goods it includes. These are the required disclosures for the Statement of Funeral Goods and Services Selected:

- The family is only charged for items they select or ones required either by law or third parties.
- Regulations surrounding embalming, such as when it is required vs. optional, are provided.
- Cash advance items that receive a markup must be recognized on the statement.

Some statements have space for the funeral director to add details regarding required selections, reason for embalming, and cash advance markups.

Requirements of the General Price List Under the Funeral Rule

The **General Price List (GPL)** is a detailed list of services and goods offered. It must be given for retention to anyone asking in person (at the office, arrangement or prearrangement conference, or transfers) about services or prices. It cannot be charged for, requested back, or shown in a manner implying it cannot be kept (e.g., in a binder).

The GPL must contain the following, excluding services not offered:

- Basic services of funeral director and staff, with a non-declinable fee that covers overhead, other staff members, and arranging, planning, coordinating, and facilitating services and documentation
- Embalming charge with separate listing for autopsies and donations
- Other preparation services (dressing, casketing, and sanitizing)
- Services and facility charges with viewing, funeral, memorial service, and graveside service listed separately
- Transportation
- Hearse, limousine, and fleet vehicles listed separately
- Ranges for casket prices and outer burial container prices listed separately
- Charges for forwarding and receiving remains listed separately
- Package pricing for direct cremations and direct burials, with separate package prices including options for an alternative container from the funeral home and one from a third party

Disclosures Included in the General Price List

The General Price List must include six clearly visible **disclosures** exactly as worded by the FTC. The disclosure topics are:

- Families may select the goods and services they want.
- The basic services fee is non-declinable and is factored into package prices (direct cremation or burial, shipping, and receiving).
- Embalming is not required by law but may be needed for some selections.
- A separate, detailed casket price list is available.
- A separate, detailed outer burial container price list is available.
- Alternative containers for direct cremations are available.

Casket Price List and Outer Burial Container Price List

The **Casket Price List** details the caskets, cremation containers, and alternative containers available or regularly offered. The document must state "Casket Price List," the funeral home name, and effective date. It must include prices and descriptions for each item, including interior and exterior features, composition (type of wood or gauge of metal), finishing, and color. It must be presented to the family when caskets are discussed. It does not have to be given for retention, and customers can be asked to return it.

The **Outer Burial Container (OBC) Price List** itemizes each OBC regularly offered to customers. The document must include the title, funeral home name, and effective date, along with prices and detailed descriptions of each item. It must include the disclosure that OBC typically are not required by law but may be required by the cemetery. It must be presented to the family anytime OBCs are discussed. It is not required to be given for retention, and customers can be asked to return it.

The Funeral Rule requires that establishments give pricing information over the phone to inquirers without demanding any information from the caller.

Business Organizations

Business law is the branch of law developed by government and enforced by agencies that defines the legal requirements for the operation of a business. A **merchant** is a person or company whose business activities involve trading goods or services for profit. A **funeral establishment** is a business organization legally formed and operated for the care and disposition of the deceased. A business can be operated as a **sole proprietorship** by one person in an unincorporated status. The sole proprietorship is one of the oldest forms of business structure and one of the most common in the US. The advantages of sole proprietorship are the low cost, ease of start-up, management autonomy, and personal profit incentive. The disadvantages are unlimited risk, limited life, and limited size due to the single manager. A **corporation** is a legal form of business organization made up of many individuals but with its own single identity under the law. Funeral homes are traditionally owned by a sole proprietor, family, or small group but are increasingly owned by larger corporations.

Forms of Partnership

A **partnership** is a form of business that exists when two or more individuals combine forces. A **general partnership** has partners that are active in the management of the business. The partners combine their goodwill, talent, capital, or management skills in a variety of ways to form a business. All are personally liable if the business is sued, and legal decisions are binding to all. The business may not be able to continue if one of the general partners dies (if there is no succession planning), and assets can be frozen if the business goes bankrupt. A **limited partnership** has both a general partner and a limited partner. The limited partner has a limited interest and liability, and the general partner actively manages the firm. A **silent partner** invests capital in a business but does not have any other involvement. A **dormant** or **sleeping partner** has no management or decision-making authority.

Types of Corporations

A **corporation** is the most advantageous legal form of business to operate a funeral home. The advantages of a corporation include limited liability for the board of directors, officers, and shareholders. There are several varieties of corporations. A **limited liability corporation** can be formed by an individual or partnership and is used to prevent personal liability; all liability is held by the business entity. A **public corporation** sells shares of ownership to the public. A **private corporation** is owned by a small number of individuals (but not the government). An **alien corporation** is established in a foreign country. An **S corporation** combines the limited liability benefits of a corporation with taxation at the personal tax rate.

LICENSURE

A **funeral provider** is any person, partnership, or corporation that provides funeral goods and/or services for sale to consumers. In all states except Colorado, a funeral director is required to apply for and obtain a license to practice. A **license** is a regulated and controlled practice of an occupational title that must be issued. An **apprentice** (intern or resident trainee) is a person actively learning the profession of funeral directing or embalming under direct supervision of a duly licensed funeral director or embalmer. **Reciprocity** is a legal principle that allows licensure in one state to be recognized in another. The conditions for funeral director license reciprocity vary by state.

AGENCY AND EMPLOYMENT

An **employer** is an individual business or person with **employees** performing duties and functions under his or her control. When hiring, funeral homes should write detailed job descriptions to establish the position's responsibilities and define the qualities necessary for success. These specifications can be used to filter out unqualified applicants. Upon hire, there should be a training period followed by an evaluation. Terminations should follow an established protocol consistent with state and federal regulations. An **independent contractor** is an individual who performs paid work for another and has autonomous control of his or her performance except for any agreed terms between the parties. An **agent** is similarly not an employee but someone who acts on behalf of the company or principal. The principal has more control over an agent's actions and may be liable for any mistakes or intentional wrongs committed by the agent. An agency may be terminated by either party, conditions in the contract, or laws rendering the contract void.

WAGE REQUIREMENTS

The Wage and Hour Division of the Department of Labor enforces the **Fair Labor Standards Act (FLSA)** to regulate minimum wage, overtime, and equal pay; this superseded the 1938 Federal Wage and Hour Act, a landmark law that first established minimum wage and overtime rules. Violations are corrected by employers with the aid of enforcement officers. Purposeful disregard for compliance could result in criminal charges. Employee complaints are resolved in civil suits. FLSA established **minimum wage**, the lowest amount an employer can pay an employee, as a federal regulation, but some states have enacted a higher minimum rate. The FLSA does not cap the number of hours an employee can work but does institute an **overtime pay** rate (1.5 × hourly rate) after 40 hours of work within the employer's designated work week. Employees that are considered professionals, administrators, executives, or managers are exempt from overtime pay laws.

TYPES OF PROPERTY AND OWNERSHIP

Property is defined as anything a person possesses. **Real property** includes land or objects that are permanently attached to the land. **Personal property** is defined as moveable possessions not designated as real property. **Escheat** refers to the case of a probate in which there are no heirs and the property of the deceased is forfeited to the state. Property may be purchased in full, purchased with a mortgage or other loan, or rented/leased. Typically, the funeral home building is owned by the individual or group that operates the business or leased with a long-term contract from a separate owner. The contents and equipment are purchased by the operators either outright or financed over time. All memorial items are purchased outright by the customer and are thus personal property.

EMINENT DOMAIN

Under **eminent domain**, the government has the authority to take control of private property for public use. Early uses of eminent domain were crucial in creating today's infrastructure. Land can be repossessed by the government to support transportation, utilities, environmental protection, defense, and waterways. While the government has the authority to take property for a just reason, they must compensate owners with fair market value.

Cemeteries can be subject to eminent domain. In some circumstances, the government can take over a cemetery, disinterring and moving decedents to another location. Cemeteries taken by eminent domain are usually no longer active and often neglected. Some states have regulations exempting cemeteries from eminent domain.

Acquisition, Ownership, and Transfer of Cemetery Plots

When **cemetery plots** are purchased, a title is issued deeding the space(s) under the purchaser's name. It includes the location, number of spaces, requirements, and purchase details. This is not a real estate transaction for property ownership but solely a title giving rights to interment in that space. To transfer the title, the owner must complete a title transfer form provided by cemetery management. Sometimes owners can list subsequent owners in the event of their death. Laws surrounding transfer of plot ownership vary by state, and the exact rules and procedures may be specific to the cemetery. Cemeteries maintain records in the event a family loses their plot deed. Ownership of **merchandise** is subject to the purchase terms. If customers order items from third parties, the customer is responsible for storing it upon delivery. The funeral home is required to use this merchandise but is not responsible for its delivery or storage. A casket ordered in advance but no longer wanted can be re-sold. In the event of lost merchandise, the supplier works with the parties involved to locate or replace the item. **Unclaimed personal property** or cremated remains are subject to state law and the funeral home's established policies.

Bailments

Property refers to the ownership interest of an individual in either real (land) or personal property. A **bailee** is an individual who receives some form of personal property from another individual (the bailor) on a temporary basis. **Bailment** is the temporary transfer of personal property by a bailor to the bailee, who has legal rights to the property for a specific purpose under an express or implied-in-fact contract. The bailor retains ownership of the property while it is in the bailee's care. The bailee is held to a standard of care that depends on the details of the bailment arrangement but always requires that the bailee treat the bailor's property with care. A funeral home is the bailee of property belonging to the decedent and his or her family.

Warranty Obligations for Funeral Directors

Uniform Commercial Code (UCC) Article 2 discusses sales contracts for transferable items and merchandise. This code is used as a template for states to create their own laws regulating topics of contract engagement, obligations, titles, and breaches. Warranty obligations are defined in both the UCC and Magnuson-Moss Warranty Act, a federal law regarding expressed and implied warranties. **Express warranties** are clearly stated guarantees for the product being sold. **Implied warranties** are assumed. Casket manufacturers provide express warranties. When selling a casket, funeral directors make an implied warranty that the casket will have functional components to successfully contain, transport, and inter the decedent without malfunctions. The manufacturer's express warranties must be clearly disclosed; otherwise, clients may interpret statements as the funeral director's warranty on the product. Some states allow funeral homes to **disclaim** warranties with approved terminology on their price list documents. The Federal Trade Commission (FTC) requires funeral homes to provide manufacturers' warranties to clients before a sale is made. This can be done by putting a printed copy of the warranty next to displayed products or a compilation of warranties in a clearly labeled, easily visible binder.

OSHA Background, Inspection, and Violation Protocol

The **Occupational Health and Safety Administration (OSHA)** was created by the Occupational Health and Safety Act, within the Department of Labor, to regulate employee safety by providing resources, education, regulations, recordkeeping, and training standards for all employers to follow. Inspections are conducted by federal or state compliance officers, who can conduct surprise or event-triggered (workplace injury/fatality or complaint) inspections. Any violations will be discussed with the employer and reported to a regional director. Recommendations are made to correct issues by a specified deadline, and monetary fines may coincide with citations. Funeral homes, as service-oriented businesses, are not required to follow OSHA's **basic recordkeeping requirements**, although some state-approved OSHA plans require it. The **General Requirements Standard** does apply to funeral homes; it encompasses general safety regulations such as fire extinguisher access, exit signage and location, electrical safety specifications, approved flooring surfaces, machine and lift user protection measures, and appropriate pictograms and signs. OSHA's Job Safety and Health poster must be displayed for employees. Employers are required to report any work-related fatalities or hospitalization of five or more employees to their regional office within 48 hours.

OSHA Standards That Apply to Funeral Homes

A funeral home must comply with numerous OSHA standards in order to maintain a safe and legal workplace. These standards include:

- General Industry Standard
- Hazard Communication Standard
- Formaldehyde Standard
- Bloodborne Pathogen Standard
- Personal Protective Equipment Standard
- Respiratory Protection Standard

Violations of these standards, or any other state or federal standards that apply, could result in financial penalties or, in cases of particularly egregious or ongoing violations, imprisonment.

Occupational Exposure Measurements

The **preparation room** is a private room designed to provide a safe and comfortable workplace for embalming and preparing the deceased. **Occupational exposure** refers to the ordinary limits of exposure from working around potentially infectious diseases or hazardous chemicals in a preparation room, most notably formaldehyde. Exposure monitoring is accomplished by sampling the air in workspaces where formaldehyde is used. **Parts per million (ppm)** measures the parts of vapor or gas per million parts of air by volume; in a solution it measures the parts of a chemical per million parts of solution. Two types of tests must be used in every funeral home that uses formaldehyde. The first is the **time-weighted average (TWA)**, which measures exposure over a period of eight hours. The **short-term exposure level (STEL)** measures exposure over a period of 15 minutes.

Formaldehyde Exposure Standard

The **Formaldehyde Standard** was enacted to regulate employee exposure to formaldehyde within workplaces, including funeral home preparation (prep) rooms. In this standard, exposure is broken down into three classifications, all measured in **parts per million (ppm)**, which measures the parts of vapor or gas per million parts of air by volume.

- **Time-weighted average (TWA):** This monitors air quality over either eight hours or the duration the embalmer is in the prep room if less than eight hours. The **permissible exposure limit (PEL)** for the TWA is 0.75 ppm.
- **Short-term exposure level (STEL):** This monitors air quality for 15 minutes during an embalming. The level of formaldehyde should not exceed 2 ppm.
- **Action level:** The level at which the funeral home needs to take action to reduce formaldehyde exposure in the prep room. If the TWA is above 0.5 ppm, formaldehyde levels must be reduced through **safe workplace practices, good housekeeping** (caps on bottles, lids on the embalming machine and garbage, and running table water), and testing repeated every six months until the TWA is below 0.5 ppm. If the TWA is above 0.75 ppm, a written exposure reduction plan, warning signs, and respirators are required.

Employer Obligations Under the Formaldehyde Standard

Employer obligations under the OSHA Formaldehyde Standard include:

- **Personal protective equipment (PPE)**: Embalmers must be provided with chemical-resistant gloves, goggles, a face shield, a bouffant, an impervious gown, and shoe covers. Contaminated PPE must be discarded or placed in labeled laundry bins.
- **Sanitization measures**: Requirements include a private facility for changing, although donning and doffing most PPE is done in the prep room; emergency "drench showers" capable of running for 15–20 minutes; eye wash stations; and first aid kits in prep rooms.
- **Emergency response**: Routine inspection of the prep room and formaldehyde storage locations ensures any issues are immediately corrected. Refer to safety data sheets for cleanup and disposal guidelines. Formaldehyde emergency response plans are required.
- **Air quality management**: Prep rooms need ventilation fans that change air 15 times per hour (every four minutes). The ideal installation location draws air downwards, away from the embalmer. Positive-pressure local exhaust ventilation systems and good workplace practices reduce exposure.
- **Employee training**: Employees working around formaldehyde must receive PPE and spill response, safe handling, and emergency response training upon hire and annually thereafter.
- **Record management**: Training, inspections, and maintenance records must be meticulously documented and stored for 30 years.

Hazard Communication Standard

The **Hazard Communication Standard** was instated to ensure employees are clearly aware of potential hazards at work. This standard contains four employer obligations:

- **Safety data sheets (SDSs)**: These replaced material safety data sheets (MSDSs) to provide vital information about chemicals and products in a simpler, universal 16-section format. SDSs are issued by chemical production, sales, and shipping companies, and they provide educational and safety resources for product composition, hazards, safe handling, and emergency response. SDSs on every chemical and product, hazardous or not, must be stored alphabetically and indexed in a binder in the prep room, with a second compilation in another location for emergency reference.

- **Safety labeling**: Although chemicals come labeled from manufacturers, secondary containers must be re-labeled with the product name, manufacturer name and address, and hazard warnings. Re-labeling is not required for secondary containers for up to 10 gallons if the contents will be used immediately.
- **Hazardous communication program (HCP)**: Funeral homes must establish, follow, and keep up to date an HCP that summarizes its protocols for compliance.
- **Employee education**: Employees must be trained on the HCP, hazardous chemicals, labeling, pictograms, emergency response, and proper PPE; this training must be documented.

The Globally Harmonized System of Classification and Labeling of Chemicals (GHS)

The Globally Harmonized System of Classification (GHS) is an international standard developed by the United Nations to guide hazardous chemical labeling, warning systems, and safety data sheets. The GHS was developed to standardize hazard warning terminology, pictograms, and safety data sheets worldwide so that international commerce could be improved and language barriers overcome. The OSHA Hazard Communication Standard includes the requirements of the GHS. All workplaces in the United States are required to have safety data sheets available on-site that conform to the GHS system and to use these in their notification and training programs.

SDS (Safety Data Sheet)

A **safety data sheet (SDS)**—formerly called a material safety data sheet (MSDS)—provides information on the physical and chemical properties of a substance as well as potential health and environmental concerns. OSHA requires that all chemicals be labeled appropriately and that SDSs be readily available in the workplace. The Hazard Communication Standard also requires that employees are trained and that the employer maintains records of the training given. The format for an SDS includes sixteen sections, of which all except 12 through 15 are mandatory (*). The sections are as follows:

I	Identification	*
II	Hazard Identification	*
III	Composition/Information on Ingredients	*
IV	First Aid Measures	*
V	Firefighting Measures	*
VI	Accidental Release Measures	*
VII	Handling/Storage Requirements	*
VIII	Exposure Controls/Personal Protection	*
IX	Physical/Chemical Properties	*
X	Stability/Reactivity	*
XI	Toxicological Information	*
XII	Ecological Information	
XIII	Disposal Considerations	
XIV	Transportation Information	
XV	Regulatory Information	
XVI	Other Information	*

Carcinogenicity

SDSs provide a number of indicators for possible health threats from a particular chemical. They are required to provide all known information regarding **carcinogenicity** (known or potential cancer-causing risks) of a substance. Carcinogenic risks are published in reports by the National Toxicology Program (NTP), the International Agency for Research on Cancer (IARC), and OSHA.

Toxicity levels are indicated by numbers called the LD_{50} and the LC_{50}. LD_{50} is the median lethal dose, or the dose at which 50% of the test subjects were killed. LC_{50} is the lethal concentration at which 50% of test subjects were killed. Dosages are typically normalized to include the mass of the possible toxin divided by the mass of the test subject. LD_{50} values may also include descriptors that indicate the mode of administration of the dose (intravenously or orally) and the timeframe for death after administration. Limits for exposure to a particular chemical are also provided. These can be measured as the OSHA permissible exposure limit (PEL) and/or the threshold limit value (TLV), which are published by the American Conference of Governmental Industrial Hygienists (ACGIH).

Chemical Protective Clothing

SDSs often recommend the use of **chemical protective clothing** (CPC). Protective eye goggles with splash guards and air vents should be used when handling chemicals. Face shields should be used when working with large quantities of a hazardous substance and are most effective when used in conjunction with safety goggles. If the mode of possible hazard exposure is through contact and/or absorption through skin, appropriate gloves should be worn. Gloves are chosen based upon their permeability by and reactivity with the chemical in use. Personal respiratory equipment may be indicated if fume hoods do not provide adequate ventilation of fumes or airborne particulates. Body protection depends on the level of protection needed and ranges from rubberized aprons to full suits that are evaluated for their permeability and leak protection. Closed-toed protective shoes should always be used when working with chemicals.

Requirements for Labels

The term *label* under GHS refers to the label on the container. GHS requires the label to contain certain elements; these requirements apply whether the label is affixed by the manufacturer or whether the chemical is placed into a smaller, secondary container in the workplace. The label must include the identification of the chemical, the manufacturer's name and US contact information, the applicable GHS pictograms, the applicable signal words (either *danger* or *warning*, as applicable), and precautionary statements (measures to reduce risk from exposure to the chemical).

Pictograms

The pictograms used in the GHS system are simple pictures used to convey hazards posed by the chemical. They are meant to be universally understandable by people with diverse language and reading fluencies. They are as follows:

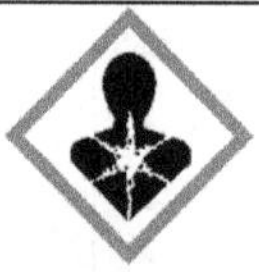 *Health Hazard*	 *Flammable*	 *Sensitizer/Irritant*
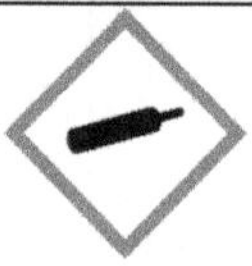 *Gas Under Pressure*	 *Oxidizer*	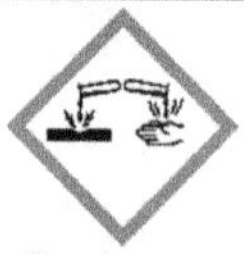 *Corrosive*
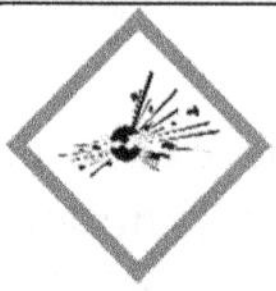 *Reactive*	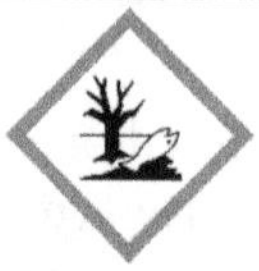 *Environmental Hazard*	 *Poison*

Signal Words

Under the GHS hazard communication and safety data sheet system, the term **signal word** is used to describe one word that summarizes the degree of danger posed by the substance. There are only two signal words: *danger* and *warning*. The word **danger** is used for more hazardous substances that present immediate hazards, such as flammability, reactivity, or poison. The word **warning** is used for lesser hazards, such as irritants, environmental hazards, and less toxic substances. The signal word is used on the label to provide a quick and easily understandable indication of the degree of hazard posed by the substance.

Bloodborne Pathogens Standard

The **Bloodborne Pathogens Standard** was initiated to reduce work-related exposure to bloodborne pathogens and potentially infectious bodily fluids and secretions. Basic requirements within the standard include:

- **Exposure control plans** address occupational tasks with exposure risks, protective measures, training, recordkeeping, and incident protocols. This plan must be updated annually.
- **Hepatitis B vaccinations** must be made available, timely and without fees, to employees upon exposure to bloodborne pathogens or other infectious materials.
- **Personal protective equipment (PPE)** must be provided to at-risk employees in line with the Personal Protective Equipment Standard. **Universal precautions,** treating all scenarios as they have exposure risks, should be standard care.
- **Employee training** includes education about bloodborne pathogens and other potentially infectious materials, transmissibility, PPE, precautions, signage, and hepatitis B.
- **Exposure protocol** requires medical evaluations and documentation of the incident.
- **Recordkeeping** consists of maintaining employee training documentation for 5 years and medical records, including exposure incidents and post-evaluations, for 30 years.

The **Needlestick Safety and Prevention Act,** under the Bloodborne Pathogens Standard, requires a needlestick exposure control plan to decrease harm from sharps (pointed instruments like needles, syringes, scalpels, and trocars) using safe workplace practices and engineering controls, including methods to separate sharps and limit direct contact risks.

Cemetery, Crematory, and Other Dispositions

Cemetery Terminology

A **cemetery** is a defined portion of real estate ground that is legally permitted and dedicated to the placement of human remains. **Interment** is the process of burying human remains in the ground. The **sexton** is the designated caretaker of the cemetery; this term originally referred to a church caretaker in the Middle Ages. A **tomb** is a site for placement of human remains. **Catacombs** are burial sites made by excavations in soft rock, originating in Roman times. **Undeveloped** cemetery land refers to the portion that has not been subdivided into graves for interment and is not for sale to the public. A **section** is a portion of the cemetery containing multiple blocks. A **block** is a portion of the cemetery that serves as a boundary for several lots. A **lot** is subdivided into one or more graves. A **grave** is a location designated for belowground burial of one or more caskets or cremated remains.

Types of Cemeteries

Areas dedicated to the burial of the dead date back thousands of years, but the cemetery as we know it today is only a few hundred years old. **Churchyard cemeteries**, also known as graveyards, arose in Europe in the 7th century and remained popular in Europe and the US until the late 18th century. At that point, in part due to concerns about the health risks of decomposition and running out of space, there was a shift to **garden cemeteries**, also known as rural cemeteries. These cemeteries often contained gardens and grassy areas where people would have picnics amongst the memorials and headstones. These practices have fallen out of favor, and cemeteries are increasingly dedicated grounds outside of cities. **Memorial parks** are modern cemeteries with flat markers and landscaped grounds. A **scattering garden** is a location, usually within a cemetery, designated for the scattering or simple burial of cremated remains. These gardens can be an alternative to releasing cremated remains elsewhere, which is illegal in many locations, and provide a place for remembrance and reflection. A **national cemetery** is specifically designed for the burial of honorably discharged veterans and eligible family members.

Cemetery Ownership Types

Municipal cemeteries are operated and maintained by a municipality (e.g., township, borough, or city). Some have restricted sections (e.g., children's, Catholic, or Jewish sections) but usually anyone can be buried within the cemetery. At **public cemeteries**, a sexton or cemetery board oversees caretaking (e.g., operations, finances, and decision-making). They may have designated sections in which only certain people can be buried; however, they are usually inclusive. They can be for-profit or nonprofit. There are also **private cemeteries**. For example, some religious organizations own and operate nonprofit cemeteries. Burials may be available to the public or restricted to members of the religion. An organization-appointed sexton or cemetery board oversees operations. For family cemeteries on private property, the section of land must be legally and indefinitely designated a cemetery. The landowner is responsible for maintenance. Some have an easement written into the deed or right of way created to allow cemetery access in the event the property is sold. Permission from the family/landowner is required for a burial. **Military cemeteries** are owned and operated by the government and reserved for veterans and their eligible family members. Some, like Arlington National Cemetery, have strict eligibility requirements, while others are open to any honorably discharged veteran.

Arranging and Preparing for a Burial

In preparing for a burial, the funeral director needs to coordinate with the cemetery, gravedigger, and vault company. All parties are notified of the service day and time and given an estimated arrival time at the cemetery. The sexton confirms the plot information or assists the family with purchasing a plot. They also notify the director of specific cemetery regulations and provide a general gravesite location. The gravedigger is coordinated by the cemetery or director. If possible, the director should drive by the gravesite prior to the service to verify that the grave was opened and plan the best route to bring the procession through the cemetery. Some cemeteries have a staff member meet the procession at the cemetery entrance and escort them to the gravesite. Upon arriving at the cemetery, the director should verify with the cemetery and vault company employees that everything is ready and discuss any last-minute issues. A visual inspection of the gravesite, tent setup, vault, and chairs evaluate safety levels for the attendees. The director provides a burial permit for a traditional burial, or a certificate of cremation for interment of cremated remains, to the cemetery.

Cemetery Equipment

A **graveside service** is the funeral committal service that takes place at the cemetery next to the burial site and includes some form of rite, such as a closing prayer and military honors, if applicable. A **canopy** (tent) is the shelter that is erected over the interment site for the attendees and is dismantled and removed following the completion of the service. The **lowering device** is a metal-framed mechanical device that sits directly above the grave and slowly lowers the casket into the grave. **Grave straps** are made of heavily woven fabric attached to the horizontal poles of the lowering device. The casket rests on the grave straps, which unroll to lower the casket. **Artificial grass** is a form of indoor/outdoor carpet with sewn edges, in various sizes, that is laid around the grave, under the tent, to provide a neat and clean surface for the chairs and guests and often to cover the pile of dirt from the open grave. A **catafalque** is a raised platform for the casket. A **casket skirt**, or casket drape, is a decorative cover for a catafalque, church truck, or other stand. These provide an attractive finish.

Memorials and Monuments

A **memorial** is an object constructed in memory of a person or event. It can be erected above ground or installed even with the ground. A **monument** is an object constructed of granite, marble, or stone, erected above ground to commemorate an event or honor the life and accomplishments of a person. A **cenotaph** is a permanent memorial, usually made of stone with inscriptions or symbols, to someone whose remains are at another location. The **base** is made of the same stone as the upper portions of the monument and provides a level surface to support them. The **die** is the separated portion of the monument above the base that includes the inscriptions, epitaphs, and symbols honoring the deceased. **Rock pitch** refers to the uneven, "chipped" appearance of stone that is frequently used on the base to minimize any damage. **Etching** refers to the process of engraving stone with a diamond-tip tool, removing the polished areas and creating a contrast for design or lettering. A **polished finish** is a diamond-polished, smooth, reflective surface. A **honed finish** is a diamond-polished, smooth, non-reflective surface. An **epitaph** is a few words or a short phrase inscribed on a memorial or monument.

Markers

A marker is a plaque made of stone or bronze mounted on stone, inscribed to designate a particular location. A **bevel top marker** is a small monument, set on a base, with a forward slanting top. A **slant marker** is placed at an angle between 45 and 90 degrees. A **flush marker** is a flat monument even with the ground. A **bronze memorial** is a flush bronze plaque mounted on a piece of stone.

Mausoleums, Crypts, Lawn Crypts, Columbaria, and Niches

Mausoleums are structures used to inter people above ground within a **crypt** (the space that houses the casket within the mausoleum) or vault for one or more people. While crypts are above ground, **lawn crypts** are double-depth interments where two people are placed in the same grave space in stacked grave liners or a specialized concrete lawn crypt with a dividing platform installed at the time of the first burial. Some mausoleums also have **niches,** small spaces to inter cremated remains. Some cemeteries (within a mausoleum or as its own structure) and churches have **columbaria**, which are specialized buildings, rooms, or walls with niches that house cremated remains. **Private familial mausoleums** are structures on cemetery grounds, built in advance, that act as a person's or family's place of rest. They are expensive to build and restricted by cemetery regulations. **Community mausoleums** are entombment structures on cemetery grounds for anyone who purchases a space; they are more expensive than in-ground burials but more economical than private ones. Mausoleums allow cemeteries to utilize vertical space. **Chapel mausoleums** (public or private) are crypt spaces inside a chapel-like setting providing lighting, seating, temperature control, and shelter from the elements. **Garden mausoleums** are exterior crypts.

Mausoleum Challenges and Preventive Measures

Mausoleum challenges occur no matter the type of mausoleum, location and environment, casket type (wood, metal, sealing, or non-sealing), pest control, and crypt-sealing techniques. Prior to entombment, the casket should be placed in a **casket protector**, which is a treated tray with an absorptive lining; covered with a specialized plastic; and then sealed to prevent leaks, control odor emissions, and keep pests out.

- **Leaking fluids**: Fluids may leak out of the casket, potentially entering other crypts and draining out of the front plates. This causes staining and requires plates to be replaced. Leaks often occur by permeating through the concrete rather than from a faulty seal. Many mausoleums are designed with a slight slope in the crypts to drain any fluids away from the front plate and into a drainage system.
- **Odor**: Crypts have vents; however, without proper airflow, decomposition smells can permeate into or be emitted from the mausoleum.
- **Pests**: Phorid flies are the most common nuisance even with proper pest treatments. They infest the sealed crypts, making eradication difficult.
- **Casket degradation**: Caskets leaking or emitting odors and pest infiltration can be a problem soon after entombment or after an extended time.

Types of Burial Vaults

An **outer burial container** is a container for the casket inside an earth grave. These containers include burial vaults, grave liners, and grave boxes. A **burial vault** is a sealed outer enclosure offering protection against the elements and the weight of the soil. **Concrete vaults** are made of formed, cured concrete and may have steel reinforcements and an interior liner of plastic resin, steel, copper, or bronze. They may also be sectional. **Metal vaults** are made of materials such as steel, stainless steel, and copper. They typically have an air seal, a flat bottom, and a dome top, with the casket placed on the bottom and the dome secured over it. **Fiberglass vaults** are made of fiberglass and are most often used as "shells" for infants or pets. **Polymer vaults** are made of durable, hardened resins; have flat bottoms and domes; and typically have an air seal. **Polypropylene vaults** are often molded from recycled materials. They are nonporous and not biodegradable. A **lined burial vault** is a concrete container with an inner lining made of copper, bronze, fiberglass, or stainless steel. It includes a gasketing material for the tongue and groove of the lid. A **grave liner** uses concrete, polymer, or fiberglass to support the soil's weight but does not seal.

Closures for Burial Vaults

Burial vaults support soil weight and pressure along with having sealing properties. Some have additional features, coatings, layers, and reinforcements to increase protection from outside elements. Concrete burial vaults can contain steel components to add strength, but some do not. They have linings—often polystyrene, asphalt, stainless steel, copper, or bronze—to provide protection from the environment. Caskets are lowered into a base, and a lid is placed on top. Metal burial vaults are distinguished by gauge and can be composed of stainless steel, steel, or copper. Caskets are lowered onto a base platform and the dome-type lid is secured to the bottom. Polypropylene and fiberglass burial vaults are also available and are constructed similarly to metal vaults, with a base capped by a dome lid.

There are three closure methods:

- **Air seal**: Dome lids lowered over the casket onto the base seal in air, creating a pressurized seal
- **Top seal**: Tongue and groove closure in which epoxy is placed
- **Double seal**: Air seal vaults that use epoxy to adhere the dome to the base as a secondary sealing measure

Cremation Options

The cremation rate across the US is approximately 60% and rising. Reasons for selecting cremation are cost, fewer religious regulations, concerns for environmental impact, and the effects of a transient society. Presenting clear cremation options helps correct the misconception that all cremations are direct cremations. Understanding why people select cremation helps funeral directors better serve families. Prior to cremation, funeral homes should require an **identification viewing** by family or an appointed family representative. Typically, sanitary care is done, features are set, and the body is reposed in a gown or selected clothing on a dressing table with sheets and a pillow. Embalming is not required for identification. Directors cannot refuse an identification viewing prior to a cremation. After the identification, the decedent is given an identification number tag. The next of kin must authorize the cremation. Some states have a "majority rule" for this authorization, which allows cremation to take place upon agreement of a majority of those within the appropriate level of kinship. However, it is best practice to secure authorizations from everyone within this level of kinship even when not required by law. The medical examiner or coroner, as appropriate, must give cremation authorization for deaths that occurred within their jurisdiction. The decedent is checked for personal effects, jewelry, a pacemaker, and radioactive implants. A suitable container of the family's choice is used to encase the body and to facilitate the cremation.

Certifications and Indemnifications to Explain to the Next of Kin

For funeral directors, there is immense liability in facilitating cremations because the process is irreversible. Funeral homes and crematories are regulated by the state; most states require the following on the authorization forms:

- Decedent information and identification acknowledgement.
- Authorizing agent declaration that the agent is the proper authorizing representative, with the paramount right as next of kin, to authorize cremation; inclusion of a disclaimer for instances where there may be a higher kinship agent who is uncontactable, estranged, or unfit to authorize (Many funeral homes will go to court to legally appoint this representative as the authorizing agent rather than risk the liability of accepting this disclaimer.)

- Medical device notice (battery-operated devices, radiation therapies, and any metal/noncombustible implants) and agreement to removal and disposal terms
- Description of the cremation and pulverization process to ensure that the authorizing agent understands the process
- Personal effects specification on what is removed prior to cremation and what is cremated with the body
- Specific instructions for disposition of the cremated remains along with a stated unclaimed cremated remains policy
- Certification and indemnification stating the information listed and provided by the authorizing agent is accurate and an acknowledgement releasing the director of liability resulting from misinformation

Explaining the Process of Cremation to a Family

Funeral directors should be prepared to explain the process of cremation to families considering this option. It is important to describe the process accurately so that families do not feel misled if they research the details on their own. The explanation could include the following: cremation is a form of disposition for human remains in which the body is exposed to extreme heat at temperatures of 1,400–1,800 °F for 1.5–4 hours, reducing it to fragile bone remnants. The temperature and duration are impacted by the size and weight of the body, condition of the body, and cremation container type. Once the cremation chamber, or **retort**, cools down, the remains are swept out into a catch pan. When the fragments are cool enough to handle, metal components are removed by hand and with a magnet. The remains are sifted into a **cremulator** (pulverization machine) to reduce them to a finer material. Cremated remains are then placed into a temporary container or the urn selected by the family. The cremation identification tag is placed inside the container. A certificate of cremation accompanies the cremated remains for travel or interments.

Treatment of the Body Immediately Prior to a Cremation

Following identification, securing authorizations, and the legal holding period, the body can be prepared for cremation. All metal, jewelry, and personal effects are removed from the body (unless they were requested to be cremated with the body). Pacemakers and battery implants are removed to prevent explosions during the cremation. The body is placed into an alternative cremation container which eases placement into the retort.

A metal **identification disc** with a cremation number and the name of the facility is placed with the body prior to cremation to act as an identifier. The disc accompanies the body through every step of the cremation process to ensure decedents, and later their cremated remains, are identifiable. Stringent records document the decedent's information with their corresponding identification number. Crematories are subject to federal and state regulations and monitoring to ensure quality care and safety.

Most units operate in the range of 1,400–1,800 °F. Many cremation units have a maximum temperature set to turn the burner off until the temperature lowers. Modern units have computerized systems to self-monitor and report progress throughout the cremation on unit monitors or remotely. The duration of a cremation is influenced by decedent factors; the usual interval is 2–2.5 hours or 1 hour per 100 lbs.

Start Sequence of a Typical Cremator

Although the control systems and sequences vary based on the type and age of the **cremator** (cremation unit), there are some commonalities in the start-up process. The technician checks or sets the temperature controls and adjusts the timer based on decedent analysis. Influential factors include size, body fat percentage, whether the decedent is embalmed, the condition of the body (e.g., extreme edema or decomposition), and type of alternative container or casket. Automated retorts calculate settings using decedent information entered into the system's computer. The cremation can begin with a cold start or, more commonly, a preheat sequence. For a cold start, the body enters the chamber before the afterburner is fired. A cold start is beneficial when the body has a high fat content or advanced decomposition; the increase in temperature as the unit heats releases bodily liquids more gradually. In preheated cremations, the **afterburner** is fired to heat the flue and warm the bricks. During the cremation, the afterburner acts as a secondary chamber, which aids in burning off gas and vapors so they aren't released as emissions. Filtration systems prevent particulates, gas, and dark smoke from exiting the stack. Once the warming temperature is reached, the blower is turned on, ensuring proper draft out of the flue (chimney stack). At this point, most units are ready for the body.

THE CREMATION PROCESS

Following the preheat, the body is placed into the chamber using cardboard rollers to transfer from the lift to the retort. Once the door is closed, the main burner is fired to begin the cremation. The container and superficial composition of the body (clothing, skin, and hair) ignite first, creating intense smoke and odor within the chamber. As the skin, fat, muscles, and tissues burn, fluid is released and evaporates under the intense heat. As organs are exposed, they dehydrate and melt away. Intense heat over an extended timeframe reduces the body to fine matter and fragile bones.

After the retort cools down, the remains are swept out into the **catch pan** using brushes and a vacuum. Personal protective equipment is needed when the remains are removed from a hot retort. Large metal pieces (e.g., surgical implants) are removed, and a magnet is used to remove metal fragments. The remains are placed into a cremulator, a cremation processor that pulverizes remaining bone fragments to create finer cremated remains. The cremated remains of an adult typically weigh between 4 and 8 lbs. Cremated remains are labeled and secured in a heavy plastic bag inside an urn or temporary container until returned to the family.

RESPONSIBILITIES AFTER CREMATION

A **certificate of cremation** is a document provided by the crematory to the family, confirming the date of disposition. The cemetery uses it to authorize the burial of the cremated remains. The **receipt for cremated remains** is a document signed by the receiving party to confirm transfer of custody (and responsibility) of the cremated remains. **Unclaimed cremated remains** are those that are never claimed from the custody of the funeral home by an authorized family member. Most funeral homes have a designated place to store and hold these remains in a secure area. In some cases, the funeral home may purchase a cemetery crypt to store them. It is important to have procedures in place if the remains are not picked up. State statutes often address this situation.

DOCUMENTATION TO HAVE AVAILABLE UPON REQUEST

Almost 40% of funeral homes operate their own crematory, a number that is rising; however, some states prohibit this arrangement. There are many state and federal regulations for operating a crematory. A **standard operating procedure manual** with step-by-step written procedures detailing facility operations, including form templates, should be available for reference. A maintenance record consisting of schedules, logs, and inspections must be retained and made available to anyone who asks to review it, including the general public. Operating permits, emissions testing, and detailed cremation logs must be maintained.

When funeral homes contract with a third-party crematory, they are liable for inspecting the facility to ensure that the operation meets state and federal requirements prior to engaging in business with them. Funeral homes may request access to the standard operating procedure manual, state operating permits/licensure, memberships, operator certification documentation, certificates of insurance, maintenance logs, and inspection records. They should also interview the crematory operations manager to gain detailed information about procedures, employees, and the equipment being used. Finally, the funeral director should perform an impromptu visual inspection of the facility and crematory. This due diligence investigation and continued periodic reviews reduce the liability of the funeral home.

Inurnment of Cremated Remains

Following cremation, the remains may be placed in a temporary container usually constructed of cardboard or plastic. They may also be placed in a permanent container, usually an urn. **Display urns** are kept at home by the family. **Sharing urns** are a set of two or more small urns. The cremated remains are dispersed among them. **Keepsakes** are small containers (jewelry, blown glass, table decorations, mini urns, river rocks, clocks, etc.) designed to encase a portion of the cremated remains. An **urn vault** is constructed of concrete, metal, fiberglass, or polymer to serve as an outer container for urns that are buried. **Inurnment** is the physical act of placing cremated remains in an aboveground niche or columbarium. A **niche** is a space specially designed for the placement of cremated remains and may be part of a larger building or structure. A niche can be constructed of concrete, plastic, glass, or other materials, with an outer door that is fitted and secured once the remains are placed inside. A **columbarium** is a structure that contains multiple niches.

Alternative Placement for Cremated Remains

Scattering is the process of spreading cremated remains over a section of cemetery ground or at sea (at least three nautical miles from shore). **Shared remains** are cremated remains that are divided and placed into separate containers that are given to two or more family members. An **ossuary** is a belowground vault for cremated remains that are mingled together and not retrievable. A **receiving vault** is a structure designed for the temporary entombment of caskets if they cannot be placed due to weather conditions or while waiting for a structure to be ready.

Disposition by Alkaline Hydrolysis

Alkaline hydrolysis, or **aquamation**, is the reduction of human remains to fine bone matter, similar to cremated remains from a cremation with flames. The decedent is placed into a metal chamber with an alkaline chemical mixture and water. The process uses a combination of mechanical elements, high temperatures, agitation, and/or pressure over 2 to 12 hours. Liquid residue is drained from the chamber. The remaining bone is pulverized into fine matter and returned to the family. Although considered eco-friendly, the process uses an estimated 300 gallons of water per person, which negates water conservation efforts.

Alkaline hydrolysis is not legal in all US states. State and local laws regulate facilities, certifications, employee safety measures, and public health considerations. Coordinating disposition by aquamation requires steps similar to those for disposition by cremation. Authorization forms must contain decedent information, identification confirmation, procedure details, personal property instructions, directives for the remains, and consenting signatures from all next of kin within the same level of kinship. Prior to disposition, a positive identification of the decedent should be made by the family or family representative. Due diligence inspection steps should be taken by the director prior to contracting services with aquamation facilities.

Disposition by Natural Organic Reduction

Natural organic reduction, or **human composting**, is disposition of a human body through accelerated, controlled natural decomposition. A few states currently allow for this method of disposition under specific regulations. The body is placed into a receptacle with organic matter (wood chips, straw, alfalfa, flowers, etc.). Decay is expedited by maintaining proper oxygen and temperature levels within the vessel to facilitate the microbial growth necessary for decomposition to occur. The resulting compound is a nutrient-rich soil that is tested to ensure safety for people, animals, and plants prior to being returned to family.

As many states do not allow natural organic reduction (NOR), families can opt to have their loved one transferred to a state that allows for disposition by this means. Prior to beginning NOR, the funeral director should proceed with authorization and disclosure forms like those needed for cremation and alkaline hydrolysis. The decedent should be identified and personal possessions removed. The next of kin authorizes disposition and acknowledges the process of NOR. The family needs to decide if they want the organic matter of their loved one back, in part or full, or if they want to donate the soil.

Embalming

EMBALMING

Embalming is a technique of using chemicals to temporarily preserve the dead by neutralizing microbial activity and decomposition, giving family and friends time to have services. Embalming chemicals bond with proteins in the body, creating firm tissue. This bond strengthens the resistance that proteins have against autolytic enzymes, bacteria, and microbes that lead to decomposition, causing temporary preservation. Once permission to embalm is obtained, the body undergoes a case analysis to evaluate conditions, characteristics, challenges, and problem areas and determine the embalming approach (including arterial selection, chemical selection, and treatment methods). The stages of embalming are:

1. **Vascular embalming**: Arterial injection of preservative, sanitization, and co-injection chemicals treats human tissue using the circulatory system to distribute fluid.
2. **Cavity embalming**: Aspiration is a technique used to remove gas and fluids from the cavity. Cavity chemicals are introduced, treating organs, tissues, and hollow spaces within the cavities.
3. **Hypodermic treatment**: Embalming chemicals can be injected directly into tissues to increase preservation in areas that received limited distribution during arterial injection.
4. **Surface embalming**: Liquid or gel chemicals can be topically applied to areas to increase preservation, bleach tissue, and cauterize leaks. Some may have immediate effect, while others soak into the tissue over time.

REASONS FOR EMBALMING

Today, embalming is performed for three reasons. The first is to **disinfect** the deceased. Dangerous pathogenic organisms can survive for long periods of time in dead tissue. Since most bodies are not buried immediately, there is potential for diseases to spread through people coming in contact with the body or through insects that may land on the body. Another purpose for embalming is to **preserve** the body prior to viewing and burial. Decomposition and putrefaction begin soon after death, and this preservation process slows the decay and decreases odors. The third purpose is to **restore** the body to a more lifelike appearance for the viewing.

EMBALMING METHODS

Four primary methods are used in embalming: vascular, cavity, hypodermic, and surface. **Vascular embalming** is the most common way to introduce embalming fluids into the body and uses the vascular system to disseminate the solutions to most parts of the body. **Cavity embalming** consists of the direct treatment of the thoracic, abdominal, and pelvic cavities, in that order, using a trocar to introduce embalming chemicals. **Hypodermic embalming** is performed on tissues with a disrupted vascular system, such as in autopsies, organ donation, and trauma cases, or in tissues where arterial fluid was unsuccessfully or insufficiently distributed during vascular embalming. A syringe and needle or a trocar is used. **Surface embalming** is done on the surface tissues using direct contact with chemicals.

EMBALMING IN ANCIENT EGYPT

The practice of embalming likely originated in Egypt more than 5,000 years ago. It is thought that Egyptians developed embalming for two prime reasons: **religion** and **sanitation**. The Egyptians believed that the soul was immortal, and as long as the body remained intact the soul would never forsake the body. Embalming was the method for the soul to complete what was called the circle of necessity: the 3,000-mile journey the soul took before it was allowed to reunite with the body. The reunited soul and body could then rise up as a whole person and live with the gods. Additionally, embalming was used because the Nile River tended to flood, which brought buried bodies to the surface. Exposure to dead bodies caused disease and death, but embalming sanitized the bodies and prevented spread of disease.

Modern Embalming with Formaldehyde

In the mid-1800s, a compound called **formaldehyde**, a substance that produces a hardening effect in organic tissues, was discovered. It could also be used to disinfect and to preserve. While embalming was not new, formaldehyde greatly improved the practice. Dr. Auguste Renouard published *The Undertaker's Manual* in 1878 with detailed embalming instructions, including the use of formaldehyde. Over the next few decades, the science and art of embalming spread. Several schools of embalming were opened, including Renouard's own US College of Embalming, which opened in 1894; it closed after World War II. Formaldehyde, which has the chemical formula CH_2O, becomes **formalin** when dissolved in water. The most concentrated formalin solutions are 37% formaldehyde. Arterial embalming fluids consist of formaldehyde, methanol, isopropanol, and other chemicals. A solid polymerized derivative of formaldehyde, **paraformaldehyde**, is a main component of the hardening compound. All forms of formaldehyde must be used with caution and proper personal protective equipment (PPE) as they can cause serious health risks, including breathing problems, headaches, and other ailments, and are considered potential occupational carcinogens.

Sanitation Considerations

Following death, the funeral director removes the decedent for transportation to the funeral home. During this time, he or she is at greatest risk and must follow certain procedures. **Sanitation** refers to the process of altering the body's condition, as the body and its immediate environment are unsanitary, with biohazardous conditions. Chemicals are applied to destroy the bacteria. **Disinfection** is the process of eliminating or inhibiting pathogens from the body or an object by chemical or physical means. **Primary disinfection** occurs during pre-embalming and includes the treatment of skin lesions and ulcerations with disinfectant and deodorant since they are a source of infection and contamination. The funeral director must also practice good **personal hygiene** by washing her or her own hands and body regularly and **environmental hygiene** by regularly cleaning all parts of the funeral home.

Protective Clothing

The Occupational Safety and Health Administration (OSHA) has set guidelines regarding the protective clothing needed when using concentrations of formaldehyde greater than 1%. An embalmer should always wear appropriate **personal protective equipment (PPE)** to prevent infectious materials (blood and body fluids) from leaking through to the skin, mouth, eyes, nose, and clothing. **Negative-pressure respirators** with approved canisters or cartridges have restricted use and are not allowed for a full work shift. **Positive-pressure air purifiers** or **self-contained breathing apparatuses** should be used to provide a measure of safety. **Protective gloves** with the least possible amount of permeation are recommended, in accordance with American Conference of Governmental Industrial Hygienists (ACGIH) guidelines. Additionally, an embalmer will need goggles or other complete **eye protection** and a **face shield** to guard against splashes or sprays (the face shield alone does not provide adequate eye protection). Clothing should be impervious to permeation. No skin should be exposed. The employer is responsible for providing employees with a private chamber for changing, an emergency shower, and an eyewash fountain.

Formaldehyde Spills

The Occupational Safety and Health Administration (OSHA) regulates the manner of cleaning formaldehyde spills. Leaking small containers should be placed in a **well-ventilated area** to prevent harmful effects. Small spills can be cleaned with absorbent materials, which should then be placed into a properly labeled container for disposal at a later time. With larger spills, either use a dike (a barrier to prevent the spill from spreading) or take other measures to contain the spill, then **remove** the contaminated product from the workplace. Each product's safety data sheet (SDS) contains instructions for cleanup, neutralization (if possible), and disposal. Some spills can be **neutralized** with a solution of sodium hydroxide or sodium sulfite; the SDS should be checked to see if the spilled chemical can be neutralized in this way. Environmental Protection Agency (EPA) rules require employers to comply with regulations regarding cleanup of toxic waste. State and local authorities must be notified as required by applicable laws. Spills greater than 1,000 lbs per day must be reported in accordance with EPA's Superfund legislation.

Legal and Ethical Obligations

Embalmers must consider several legal and ethical obligations. The embalmer is charged with **judicious counseling** on funeral preparation for the deceased person's family members. The embalmer must also observe all **regulations and rules** pertaining to the handling of the deceased. These include properly identifying and handling the deceased, protecting the health of the public through control and sanitation of the deceased, and assisting the family with viewing the deceased family member or with organ donation requests. An embalmer should not **misrepresent** his or her credentials or make **derisive statements** about other embalmers. He or she should **maintain credentials** through further education and training. Professional conduct should be maintained at all times, including when caring for the deceased and when dealing with members of allied professions or the general public.

Death and Postmortem Changes

Types of Death

The following are several types of death:

- **Necrobiosis** is the death of cells over the lifespan of a living organism. The dead cells are continuously replaced by living ones.
- **Necrosis** occurs when many cells die in a particular organ or part of an organ.
- **Clinical death** occurs immediately after brain activity, breathing, and circulation cease. There is a small possibility that this can be reversed if immediate life-saving measures are taken.
- **Brain death** occurs when the brain is starved of oxygen for three to seven minutes. The brain will be the first organ to die if respiration or circulation ceases. After this happens, the brain cannot be brought back to life.
- **Somatic death** is the death of the organism as a whole. This generally occurs after brain death.

Antemortem Changes

Death will usually follow a sequence of events known as the antemortem period, agonal period, and somatic death. The **antemortem period** sets the stage for life to cease. The **agonal period** occurs just prior to death, leading to the body's cessation of the metabolic and physiological activities that are necessary to sustain life. During the agonal period, a number of things happen. Circulation changes and the blood thickens (agonal coagulation). Respiration and circulation slow, causing agonal hypostasis. Coagulation causes agonal capillary expansion, in which the capillary walls swell and rupture due to the thickened blood. Blood serum escapes from the intravascular system to extravascular locations, causing agonal edema. There will also be a loss of moisture and fluid to the environment, eventually causing agonal dehydration. **Somatic death** occurs when all functions that sustain life have ceased and the body's cells are dead. Signs of death include the cessation of breathing and circulation, flaccidity of muscles, and eye changes (cornea cloudiness, flattening of eyeballs, and dilating of pupils). Postmortem lividity sets in, followed by rigor mortis, algor mortis, and eventually decomposition.

Postmortem Changes

An embalmer should be aware of several postmortem changes that affect the human body. These include algor mortis, liver mortis, dehydration, hypostasis, thickened blood, rigor mortis, postmortem stains, pH changes to the body, and eventually decomposition. **Decomposition** involves two major changes to the body tissues. One is **autolysis**, which usually starts in the pancreas. Digestive enzymes in the cells break down the proteins and carbohydrates. Autolysis is a minor component of decomposition. **Putrefaction** is the main component of decomposition. Bacterial activity leads to gas and bloating; hydrogen sulfide gas causes a brown-black discoloration in the blood vessels, which appears as **marbling** on the skin. In adults, decomposition usually first appears in the lower right quadrant of the abdomen, and this area will take on a green discoloration. In babies, decomposition usually begins in the brain. Finally, the skin will blister and slip, and the nails and hair will be lost.

Algor Mortis

One postmortem change is **algor mortis**, which is the cooling of the body after death. The body will start to cool until it reaches ambient room temperature. A number of factors influence the rate of algor mortis, including illness or infection prior to death, high room temperature, activity just prior to death, and decomposition. These variations are usually small enough that the temperature of the body can be used to roughly approximate when the person died. For the first 12 hours, the body temperature will drop about 1.5 °F per hour, and for the next 12 hours, the temperature will drop about 0.7 °F per hour. Therefore, in the first 12 hours, the **Glaister equation** can be used to determine the approximate time of death:

$$\text{hours since death} = \frac{98.4 - (\text{rectal temperature in } ^\circ\text{F})}{1.5}$$

There are rare exceptions to this pattern. After some deaths, including those from septicemia, asphyxia, fever at time of death, and alcohol poisoning, the body's temperature may rise by about 3.6 °F in the hours immediately following death before beginning to cool. This phenomenon, which is poorly understood but attributed to bacterial activity and/or cellular oxidation, is known as **postmortem caloricity**.

Rigor Mortis

Rigor mortis occurs gradually after death and refers to the onset of rigidity to the body, caused by conversion of glycogen stores into lactic acid. The muscles are not shortened during this process. The excessive lactic acid causes a cross-linking of actin and myosin. **Rigor mortis** is accelerated by heat, acidosis, uremia, and certain other medical conditions that lower the pH of the body. It will usually dissipate within 12 to 36 hours after death. Rigor mortis affects the amount of fluid absorbed by the tissues, and injection of fluid under high pressure during rigor mortis may cause **tissue swelling**. Tissue absorbs embalming fluid at different rates. Arterial walls and skin have the lowest uptake of fluid, while muscle and viscera have the highest. When rigor mortis sets in, the blood vessels contract, restricting the flow of fluid to the tissues. This makes it difficult to inject enough embalming fluids. If the body is embalmed at the beginning of rigor mortis, the embalmer may incorrectly assume that enough fluids have been injected into the tissues.

Livor Mortis

Livor mortis (postmortem lividity or cadaveric lividity) is discoloration caused by the postmortem settling of blood to dependent areas within the vascular system. Blood volume and thickness impacts lividity: less blood causes less discoloration, and thicker blood restricts gravitational settling, resulting in less discoloration. Lividity begins as reddish-pink patches along dependent tissue. As the blood pools, discolorations darken and begin to take on a purple hue. Lividity can be observed along the back, buttocks, and fingernails of a supine person (on their back with arms at their sides). If the head is below the chest or tilted to one side, lividity can be seen in dependent facial areas. **Contact pallor** will be noticed in dependent areas subjected to pressure. These light areas, surrounded by livor, are seen where the body's weight is resting on the embalming table, or on the face under medical equipment (such as endotracheal tubes and tape) when the head is lower than the chest. This discoloration can often be cleared during arterial injection. Livor mortis can eventually turn into postmortem stains as the hemoglobin leaches out of settled blood, permanently discoloring the extravascular tissue it soaks into. Extravascular changes such as Tardieu spots (caused by ruptured blood vessels), like ecchymoses, do not clear with arterial injection.

Labeling the Body and Inventorying Personal Effects

When a decedent is transferred into the care of the funeral home, an **identification tag** needs to be placed on the person. This should have, at minimum, the person's name on it; additional information can include the funeral home, date, place of death, and disposition method. The funeral director obtains permission (oral or written) to embalm from the next of kin. Prior to beginning treatment, identity is verified using the identification tag. All personal effects, including bedding, clothing, accessories, and jewelry, are removed from the body and detailed on a personal possessions inventory document. When detailing jewelry, it is important not to assume the material content (gold, silver, diamond, etc.) or brand (unless it is clearly indicated) of items for liability purposes. For example, a ring is detailed as having a yellow-colored band with a clear or white stone rather than "a gold ring with a diamond." Items are sanitized or laundered as needed and secured in a labeled bag to await instructions from the family. Any items that are soiled beyond the scope of cleaning are documented and disposed of as biohazard waste. Funeral homes should have written protocols and policies for identifying decedents and handling personal effects.

Linear Guides, Anatomical Guides, and Anatomical Limits

Linear guides (LG) are imaginary lines visualized on the skin to indicate the location of a structure within the body. **Anatomical guides (AG)** are structures within the body used to locate other surrounding structures. **Anatomical limits (AL)** are the beginning and end of a structure relative to other close structures.

Common Carotid Arteries

Common carotid artery: The right common carotid artery branches off the brachiocephalic artery, and the left common carotid branches off the arch of the aorta. They each bifurcate into the internal and external carotids. The common carotid is located medial and deep to the jugular vein, with the vagus nerve running between.

- LG: the anterior base of the earlobe down to the sternoclavicular articulation
- AG: posterior and medial to the sternocleidomastoid muscle

- AL: begins at the sternoclavicular articulation to the superior margin of the thyroid cartilage, with the left common carotid beginning at the second costal cartilage, running up to the superior margin of the thyroid cartilage

Axillary, Radial, and Ulnar Arteries

Axillary artery: an extension of the subclavian artery located lateral and deep to the axillary vein

- LG: extends along the axillary space of the outstretched arm, from the base to the lateral border of the axillary space
- AG: posterior to the medial border of the coracobrachialis muscle
- AL: begins at the lateral margin of the first rib and ends at the lower margin of the tendon of the teres major muscle

Radial artery: a bifurcation of the brachial artery located between two radial veins

- LG: midline of the antecubital fossa to the midline of the index finger
- AG: lateral to the flexor carpi radialis muscle's tendon and medial to the brachioradialis muscle's tendon
- AL: begins an inch lower than the interior elbow and ends at the thumb's thenar eminence

Ulnar artery: a bifurcation of the brachial artery located between two small veins

- LG: midline of the antecubital fossa down between the pinky and ring fingers
- AG: lateral to the flexor carpi ulnaris muscle's tendon
- AL: begins an inch below the interior elbow and ends at the pisiform bone, one of the lateral carpal bones

Femoral Arteries and Other Arteries

Femoral artery: extends off the external iliac artery, lateral and superficial to the femoral vein

- LG: middle of the inguinal ligament to the middle of the medial condyle of the femur
- AG: within the femoral triangle, which consists of the inguinal ligament at the base, the sartorius muscle at the medial border, and the adductor longus muscle at the lateral border (The femoral artery is medial to the sartorius and lateral to the adductor longus.)
- AL: begins at the inguinal ligament and becomes the popliteal artery as it enters the adductor magnus muscle

Additional arteries that can be used to inject the leg:

- **Popliteal artery**: located between the popliteal surface of the femur and the oblique popliteal ligament, extending from the adductor magnus muscle to the inferior border of the popliteus muscle
- **Anterior tibial artery**: located between the tibialis anterior muscle and hallucis longus muscle's tendon, extending from the popliteus muscle to the center, anterior joint of the ankle
- **Posterior tibial artery**: located between the posterior tibia and calcaneus tendon, extending from the popliteus muscle down between the medial malleolus and calcaneus bones

Selecting Arteries for Injection in Unautopsied Bodies

In unautopsied bodies, the selection of arteries is based on decedent condition and arterial quality. Commonly selected arteries for **primary injection sites** are the common carotids, femorals, and axillaries. These major arteries are used first, and then smaller ones are selected as needed to evenly distribute fluid. The embalmer needs to evaluate the artery's location, size, proximal structures, and accessibility, as well as the necessary incision site. Bodily conditions of the deceased that influence arterial selection include age, gender, size, cause and manner of death, malformations, trauma, and disease.

Techniques for **raising vessels** can vary slightly based on the specific vessel; however, there are general standards of practice for all locations. Ensure instruments are clean and functioning properly. Pinpoint the incision site using the linear guides for the artery selected. Incise the skin and locate the vessels using anatomical structures and guides. The superficial vessel should be raised first, followed by the deep vessel. Use ligature to secure the vessels. Instruments should be placed into the deep vessel prior to preparing the superficial one. Select arterial tubes based on the size of the lumen. Coagulations should be removed prior to inserting the cannula.

Rate of Flow and the Different Types of Pressure

Centrifugal pump embalming machines are the primary choice for arterial injection. They vary in components and features. Prior to injecting arterial solution, the pressure and rate of flow must be adjusted appropriately. **Rate of flow**, the quantity of embalming mixture injected within a specific amount of time, is measured in ounces per minute. **Pressure** is measured in pounds and is defined as the intensity at which fluid is circulated through the vascular system. **Potential pressure** is the pressure level maintained in the tubing when the embalming machine is on and the stopcock or rate of flow valve is closed. **Actual pressure** is the gauge measurement during injection (with the rate of flow valve and stopcock opened). **Differential pressure** is calculated by subtracting the potential pressure from the actual pressure. This value equals the rate of flow, so it can be calculated this way when the embalming machine does not have a rate-of-flow gauge. Differential pressure accounts for pressure loss as fluid travels through the tubing and encounters vascular resistance; the pressure gauge does account for this loss, so it does not reflect the actual pressure within the body. **Injection pressure** is the level of pressure required to counter vascular resistance.

Restricted Cervical Injection

A **restricted cervical injection**, often simply called a **restricted cervical**, is a technique where both the right and left common carotid arteries are raised. The right internal jugular is typically used for drainage. The left common carotid is incised and tied below the incision. The arterial cannula is inserted down the right common carotid to inject the torso, arms, and legs. The ligation on the left side limits distribution to the face but allows drainage to exit the head through the incision. While injecting down, collateral circulation allows arterial fluid to enter the head via the right and left vertebral arteries. Injecting up the left common carotid, followed by the right, treats the head.

This technique allows for control over the arterial fluid, pressure, and rate of flow entering the head. Arterial fluid specific for the head can be used rather than using the same solution as the body. Emaciated edema cases are examples of when a higher-strength fluid with edema-treating chemicals is used for the body and a less harsh solution with humectants is injected up the head. This technique is also useful in cases of jaundice, facial trauma, anticipated facial distension (due to freezing or decomposition), burned or drowned victims, eye enucleations, distribution problems, or delayed viewing cases.

Components of an Arterial Solution

During the initial pre-embalming case analysis, the embalmer evaluates the condition of the body, factoring in service timeframes and other known information to formulate an injection solution and plan. A **preinjection solution** is injected to condition the body before injection of a preservative-based mixture. **Co-injection fluids** are mixed into the preservative mixture to aid arterial fluid in preserving and treating the condition of the body.

- **Active dyes** are mixed into the arterial solution to distribute a cosmetic color through the arterial system and tissue.
- **Inactive dyes** are noncosmetic coloring in the chemicals. They do not affect injected tissue but rather aid in visual differentiation between chemicals.
- **Water corrective fluids** help correct water components and contaminants and may help to counter medicinal and chemical influences in the decedent that can impact the effectiveness of arterial fluid.
- **Humectants/restorative fluids** assist in preserving moisture within tissue, minimizing the dehydrating effect of the preservative.
- **Edema co-injection fluids** increase the dehydrating properties of arterial fluid and pull edema out of the tissues.
- **Jaundice fluids** are low-index or formaldehyde-free chemicals that aid in removing bilirubin discoloration.
- **Index** refers to the percentage of formaldehyde gas present in the solution. Arterial fluids vary in index.

Cavity and Arterial Fluids

The purpose of cavity fluids is to preserve and de-germ the interior of the body cavity. For this reason, the cavity fluid will contain high concentrations of disinfectants and preservatives. The fluids generally lack any dyes, deodorants, or modifying agents as there is generally no need for cosmetic treatment to the thoracic and abdominal cavities and their organs. The composition of the cavity fluid has a higher **acidic** (4.5 to 5.2 pH) content, so it will react with the tissue proteins. **Arterial fluids** are dyed for aesthetic or cosmetic reasons. Deodorants, previously called reodorants, are responsible for masking the harsh chemical smells from the other treatments received by the body. Surfactants, surface wetting and surface-tension reducing agents, help the flow and diffusion of the embalming fluids. Other arterial fluids include modifying agents, germicides, preservatives, and anticoagulants. The **index** of a fluid refers to the percentage of pure formaldehyde gas dissolved in 100 milliliters of a solution.

Preservatives in Embalming Fluids

The preservatives used in embalming fluids are aldehydes, alcohols, phenolic compounds, and germicides. **Aldehydes** are cross-link proteins. One of the most common preservatives is formaldehyde, a lower aldehyde that provides many more cross-links. These help with tissue firmness and provide a barrier to decomposition. **Alcohols** such as methanol, ethanol, and isopropyl alcohol are sometimes used in conjunction with aldehyde in the embalming process. Methanol is most common because it is both a preservative and an anti-polymerizing agent. Ethanol and isopropyl are germicides. Isopropyl is more common because it is less expensive. **Phenolic compounds** preserve and disinfect due to their ability to precipitate protein. Phenols are used as bleaching agents and create a putty-gray color when used with aldehydes in the embalming process. Quaternary ammonium is a preservative used as a surface disinfectant. Another preservative, glutaraldehyde, has been labeled the "cold chemical sterilant."

Modifying Agents

Modifying agents are required in embalming fluids due to the caustic nature of disinfectants and preservatives, which can scorch delicate capillaries and cause a fluid diffusion problem. Modifying agents delay the actions of the disinfectants and preservatives until the tissues have soaked up adequate fluid. **Humectants** help the tissues retain moisture so the aldehydes and alcohols do not dry them out. Humectants include glycols, glycerols, sorbitols, other polyhydroxy alcohols, and soluble lanolin compounds. **Buffers** are stabilizers that resist any changes in pH. Formaldehyde polymerizes in acidic conditions and decomposes in alkaline conditions. Examples are borax, sodium phosphate, citrates, and sodium salts. Methyl alcohol is routinely added to arterial fluids to combat polymerization of formaldehyde.

Accessory Chemicals

Autopsy gels are surface preservatives for necrotic areas. They are often applied after enucleating an eye or may be poured over viscera in the abdominal/thoracic cavity. A **tissue builder** is injected with a hypodermic syringe after embalming. **Hardening compounds** treat cavities and organs from an autopsied body, as well as decubitus ulcers or amputated limbs, to avoid leakage in the bottom of the casket or body bag. **Cement** is a liquid material that glues the tissue together. It is used in incisions, lip or eyelid closure, etc. **Sealing agents** (sealers) are liquid solutions that begin to dry tissue immediately upon application, leaving a hardened coating and stopping the movement of body fluids and moisture. **Humectants** are chemicals that help tissues maintain moisture. A **surface pack** (compress) is a piece of cotton that is saturated with a chemical agent and applied directly onto the surface of the skin to treat a specific area. Gauze may be used in a surface pack, but it should not be used on visible areas such as the hands or face because it leaves indentations. **Perfuming agents** (masking agents) are added to arterial fluid to mask foul-smelling odors. **Mold inhibitors** are chemicals that prevent mold growth. A **pediculicide** is a chemical agent used to exterminate lice.

Drainage

During the pre-embalming case analysis, the embalmer selects a vein to drain from. Primary selections for drainage are the right internal jugular and femoral veins. The left internal jugular and axillary veins can be used, but there are more bifurcations between them and the right atrium, potentially complicating drainage. The right atrium can be trocarized above and to the left of the umbilicus for direct gravity drainage.

Drainage instruments include:

- **Angular spring forceps:** These are inserted into the vein to facilitate open, free drainage. They can be used to remove and break up clotted matter. Using forceps for drainage can be messy and reduces the ease of intermittent drainage.
- **Drain tube:** When inserted into the vein, a drain tube allows for open or closed, continuous or intermittent drainage options. The interior rod can be used to break up clots. Tubes can leave facial indentations and puncture the vein, and drainage is restricted to the diameter of the tube.

Methods of drainage include:

- **Alternate**: Injection and drainage are not simultaneous. The embalmer alternates between injecting arterial solution and draining.
- **Concurrent:** Injection occurs while drainage flows openly.
- **Intermittent**: Throughout the injection, drainage is opened and closed as needed.

Contents of Drainage and Complications That Impact Drainage

Embalming drainage contains blood and its components, bodily fluids, and arterial solution. Drainage flows through the veins towards the heart as the arterial fluid is injected and displaces bodily fluids. When injection begins, there can be a delay before drainage emerges. At first, drainage has a high blood content, but this dilutes into a lighter-colored fluid as the arterial fluid pushes blood, lymphatic fluid, and interstitial fluid through the body. Postmortem, the blood coagulates, becoming thicker and settling into dependent areas creating **livor mortis.** Blood clots that are removed with drainage all originate from inside the heart or venous system; arterial clots are unable to enter capillaries because of their size, making it impossible for them to enter drainage fluid.

The amount of drainage does not always coincide with the amount of fluid injected; it is also dependent on the cause and circumstances of death (trauma, surgeries, autopsies, and organ donation all reduce vascular blood volumes).

Other potential drainage challenges are created by the body size and weight being subjected upon the vascular system. Increased arterial injection pressure may be needed to counteract this internal pressure.

Cavity Embalming

Cavity embalming consists of aspirating hollow viscera and organs and then injecting a preservation chemical. This step is essential for removing the contents of organs to prevent the accumulation of gases, fluid, and odors within the torso. Injecting cavity chemicals treats areas within the thoracic, abdominal, and pelvic cavities that may not have received sufficient preservation via arterial injection. This includes visceral organ walls, contents, and hollowed spaces.

Hollowed viscera and their contents include:

- **Lungs, trachea,** and **bronchi**: blood, edema, gases, and infectious fluids
- **Heart, ascending and descending aorta,** and **superior and inferior vena cavae:** blood and fluid
- **Stomach**: food, blood, gases, gastric acid, and hydrochloric acid
- **Small and large intestines**: blood, undigested and digested foods, gases, and in the large intestine, fecal matter
- **Urinary bladder**: urine, fluid, blood
- **Gallbladder:** bile
- **Kidneys**: urine, blood, and fluid

Solid organs include the pancreas, spleen, liver, and brain. The lungs and kidneys have solid portions in addition to their hollow cavities.

Abdominal Divisions Layout

The embalmer can mentally picture gridlines over the abdomen to help in remembering the contents of each section. Knowing the contents of each abdominal section allows for thorough cavity treatment. There are two sets of gridlines used: the four-region method and the nine-region method.

Four-region method: Visually section the abdomen into four regions by imagining a horizontal midline intersecting a vertical line through the umbilicus. The sections formed are the right upper quadrant, left upper quadrant, right lower quadrant, and left lower quadrant.

Nine-region method: Visually section the abdomen into nine sections by imagining two vertical lines from the center of each clavicle down the abdomen. The first horizontal line runs inferior to the tenth costal cartilage. The second horizontal line runs between the protrusions of the iliac tubercles.

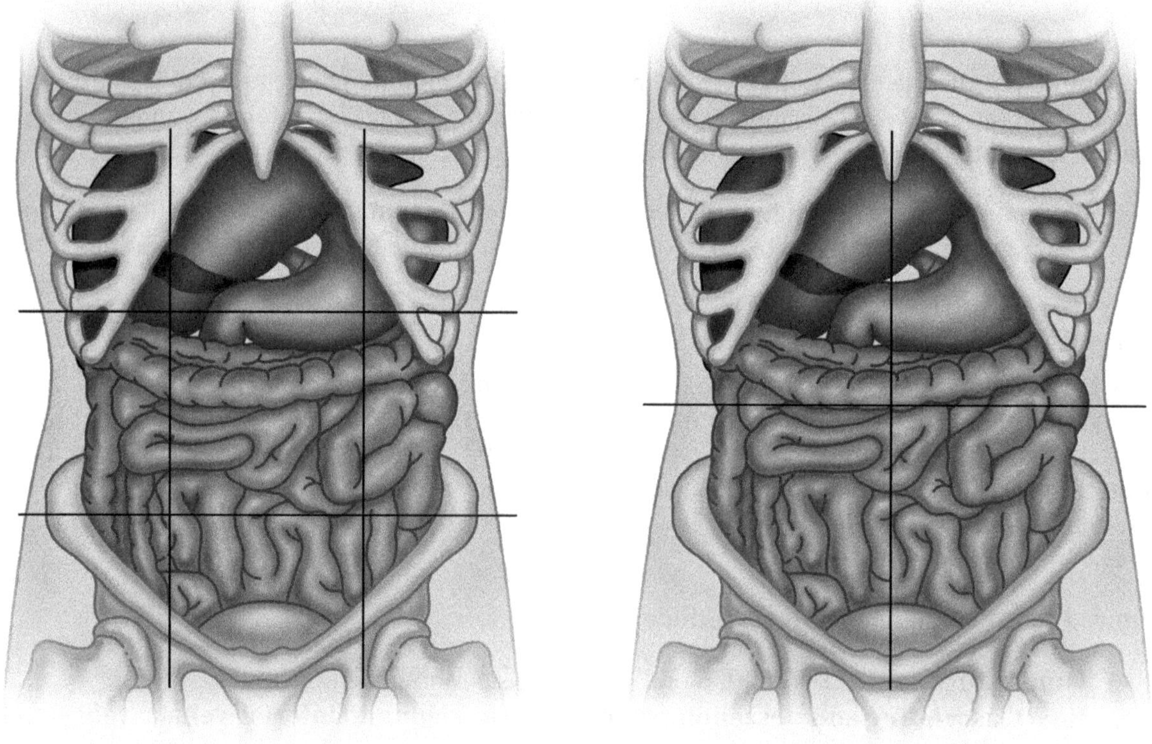

Contents of Each of the Nine Regions of the Abdomen

The nine abdominal regions and their contents are:

- **Right hypochondriac (upper right)**: gallbladder and portions of the liver, right kidney, greater omentum, and small intestine
- **Epigastric (upper center)**: stomach (including cardia and pylorus openings), suprarenal glands, and portions of the liver, kidneys, greater omentum, duodenum, and pancreas
- **Left hypochondriac (upper left)**: portions of the liver, left kidney, and greater omentum, along with the pancreas tail, spleen, and left colic splenic flexure
- **Right lumbar (middle right)**: portions of the liver, right kidney, small intestine, and greater omentum, along with the right colic hepatic flexure and ascending colon
- **Umbilical (center)**: transverse colon, abdominal aorta, inferior vena cava, and portions of the kidneys, duodenum, small intestine, and greater omentum
- **Left lumbar (middle left)**: portions of the left kidney, descending colon, small intestine, and greater omentum
- **Right inguinal (lower right)**: cecum, appendix, and portions of the small intestine, ascending colon, and greater omentum

- **Hypogastric (lower center)**: portions of the small intestine and greater omentum; during pregnancy, the expanded bladder and uterus extend from the pelvic cavity into the abdominal cavity
- **Left inguinal (lower left)**: sigmoid colon and portions of the descending colon, small intestine, and greater omentum

Instruments Used for Cavity Treatment

- **Trocar**: A long, hollow (18" long × 5/16" bore) metal instrument with a detachable point, a trocar is used to remove fluids and gases within the cavity. It is additionally used for injecting cavity fluid. **Infant trocars** (12" long × 1/4" bore) are used for treating infants and children or as a hypodermic needle.
- **Tubing**: 3/8" to 1/2" diameter plastic or rubber hose connects the aspiration machine to the trocar and drainage system. Clear or translucent tubing allows for visual monitoring.
- **Autopsy (post) aspirator**: A hollow metal instrument (8–10" long × 3/8" bore) with a head attachment, this instrument is designed to prevent fat, tissue, and large coagulants from entering the tubing.
- **Nasal tube aspirator**: This hollow (10" long × 3/16" bore) instrument with a rounded 90° curve is used for aspirating the nasal and oral cavities.
- **Gravity-fed injection tube**: This connects the trocar to the bottle of cavity fluid. Machine injectors may be used instead.
- **Aspirators**: **Hydro aspirators** are water-based suctioning systems. The pressure of the water source creates a vacuum which allows fluids to be removed from the body through the trocar and tubing into the drainage system (flush sink, drain line, and treatment holding tank). **Electric aspirators** have an impeller spun by an electric-powered motor which generates suction.

Aspiration Techniques for Cavity Treatment

For cavity treatment, the **standard trocar entry point** is two inches above and two inches to the left of the umbilicus. The location may need to be adjusted based on the size and characteristics of the decedent; however, in most cases, from this point the trocar can reach all locations within the thoracic, abdominal, and pelvic cavities, including into the tissues of the neck.

Tips:

- Knowing the location and basic physiological function of the organs and viscera allows the embalmer to properly treat the cavity contents.
- Listening to the suctioning sound while aspirating can indicate whether the system is working. Sound changes can suggest the system flipped: rather than suctioning, water is being flushed through the tubing and trocar to clear a blockage.
- The recommended technique for thorough treatment of the cavities is **fanning**, or moving the trocar right to left in a fanlike pattern, at varying depths.
- Continuous movement helps prevent the trocar from sucking up large amounts of fat or tissue that could cause system blockages. When a fluid pocket is found, the trocar can be held stationary to evacuate it before moving on.
- Periodically remove the trocar from the body to rinse it or allow air into the system.

Trocar Guides for Accessing the Heart, Stomach, Cecum, and Bladder

Trocar guides for accessing the heart stomach, cecum, and bladder are as follows:

- **Right side of the heart**: Align the trocar from the left anterior iliac spine across the torso pointing towards the right earlobe.
- **Stomach**: Align the trocar with the left fifth intercostal space pointing towards the midaxillary line.
- **Cecum**: Align the trocar a quarter of the distance from the right anterior superior iliac spine to the pubic symphysis; remain superficial until approximately 4" from the iliac spine, then lower 2" into the large intestine.
- **Urinary bladder**: Align the trocar midline with the pubic symphysis; once tapped, pull back and lower the trocar to insert it into the bladder.

Embalming after Autopsies

Embalming Treatments for Cases with Cranial Autopsies and Vertebral Autopsies

A **cranial autopsy** removes the brain from the cranium. A restricted cervical can be used to inject arterial solution down into the body while draining from the right jugular vein. Alternatively, the right femoral artery and vein can be used. During injection, the vertebral arteries should be clamped inside the cranial cavity. Inject the head via the left then right common carotids. Leaking vessels inside the cranium need to be clamped, including the left and right internal carotids and superior thyroid arteries. Cranial treatment steps include removing pooled fluid, applying topical preservatives, and packing with cotton; securing the cranial cap; treating the incision; and suturing right to left.

A **vertebral or spinal autopsy** is performed to examine the vertebral column. A wedge section of the spinal cord can be removed ventrally from the inside as part of a full or partial autopsy. Treatment is conducted in concert with treating the cavity. A **dorsal spinal autopsy** removes a section of the vertebrae or the entire spinal column dorsally. A loose, temporary suture can hold the affected tissue together for arterial injection. Post-injection, the sutures should be removed, the tissue treated with preserving gel and powder, and the incision re-sutured with a tight baseball stitch.

Embalming Treatments for Cases with Thoracic Autopsies and Abdominal Autopsies

Thoracic autopsies involve the removal of at least one organ within the thorax. Injection via the lower thoracic aorta (posterior to the diaphragm along the vertebrae) distributes fluid to the abdominal cavity and legs. The arms are injected from the left and right axillary or subclavian arteries. The head is injected using the left and right common carotids. The thoracic cavity is dried, treated with preservative gels or powders, and packed with absorptive materials soaked with cavity fluid. The breastplate is repositioned and the incision sutured. The abdominal and pelvic cavities should be aspirated and treated with cavity fluid.

Abdominal (abdominopelvic) autopsies involve the removal of abdominal organs or contents for examination. The left and right external iliac arteries can be used to inject the legs. The thoracic cavity, arms, and head are injected with the abdominal aorta, posterior to the diaphragm along the vertebrae. Alternatively, the right common carotid (or restricted cervical) can be used, injecting down first with a clamp on the abdominal aorta and then up into the head. The inferior vena cava is used for draining. The cavity is treated by drying, coating with preservative gel or powder, packing with absorptive materials or returned viscera, and suturing the incision.

Organ and Tissue Recovery

Impact of Viable Organ Donation on the Embalming Procedure

Viable organs are procured via a midline thoracic or abdominal incision or a T incision arcing along the base of the ribcage and down the abdominal midline. Location and length vary depending on the organs being procured. Arterial injection is approached similarly to that of partial autopsies and is based on the organs donated. The embalmer analyzes the situation and finds the most practical and feasible means of injection.

For **full organ donations** (when heart, lungs, liver, kidneys, pancreas, and intestines are procured), the common iliac arteries are used to inject buttocks, genital areas, and legs; the subclavian or axillary arteries are used to inject the arms; and the common carotid arteries are used to inject up the head. The cavity spaces are dried; hypodermic treatment of the thoracic tissues, abdominal walls, and buttocks is recommended; preservative gel and powders are applied; absorptive materials soaked with cavity fluid can be used to fill and restore the natural look of the areas; and the incision(s) sutured.

Impact of Eye Enucleation and Skin Donation on Arterial Embalming

Eye enucleation or cornea donation: Enucleations cause vascular disturbances and increased risk of orbital swelling and ecchymosis. Preinjection treatment consists of removing the procedure packing, treating the cavity with a preservative gel or cauterant, and rebuilding the eye with cotton to restore a natural appearance. A restricted cervical, increased solution strength, and monitoring injection pressure and rate of flow are recommended. Post-injection, the eye cavities should be cleaned, treated with powder, built up with cotton or putty and eye caps, and glued shut.

Skin donation: Donor skin can be removed in thin layers or thick, extracting all three layers of integument. Skin shavings are procured with a **dermatome** and taken from the thighs, calves, or back. Deep skin procurements are typically from the back of the torso. The body should be positioned on blocks so there is adequate air flow underneath. Following arterial injection, the areas of procurement can be treated immediately or left to dry out prior to treatment. A cauterant and preservative gel can be applied to the area to ensure preservation and minimize leakage. Adsorptive pads and powders can be used inside plastic garments to provide additional treatment and prevent leakage.

Impact of Long Bone Donation on Arterial Injection

Long bone donation entails extracting the femur, tibia, fibula, and hemipelvis from an incision from the iliac crest down to the metatarsals. The humerus and humeral head can be procured, although this is not as common as long bone. Long bone procurement is often accompanied by simultaneous procurement of veins, cartilage, tendons, and ligaments. These procedures significantly disrupt the vascular system. Two methods can be used to embalm these bodies:

- Remove recovery sutures and prosthetics; clamp broken vessels; inject up the right femoral artery or down the right carotid; inject up and down radial or ulnar arteries in cases of humoral donation; inject down both femoral arteries; hypodermically treat remaining tissue; replace prosthetics; coat tissue with preservative gel or powders; suture incisions.
- Leave the recovery sutures in place for the primary injection via the right common carotid artery or a restricted cervical, allowing fluid to **free flow** into the legs. The fluid will enter intact vessels and freely flow out of disrupted vessels, allowing for a saturation into remaining tissues that cannot be reached by vascular injection. After arterial injection and cavity treatment, sutures can be removed and excess fluid drained. This is followed by hypodermic treatment, powder or gel, and sutures.

NBE Sciences

Special Cases in Embalming

Infants and Children

For infants and children under 4 years old:

- Babies typically have a very high moisture content, which can increase with organ failure, disease, and medical interventions. Preinjection is not recommended, but index does not necessarily need to be reduced for an infant.
- Delicate skin and structures react more sensitively than adult tissues.
- A muscular suture or adhesive compound should be used instead of needle injectors to secure the mouth. If the mouth is left open, massage cream can prevent dehydration.
- The small vascular system requires smaller instruments and cannulas. All arteries are usable, just smaller in size. Autopsy vascular selection is the same as an adult. For unautopsied bodies, the common carotid and femoral are useable. Although harder to access, the abdominal aorta (along the spine, beneath the intestines) and ascending aorta (in the chest, under the sternum) can be selected for injection.
- An infant trocar is used for aspiration and cavity injection.

For children 4–12 years old:

- Similar to adults, the common carotids and femoral arteries are primary selections.
- Index, type, and amount of fluid are based on the condition of the body (e.g., disease, trauma, and size).
- Rate of flow should be reduced.

Deformities and Malformations

Special consideration is needed to determine the best course of treatment in cases of **deformities** and **malformations**. Some must be addressed prior to arterial injection, while others can be treated post-embalming.

Severe spinal curvatures and physical contortions can be softened prior to embalming by using blocks and body positioning techniques to establish a more natural resting position. Facial abnormalities (protruding teeth or distorted mouth) can be adjusted when setting features. The embalmer will not always be able to completely rectify all of these conditions; however, restoring a peaceful and natural look based on the decedent's normal appearance is appropriate.

Post-embalming, there are adjustments that can be made in cases of skin malformations, growths, tumors, and disfigurations. By request or with the permission of the family, these can be removed and treated. Excise growths and use chemicals and cauterants to achieve a clean, dry, and firm surface. Once preserved, restoration can begin to rebuild and normalize the decedent's appearance. Features can be built up using tissue builder or wax. A tissue reducer can be used to help remove and displace facial edema.

Obesity

An obese decedent should be placed on blocks with the elbows close to the body to be as narrow as possible. A stronger solution ensures preservation and fixation, which helps with moving, dressing, and lifting the body later. Using higher pressure can counteract bodily resistance upon the vascular system, particularly the weight of the viscera pushing down directly on the vessels within the cavity. Femoral arteries are more difficult to raise because they are deeper, under substantial layers of fat. Bodily pressure creates purge, pushing fluid out of the nasal and oral cavities. Gases tend to build up more because **algor mortis** takes longer because these bodies retain heat. Trocar insertion points may need to be altered to aspirate and treat the entire torso. Additional cavity fluid may be needed to achieve preservation. Reaspiration is performed to remove purge, gas, and pressure. Aesthetically, the jowls and cheeks appear larger when the person is lying down, often completely hiding the neck. This makes positioning in the casket more challenging. Always position the body so the head is elevated the highest, the chest is elevated above the buttocks, and the buttocks above the legs. This helps prevent purging.

Jaundice

Jaundice is when the skin, sclera, mucus membranes, and body tissues appear yellow as bilirubin, a yellow-colored fluid, builds up within the blood and seeps out of the circulatory system. The body produces bilirubin when red blood cells deteriorate. Bilirubin is filtered out of the blood by the liver and used to create bile (which breaks down food in digestion). **Jaundice** is a symptom of a disease that is causing rapid red blood cell breakdown or liver malfunction. These diseases include cirrhosis, alcohol-induced liver damage, hepatitis, cancer, and some autoimmune diseases. Bile duct occlusion, viral infections, operations, liver injury, and other cancers (e.g., lymphoma, pancreatic, and gallbladder) can also result in jaundice. The underlying cause needs to be diagnosed and treated to improve patient color. Conditions seen in conjunction with jaundice include dark urine, fever, weight loss, and edema.

Jaundice can impact embalming because excessive amounts of bilirubin within the circulatory system causes an acidic environment. Oxidation of acidic, quick-acting arterial fluids causes bilirubin to turn into the green-colored biliverdin, turning the decedent green over time as the chemicals interact. Specialized jaundice fluids have lower levels of formaldehyde and buffers to neutralize pH to reduce this chemical reaction.

Methods of Treating Jaundice

All body conditions (e.g., weight, edema, and decomposition) must be considered in jaundice cases. Establishing preservation is more important than preventing discoloration; biliverdin (green) can be covered by cosmetics when tissue is firm and dry. Restricted cervicals are recommended.

Method options include:

- **Jaundice fluid**: This is a specialized, low-index fluid with buffers and active dye.
- **Preinjection**: Preinjections (with or without adding dye) flush blood out, reducing bilirubin levels. This is followed by normal arterial solution to achieve preservation (not for decomposition or edema).
- **Cavity fluid**: A few cavity chemicals (read the label) can be injected arterially to bleach and preserve.
- **Mild arterial fluid**: Vast amounts of fluid are needed to ensure preservation but can result in swelling and underembalming.
- **Bleaching co-injections**: Traditional arterial fluid is mixed with co-injections formulated to bleach discolorations.
- **Relative counterstaining**: This is a combination of methods to counteract jaundice using red dye, water conditioners, anticoagulants, and selected arterial fluid. Mix and inject one gallon at a time. The first gallon consists of accessory chemicals, 4 oz of arterial fluid, and 12 oz of dye; for each subsequent gallon, use co-injections but increase arterial fluid and decrease dye (based on coloration). Edema fluid or humectants can be added to treat conditions as needed.

Edema

Edema is an excess accumulation of fluid in tissue and/or serous (hollow) cavities. Fluid moves from the capillaries into interstitial space (tissues) and then back into the capillaries. Edema begins to accumulate when more fluid exits the capillaries than is absorbed back into them. Fluid accumulation can be **intracellular** (in cells), **intercellular** (between cells), and in serous body cavities. Edema is considered **localized** when a specific area of the body is affected and **generalized** when seen throughout the body, especially in dependent tissues. Edema can be caused by surgery; trauma; reduced cardiac function; renal, liver, kidney, and lymphatic diseases; and drugs or medications like steroids. Understanding the cause of edema helps in treating it.

Classifications of edema are:

- **Cellular (solid) edema** occurs when individual cells retain too much fluid, causing firm, swollen tissue. This doesn't **pit** (indent) when touched and won't be reduced by injection chemicals. Tissue must be excised in attempt to drain fluid. This is commonly seen in facial tissue following intense corticosteroid use.
- **Intercellular (pitting) edema** occurs when excess fluid is retained between cells.

Possible locations of edema are:

- **Ascites**: abdominal or peritoneal cavity
- **Hydropericardium**: pericardial cavity
- **Hydrothorax**: pleural cavity
- **Hydrocephalus**: cranial cavity
- **Hydrocele**: surrounding the testicles within the scrotum
- **Anasarca**: generalized throughout the body

Embalming Methods for Edema Cases

Restricted cervicals are recommended in cases of edema, allowing control over the head and giving the option of injecting different strength fluids into the body than the head. Specialized edema arterial fluids have a high index to counteract dilution that occurs as it enters the circulatory system and tissues **(secondary dilution).** Alternatively, a high-index arterial fluid can be used in conjunction with an edema co-injection fluid. These contain salts and large colloidal molecules to draw fluid out of tissues and into the vascular system, allowing it to drain out. Alternatively, Epsom salts can be dissolved in water and added to a normal arterial solution to create a hypertonic solution to reduce edema. Reducing the amount of water mixed into the arterial solution can help with reducing secondary dilution.

Waterless embalming consists of reducing (not eliminating) the amount of water added to arterial solutions and increasing the accessory chemicals (water-treatment fluids and vascular conditioners) used, which makes the arterial fluid more effective. Accessory chemicals dilute the solution while adding treatment capabilities. This technique can be used in many extreme cases (gas, gangrene, edema, decomposition, trauma, emaciating, drownings, and dehydration), tailoring the chemical concoction to meet the specific needs of the case.

Techniques to Treat Edema in Specific Areas of the Body

- **Facial edema**: Manual pressure expresses and manipulates fluid from the tissue. Use the trocar to create channels into neck tissue, allowing fluid to drain down into the torso. Gravity reduces fluid from the head and neck when the head is positioned higher than the shoulders and shoulders above the torso.

- **Trunk**: Hypodermic injection can treat dependent areas (shoulders, buttocks, sides). Aspiration reduces fluid within serous cavities.
- **Ascites**: This causes secondary dilution for cavity fluid rather than arterial fluid; reduce with aspiration.
- **Hydrothorax**: Aspiration reduces fluid.
- **Hydrocephalus**: Post arterial injection, insert a hypodermic needle into the nose and through the cribriform plate to drain. Injecting cavity fluid increases preservation.
- **Hydrocele**: Create drainage channels with the trocar by passing over the pubic symphysis into the scrotum, retract the trocar, and use manual pressure to push fluid into the pelvic cavity. Cavity fluid can be injected this way. Avoid rupturing the scrotum.
- **Legs**: Raise femorals to inject arterial solution; use the trocar to create a channel from the cavity to the thighs, then elevate the legs at the ankles. Gravity will pull fluid down into the cavity. Hypodermically treat as needed.
- **Arms**: Inject separately and elevate the hands to reduce fluid.

Special Circumstances

Standards for Embalming in Anticipation of a Delayed Viewing

In cases where viewing or disposition will be delayed, embalming involves a different choice of fluids, and the body must be stored properly.

Injection: High-index and 2–3% concentration with water conditioners, anticoagulants, mold inhibitors, humectants, and water should be injected into the body through a 6-point injection, when possible, to achieve the best distribution.

Storage:

- Keep the body positioned on blocks to allow airflow.
- Use massage cream on the face and hands.
- Cover the body with a sheet or gown but leave face uncovered.
- Spray body with wetting agent containing humectants and mold inhibitors.
- Place in cool area.
- Reaspirate as needed and treat problem areas as they occur.

An embalmed body may be kept refrigerated, where allowed by law, for several weeks. However, there may be a legal limit on the length of time that a body may be stored without state or local governmental permission. The limit and procedures for obtaining an extension vary by jurisdiction.

Embalming Considerations for Disaster Cases

Disasters resulting in mass casualties pose several challenges to death care professionals, and normal procedures may not be possible.

- **Disaster Mortuary Operational Response Teams (DMORT)** provide local support, resources, and structure to death care professionals in the event of disasters to efficiently identify and process remains to return to families.
- Bodies should be prepared per the direction of the next of kin. Embalming preparation standards are case-specific with considerations for cause of death, trauma, decomposition, and environmental factors (water, cold, heat, and animal activity, including flies or maggots) while factoring in the potential for delayed viewings if remains are potentially viewable.
- If the body is able to be preserved, restoration efforts can be attempted.

Priorities of a Response to a Mass Fatality Involving Radiation

In the unlikely event of a mass fatality involving radiation, such as detonation of a nuclear "dirty bomb," mortuary response teams must prioritize **radiation safety**. This includes minimizing both personal exposure to radiation and the spread of contamination through prudent handling of disposition. All personnel should be equipped with dosimeters and personal protective equipment (PPE) appropriate to the circumstance. Exposure should be limited to 50mSv or a lower limit determined by radiation protection professionals. Bodies should be removed from the **hot zone** of high radiation, decontaminated in a warm zone of moderate radiation, and finally moved to a field morgue in an uncontaminated area. Decontamination consists of removing the decedent's clothing and personal items and washing localized areas of contamination on the body. Autopsy, embalming, and disposition options depend on the level of contamination; radiation protection professionals should assist in making these determinations. If a decedent is highly radioactive (greater than 1 mSv/hr at 30 cm), autopsy, embalming, and public viewing are not recommended. These decedents should be buried in a sealed casket to delay the release of radioactive material into the environment; in some cases, a shielded casket is recommended.

Post-Embalming Analysis

Once the initial embalming (vascular, cavity, hypodermic, and surface embalming) is complete, there is a waiting period to allow the chemicals to work. Chemicals will further saturate tissue, ideally giving the body a firm, fixated feel. Some chemicals will further dehydrate tissues (edema treatments) while others prevent dehydration (humectants). Surface embalming treatments need time to penetrate and soak into the tissues to preserve, dehydrate, or cauterize. Once the body sets (at least 30 minutes; however, longer is better, so 12–24 hours is preferred), post-embalming care can begin. A **post-embalming analysis** evaluates the condition of the body and develops additional treatment plans. The body may need additional care to treat any areas of trauma, disfigurement, wounds, or holes from medical equipment. Tissue should be firm and dry.

Additional Treatments Prior to Dressing and Casketing the Decedent

Any tissue that is not firm and dry after embalming can be treated with cauterants, preservative gels, wraps and packs, preservation or absorptive powders, and plastic garments. The body should be **reaspirated** if there are signs of abdominal distention from fluid or gas buildup, if there is oral or nasal purge, or if the body is being transferred. Areas that begin to show signs of decomposition or tissue degradation should be treated immediately to prevent further deterioration. Chemical gels and powders can be applied to increase preservation. Features can be restored to a natural appearance with hypodermically injected feature builder, tissue reducer, and wax. Plastics are used on problem areas to reduce the risk of leakage. Powder can be added inside plastics to add in preservation and absorption. Additional preservation can be added with a hypodermic needle or with a topical application of gels and dehydrating chemicals. In cases of emaciation, with permission of the family, sunken features can be built up and filled in with either firming or normal feature builder. Reconstruction in cases of trauma can be further built up with wax to restore a normal appearance. Once the body conditions are treated, dressing, casketing, and cosmeticizing can begin. Once the decedent is in the casket, facial trauma reconstruction can be finalized.

Restorative Art

Physical Anthropology and Physiognomy

Physical anthropology is the study of humans as a biological species, with emphasis on evolutionary adaptations and modern variation. As early humans spread around the globe, local populations developed differences in physiology based on the local conditions, such as high altitudes, extreme temperatures, and available food sources. **Physiognomy** is the study of the structural configuration and exterior markings of the face and features. This craniofacial morphology varies by sex and race, with variations in skull shape, facial shape, and nasal index that cause differences in the slope of the eyes and shape of ears and lips. Physiognomy was once purported to be a science that "proved" inferiority of particular groups or could be used to identify criminals but today is merely descriptive of general trends in face shapes in various groups. A **norm** is a typical or standard appearance or condition.

Restorative Art

Restorative art is the application of either minor or major restoration techniques to reconstruct natural form and color on the decedent. Embalming is one type of restoration. Injection of the proper embalming chemicals can restore facial tissues, decrease facial swelling, remove postmortem intravascular discolorations, reduce extravascular blood discoloration, and restore natural facial coloration. **Joel Crandall** is considered the "father" of restorative arts. He developed techniques, special waxes, and cosmetics, and he educated morticians on restorative techniques. The major reason for restorative art is the psychological benefit to the family. **Minor restorations** require subtle alterations, modifications, or corrections. **Major restorations** are extensive procedures that require considerable time and technical skill. Written permission must be given before a major restoration.

Securing Permission from the Next of Kin to Perform Restorative Care

Embalming authorization by the next of kin includes authorization to perform **restorative care** because restoration and embalming coincide and overlap. For example, if a decedent does not have teeth or dentures available, a mouth former and cotton are used to build out and restore the natural form of the mouth. Oral permission for these can be given but should be followed by signed written authorizations. In the event of major restorations, specific permission can be notated on the original embalming authorization form, or a separate form can detail the agreement. A director should not promise, guarantee, or even allude to the possibility of a viewing for someone he or she has not seen. The extent of the trauma and condition of the body need to be evaluated prior to discussing options with the family. Caution the family that although every effort will be made to meet their wishes, it may not be feasible to accomplish a restoration that will provide them with a quality or therapeutic viewing experience.

Terms of Form

A **margin** is a borderline or edge. An **arch** is a curved structure. To **abut** is to adjoin, as in the line of eye closure. A **depression** is a concave region or the lowermost section of a part. **Distension** describes a condition in which the tissue expands or swells. A **taper** (feather) is a shape that gradually grows narrower toward one end. The **termination** is the tip or end of something. A **projection** is a part that sticks out beyond the level of other nearby parts. A **protrusion** is something that is forward or outward from its normal or typical position; the opposite is a **retrusion**. The term **radiate** refers to branching out from a central point. An **inversion** is the condition in which tissues curve in an opposite direction or fold inward.

The Cranium

The Occipital and Parietal Bones of the Cranium

The **cranium** is the portion of the skull that surrounds and protects the brain. The **occipital bone** curves under the cranium at its base and serves as the cradle for the brain. The **foramen magnum** is the opening in the occipital bone, halfway between the two mastoid processes, for the spinal cord. The **parietal bones** are the widest part of the cranium on the superior portion of the sides and back, and they cover two-thirds of the posterior roof of the cranium. The **parietal eminence** is superior and posterior to the ears and is convex in form.

The Temporal Region of the Cranium

The **temporal bone**, located on the sides and lower part of the cranium, consists of four bone segments: the tympanic, petrous, and mastoid below the temple and the squama temporalis, which forms the upper front part of the temporal bone. Together these four parts define the **temporal cavity**. This region contains the **temporalis muscles**, the powerful muscles for chewing. The **zygomatic arch** is the thin, arched process extending anteriorly from the lower part of the squama to the zygomatic bone. The **zygomatic bones** (cheekbones) are located inferior to the eye socket and represent the widest part of the cheek.

Frontal Surface Bones of the Cranium

The **mandibular fossa** (glenoid fossa) is the depression in the temporal bone that articulates with the mandible, forming the temporal mandibular joint (TMJ). The **mandible** is the lower jaw. The **mastoid process** is the curved protuberance of the interior portion of the temporal bone just medial to the earlobe. The **condyle** (jaw hinge) is a curved prominence at the end of the bone, creating the articulating posterior process of the mandible ramus. It is posterior to the **coronoid process**, which is the non-articulating process at the top front corner of the **ramus** (the perpendicular portion of the mandible where the temporalis muscle is inserted). The **submandibular** area refers to the portions inferior to the mandible.

Surface Bones of the Face

The **mental eminence** is the point of the chin on the inferior portion of the anterior mandible. The **maxilla** is the upper jaw that covers much of the superior face, including both sides of the nasal cavity and the roof and floor of the mouth. The **incisive fossa** is a naturally formed depression in the maxilla above the incisor teeth and below the nose; the same term also applies to the depression in the palate just behind the incisors. The **alveolar process** is located at the edge of the maxilla and mandible bones (which have tooth sockets). The **glabella** is a region of the frontal bone and the skin over it, located between the superciliary arches above the root of the nose.

Variations in Skull Shape and Form Based on Age and Gender

The **cranium** is composed of bones joined together by sutures. Proportionally, babies have a 1:8 facial-to-cranial proportion, while adults have a 1:2 proportion. Babies are born with fontanelles, spaces between the bones that allow for flexibility during birth and growth afterwards. The anterior fontanelle closes when the child is 7–19 months old. Throughout childhood, the sutures remain soft to allow for growth while protecting the brain. A second cranial growth spurt occurs around puberty, after which cranial sutures ossify. With age, cranial alterations include changes in jaw size, shape, and length from dental alterations. Facial musculature and integument changes are also notable.

Skull standards dictate an oval shape two-thirds as wide as it is long. In reality, skulls vary in shape, size, and dimension, allowing for individualization. Gender variations are noticeable after puberty; female skulls are smaller and thinner, while males have thicker skulls with more pronounced musculature and eminences, though the eminence of the forehead in some women is more accentuated.

Prominences and Cavities

There are several prominences in the facial region. The **frontal eminences** are outwardly curved prominences located on the frontal bone, superior to the supraorbital margin. The **frontal nasal prominence** forms the forehead region. The **nasal placodes** include the nostrils and form both medial and lateral prominences. Finally, there are the **medial and maxillary prominences**, which when fused together comprise the upper lip, and the **mandibular prominence** forming the lower lip and jaw. A **cavity** is a depression or recessed area forming a hollow region. The **buccal cavity** is the region between the inner cheeks, teeth, gums, and lips. **Buccal depressions** are the naturally formed facial depressions curving slightly inward below the cheekbone.

Facial Muscles Impacting Form and Expression

Facial muscles contribute to the form of the face. Their movements create expressions. As muscles flex and extend repeatedly over time, wrinkles, folds, depressions, and furrows are created.

- **Occipitofrontalis**: This muscle extends from the occipital bone to the eyebrows. When flexed, the scalp moves, raising and lowering the eyebrows, creating furrows along the forehead.
- **Procerus**: This muscle extends from the nasal bone's inferior margin up to the inferior forehead, joining the frontalis muscle. When contracted, the medial eyebrows lower, wrinkling skin horizontally over the nasal bridge.
- **Corrugator**: A triangle-shaped muscle originating at the nasal root, it extends laterally towards the center supraorbital margin. When contracted, the medial eyebrow lowers, producing vertical wrinkles.
- **Buccinator**: The primary muscle of the cheek and lateral mouth wall, this muscle moves the cheek and creates the bucco-facial sulcus.
- **Risorius**: This superficial muscle runs along the cheek from the mouth, atop the masseter muscle; it pulls the mouth and creates a smile.
- **Triangularis/depressor anguli oris**: This muscle extends from the chin up to the superior corner of the mouth, and it contracts, pulling the mouth down, and creates the angulus oris eminence.
- **Quadratus/depressor labii inferioris**: Extending from the chin up to the bottom of the lip, this muscle contracts to pull the lip down and toward its respective side.

Restoration of the Skin

Dermis (derma, corium) is the dense skin layer below the epidermis. **Epidermis** is the external layer of skin surrounding the dermis. Preservative treatments for desquamation include a hypodermic injection and application of a cavity pack to seal the skin back into place. **Hypodermis** is the tissue at the lowermost point of the integumentary system, deep underneath the outer skin; it was formerly called the subcutaneous layer. **Excision** is the process of reducing or eliminating tissue by surgical cutting. For example, wrinkled eyelids are treated by excising the wrinkled eyelid, creating a wax replacement, and applying cosmetics. **Surgical reduction** is the process of removing distended or swollen tissues. An **undercut** is a form of excision made at an angle on the excised borders to allow skin to extend beyond the deeper tissues. A **laceration** is torn tissue, similar to a cut but with jagged edges. An **abrasion** is a skin surface condition characterized by losing a portion of the epidermis due to friction, such as a **razor burn**. An embalmer should treat a moist abrasion by covering the area with a compress of undiluted cavity fluid or autopsy gel.

Facial Markings

The four primary factors influencing facial markings are age, environment, position of the body, and condition of the body. **Grooves** are long creases or lines within an otherwise flat, smooth surface. **Furrows**, also called wrinkles, are creases. **Folds** are extended depressions. These are all created over time from repetitive facial movements and expressions. These terms are often used interchangeably. A **sulcus** (plural: sulci) is a profound, thin furrow or groove with depth. A **fossa** is a depression or concavity. A **sunken** surface is an area that is depressed more than its surrounding area. A **line of closure** is the thin line or marginal slit at the point of contact of upper and lower mucous membranes, such as the eyes and lips.

Facial Markings Present at Birth

The **philtrum** is a groove that runs straight up the middle of the superior lip below the nose. The **nasolabial fold** is a natural eminence on the cheek adjacent to the mouth, running from the posterior margin of the nasal wing to the side of the mouth. The **nasal sulcus** is located at the angular region between the posterior margin of the wing of the nose and the nasolabial fold. The **oblique palpebral sulcus** is an elongated groove below the eye, bending from the inner canthus. The **angulus oris eminences** are the small, raised folds on the side of the mouth line of closure. The **angulus oris sulcus** is the straight, elongated depression at each corner of the mouth line of closure. The **labiomental sulcus** is a deep, narrow furrow between the lower integumentary lip and chin. The **submental sulcus** is a narrow furrow at the connection between the base of the chin and the submandibular area. **Dimples** are small and rounded or vertical superficial hollows on the chin or cheek.

Facial Markings Acquired by Age

People use certain muscles repeatedly (for squinting, etc.) throughout life, which create **acquired facial markings**. The **nasolabial sulcus** is the furrow located medial and adjacent to the nasolabial fold. The **transverse frontal sulci** are the horizontal furrows on the forehead. The **superior palpebral sulcus** is the long furrow of the upper eyelid's superior border. The **inferior palpebral sulcus** is a narrow groove attached to the lower border of the eyelid. The **interciliary sulci** are upright furrows between the eyes and eyebrows. The **optic facial sulci**, often called "crow's feet," are the narrow grooves extending from the corner of the eyes. These are typically the first facial markings to be acquired. The **bucco-facial sulcus** is a furrow characterized by two curved lines of different lengths, extending downward toward the line of mouth closure. The **mandibular sulcus** is a narrow groove rising from below the jawline to the nasolabial fold. **Platysmal sulci** are the shallow or deep crevices in the neck, ending below the ears. The **cords of the neck** are ridges formed by sagging muscle tissues. The **labial sulci** are narrow grooves originating from the upper and lower integumentary lip, called "the furrows of age."

Facial Proportions

Several values are used to measure facial proportions. The **angle of projection** refers to the degree from vertical at which the plane(s) of the feature of interest extends outward. These include imaginary **horizontal lines** to establish alignment and proportion. One such line aligns the eyebrow and the top of the ear on the same horizontal plane. Another horizontal line can be imagined from the vertex of the cranium to the line of eye closure—this is half the length of the head. Several **vertical lines** also serve to provide references for facial proportions. A vertical line extended from the medial end of each eye to the wing of the nose can be useful, as can a vertical extension from the middle of each eye to the corners of the mouth.

Classic Proportions of Facial Length

The face (and photographs of the face) can be visually dissected vertically into equal sections to help restore features accurately. When measuring length from the top of the head to the bottom of the chin, the eyes are central. **Facial length** can be divided into three equal sections between the hairline and chin:

- The natural hairline on the forehead to the superior margin of the eyebrows.
- The superior margin of the eyebrows to the inferior base of the nose. This measurement equals the ear's length because the superior margin of the ear is at the same level of the eyebrows and the inferior margin of the ear is at the same level as the base of the nose. It also equals the distance between the lateral margin of the eye and the ear's tragus.
- The inferior base of the nose to the inferior margin of the chin. This section can be divided into three equal subsections:
    - Base of the nose to the natural lip line
    - Natural lip line to the superior margin of the chin
    - Superior margin of the chin to the inferior margin of the chin

Facial Widths in Relation to the Width of the Eye

Facial width, ear to ear, is visually dissected using the width of an eye as the standard of measurement. The following are measured in relation to the eyes as:

- Face: 5 eyes wide
- Between the eyes: 1 eye wide
- Nose: 1 eye wide at the base
- Mouth: 2 eyes wide

Other useful facial proportion guides that can aid restorations include:

- A visual line straight down from the **inner canthus**, (the medial corner of the eye) intersects with the lateral margin of the wing of the nose. An instrument can be held vertically at the canthus and touch the lateral edge of the wing.
- A visual line from the center of the eye, extending down, intersects with the lateral corner of the mouth.
- Commonly, the following distances are equal (excluding obese or emaciated cases):
    - Left tragus to right tragus
    - Superior, medial margin of the eyebrow to the chin
    - Nasal tip to either tragus
- The ear is two eyes long.
- The face is three ears long.

Importance of Photographs

Photographs are invaluable when it comes to preparing a decedent for their viewing. They show facial characteristics and traits unique to each person rather than strictly following the **canon of beauty**, proportional aesthetic standards. Useful photographs are recent and relevant; a high school graduation photograph isn't an ideal resource for someone in their eighties. The photographs can be professional or snapshots. Professional photos are more consistent, with good lighting and standard angles, while snapshots may provide information about the decedent's everyday appearance and show details such as freckles or scars that may have been edited out of professional photos. Snapshots are also more likely to be recent. Evaluate the quality of lighting in the photograph along with any alterations that could affect the person's natural characteristics and skin tone. If the photographs are from a major life event, the person may be wearing their hair and cosmetics differently from their everyday style. Review pictures with the family prior to use, discussing hair (style, cut, and coloring) and cosmetics, to avoid confusion on viewing expectations.

Three-Quarter, Profile, and Frontal View Photographs

For extensive restoration, multiple photographs taken from various angles allow for a more accurate reconstruction. **Profile views** (side shots) show projections and depressions; **frontal views,** straight-on shots, show direct facial characteristics; **three-quarter views**, with the head turned at a 45° angle, depicts the proportions of the cheeks. **Highlights** are the portions of a surface that are located at right angles to the source of light and appear brighter because of the reflection. A **shadow** is a poorly lit region that appears darker than nearby regions because of blocked light. **Inverting** the photograph allows the eye to pick up on previously unnoticed aspects of the face and the person's unique asymmetry.

Facial Profiles

There are three basic forms of a facial profile. The **vertical** form is when the forehead, base of the nose, and chin all protrude the same distance from the face. A string held in front of someone with a vertical profile would hang straight down, touching these three points without bending or curving. In the **concave** form, the nose is recessed while the chin and forehead protrude, creating an inward curve. This facial profile is sometimes referred to as infantine or childlike in appearance, and it is the least common of the three basic types. The **convex** form is an arched shape similar to a segment of a sphere. The convex facial profile is the most common facial profile.

Facial Profile Combination Types

Facial profiles are often more complicated than the three basic types. A **convex-concave** profile has an outward curve at the chin that protrudes beyond the upper lip while the forehead recedes from the eyebrows. A **concave-convex** profile is characterized by a forehead that protrudes past the eyebrows and a receding chin. In a **vertical-convex** profile, the forehead is on a vertical plane but the chin recedes. In a **vertical-concave** profile, the forehead is on a vertical plane and the chin protrudes. In a **convex-vertical** profile, the forehead protrudes farther than the eyebrows, and the upper lip and chin evenly extend to an imaginary vertical line. In a **concave-vertical** profile, the forehead protrudes and the chin is on a vertical plane. In a **concave-nasal** profile, the forehead and chin protrude while the nose is *retroussé* (turned up).

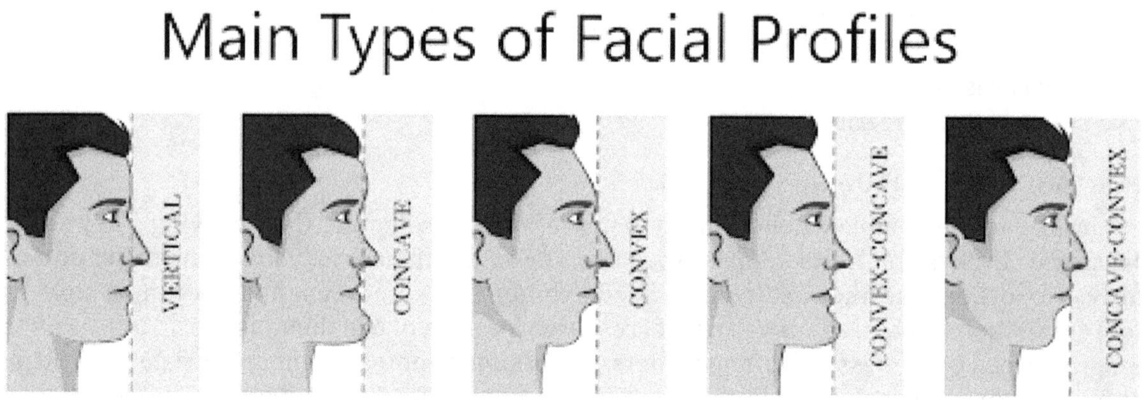

HEAD FORMS (FRONTAL VIEW)

Oval is the most common head shape form and is characterized by generally rounded curves and cheekbones that are wider than the skull, giving an egg-shaped appearance. **Round** (infantine) is a shorter head shape with full, rounded cheeks and skull and a full jawline. A **square** (strong) head shape has straighter edges, with the forehead, cheek, and jawline similar in width. A **triangular** head shape is characterized by a wider jawline and narrower forehead, with the eyes close together. An **inverted triangular** head shape is characterized by a wider forehead and cheekbone and narrow jawline. A **diamond** head shape has wide cheekbones and a narrower forehead and jawline. **Oblong** is a narrow, elongated head form with a round or square chin and (often) a longer nose.

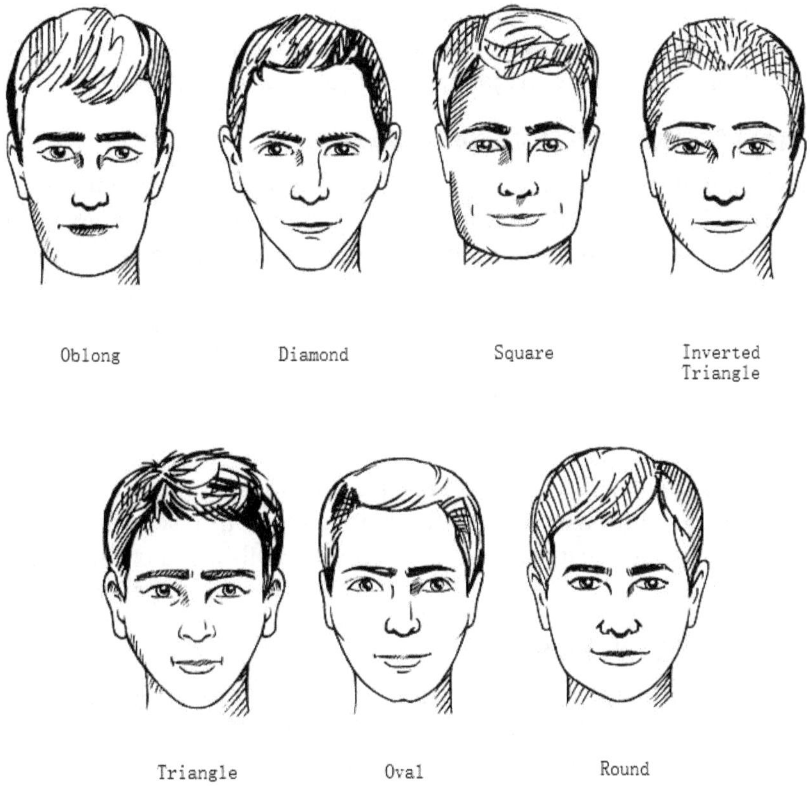

BILATERAL FORMS OF HEAD AND FEATURES

The term **bilateral** refers to something that has two sides, often symmetrical or similar. In the case of the human head, the key is the prominence of the cheekbones and the distance between them. As the embalmer looks at the face, all structures and features can be seen to radiate from the arch of the cheekbone. An **arch** is a rounded, half-circle form. The **superciliary arch** is the outline of the curved bone ridge where the eyebrow (supercilium) originates. The cheekbone serves to separate the front plane of the face, below and above the eye, from the side of the face. **Asymmetrical** features are similar but lack identical proportions. In the human face, ears exhibit the greatest amount of asymmetry, but the eyelids, eyebrows, cheeks, nose, and mouth can also be asymmetrical.

Bilateral Curvatures for Facial Features

Bilateral curvatures are facial features that have two sides. **Bilateral differences** are the variances between the two sides that create the natural asymmetry of the face. An individual's bilateral form can be examined by standing above the head and looking directly down the face. The inferior bilateral view provides another perspective from the opposite vantage: looking directly up at the face from a position directly inferior to the chin. These views show the projections, recessions, curvatures, margins, similarities, and asymmetries of the individual's unique facial features. Although the cheeks are the focal point of bilateral form, the forehead, eyes, nose, mouth, and chin all have important bilateral curvatures and characteristics.

These views can be used to ensure that features are set accurately and to monitor facial swelling during arterial injection. Photographs portray a person's unique characteristics and natural asymmetries. Features can be measured and mathematically scaled from the photographs to recreate the features on the decedent. Wax can be used to rebuild damaged areas while using intact features to guide the scale, placement, projection, and curvature of waxed features.

Types of Wax and Methods of Coloring Wax

Restorative wax is available in different colors and consistencies. Consistency is selected based on the type and depth of restoration while factoring in environmental influences (temperatures and humidity). Soft wax known as **surface restorer** is used for minor imperfections (such as superficial abrasions, razor burn, or sutures) that require a thin application of wax to restore the skin's surface. Medium-density **restorative** or **derma-surgery wax** is a thicker, slightly firmer wax used for either surface or shallow restorations. Firm **wound filler** is a hard, dense, clay-like wax recommended for large restorations. A **filler** is a mix of plaster of paris, cotton, and liquid sealer that is used to fill a large cavity.

Translucent wax is available in a few color tints. **Opaque wax** has starch and color additives, which decrease adhesion. Cream-based cosmetics can be mixed into wax prior to use. Wax can be applied over cosmetics for minor restorations, or cosmetics (oil-based creams, sprays, and liquids) can be applied afterwards.

Basic Wax Modeling Techniques

Modeling is the technique of shaping wax to create a more natural appearance. Surfaces must be firm and dry before applying wax. Wax can be heated with body heat to increase malleability or heated with a hair dryer to soften. Instruments can be heated rather than heating the wax. To prevent the wax from peeling when smoothing and finishing the area, apply light pressure with fingers or a brush slightly dampened with water or massage cream. **Stipple** with a brush, gauze, or paper towel to create pores.

Techniques Used to Create Facial Furrows, Grooves, and Folds

A variety of techniques can be used to recreate facial markings like furrows, grooves, and folds using wax and tools. Wrinkles and grooves can be made by pressing a blunt instrument into the wax and drawing it along the surface of the wax to create a crease. A piece of damp ligature can also be pressed into the wax to create a thin indented line. Once the depth is created, the edges should be softened to make them look more natural. To create a deeper furrow, rather than indenting the wax further, a strip of wax can be placed on both sides of the crease to create the necessary depth. These strips of wax can be feathered and smoothed to create a natural-looking furrow. Gentle stippling can add a natural pore-like texture to the skin. Cosmetics can be applied to the wax or sprayed on after these characteristics are created, or the wax can be tinted with cosmetics prior to its application.

Structures of the Outer Ear (Pinna)

The ear consists of three parts, all of which are associated with hearing: the external ear (pinna), middle ear, and inner ear. The **pinna**, as the visible portion of the ear, is of most interest in restoration. The **helix** is the pinna's outer boundary, rising from the lobe and curving forward and inward to the cheek. The **external auditory meatus** is the opening to the ear canal, serving as an anatomical guide to correctly position the ear. The **tragus** is a piece of cartilage that arises from the posterior margin of the lateral cheek and protects the external auditory meatus. The **concha** is a shell-shaped depression next to the external auditory meatus. The **crus** is the lowermost portion of the helix, above the tragus, in the flat region of the concha. The **lobe** or lobule is the lowermost portion of the ear, hanging freely from the **antitragus**. The **crura of the antihelix** are the portions of the antihelix that divide outward into an upper and lower region. The **crus of the helix** is the flat portion of the concha, just above the tragus, where the helix begins.

Nose Classifications and Profile Descriptions

A **leptorrhine** nose is characterized by an elongated, slender shape and a high bridge typical of people of Western European descent. A **mesorrhine** nose is characterized by a medium-wide shape and a medium to low bridge typical of Asian descent. A **platyrrhine** nose is characterized by a short, wide shape and a flattened bridge typical of African descent. A **straight nasal profile** (Grecian) is the most common nasal profile, characterized by a straight dorsum from top to bottom. A **convex nasal profile** (Roman) has a characteristic hump on the bridge just below the root; this is also called an aquiline profile. A **concave nasal profile** (infantine) has a characteristic dip in the bridge and is turned upward at the end, which can give it a childlike appearance, as if it has too much adipose tissue. A ***retroussé*** nose is one that bends upward at the tip.

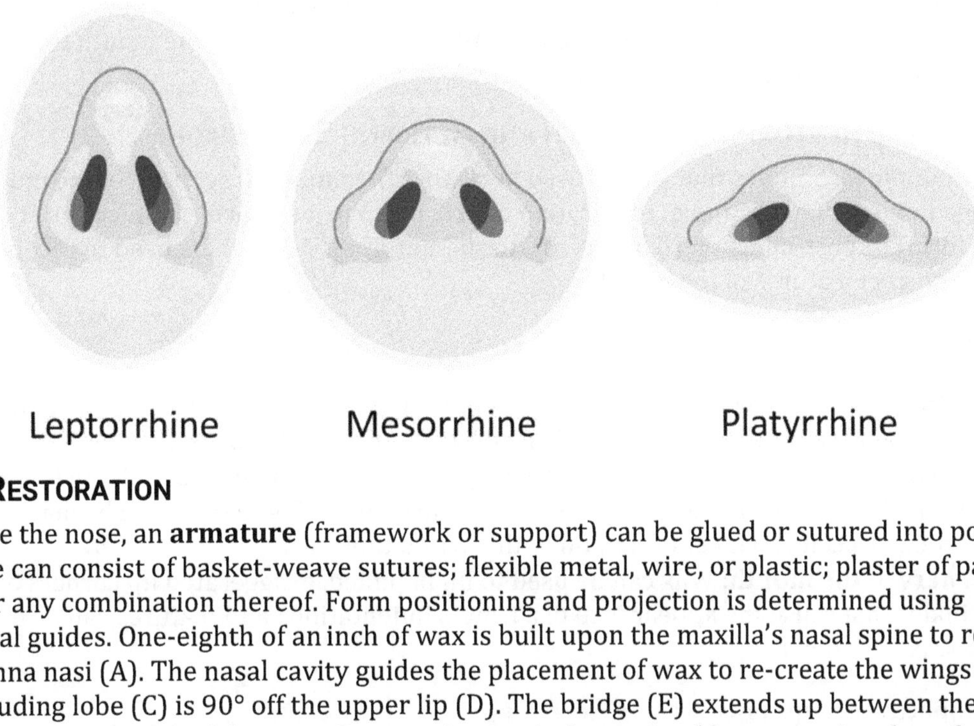

Nasal Restoration

To restore the nose, an **armature** (framework or support) can be glued or sutured into position. Armature can consist of basket-weave sutures; flexible metal, wire, or plastic; plaster of paris; cotton; or any combination thereof. Form positioning and projection is determined using anatomical guides. One-eighth of an inch of wax is built upon the maxilla's nasal spine to recreate the columna nasi (A). The nasal cavity guides the placement of wax to re-create the wings (B), and the protruding lobe (C) is 90° off the upper lip (D). The bridge (E) extends up between the eyebrows to the root (F) of the nose. Root projection is determined by comparing that of the glabella (G), upper lip, or posterior border of the nasal wings. The tip (H) is added in proportion to the protruding lobe. The dorsum (I) incline is created, adding concave or convex features, ensuring that wax extends into the cheeks to fill the nose out. Using the bilateral aspect (inferior or superior vantage) and profile, the wings are created and shaped to meet the face, upper lip, and protruding lobe. The arch of the wing (J) is shaped, and the anterior nares (nostrils; K) are formed. Final details are etched in, and all viewpoints are scrutinized to ensure accuracy.

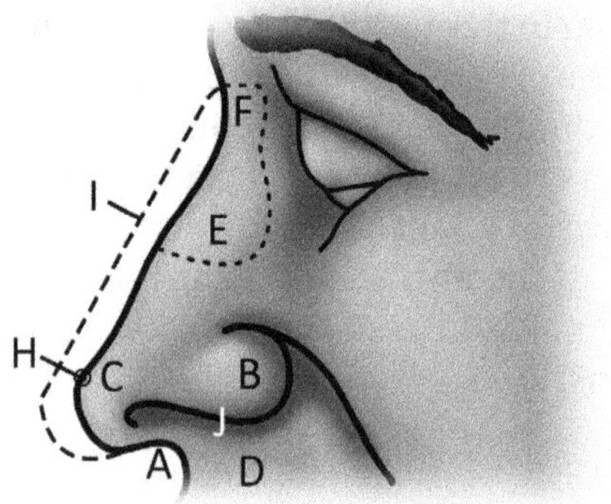

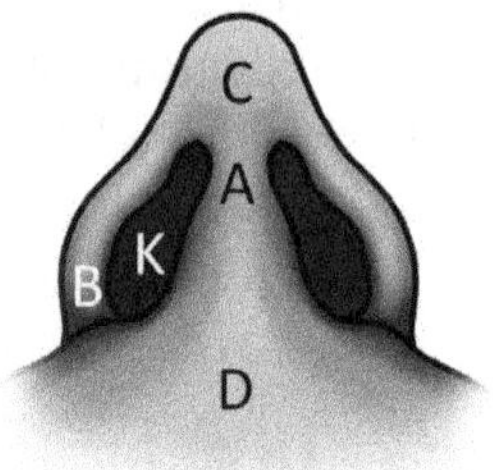

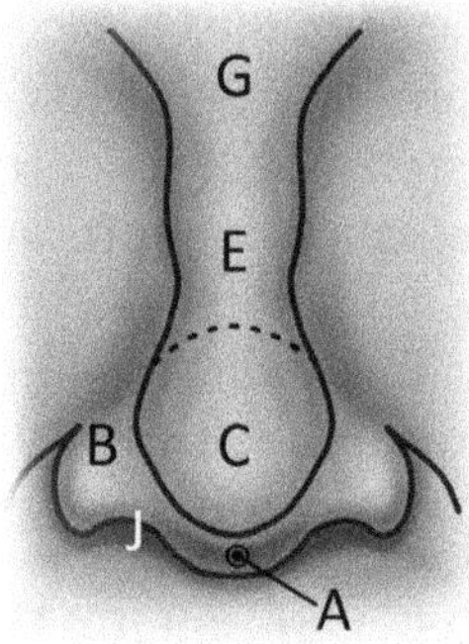

Restorative Art Features of the Mouth

The **integumentary lips** (upper and lower) consist of an upper (superior) portion, which is attached to the upper mucous membrane at the base of the nose, and a lower (inferior) portion, which is attached to the lower mucous membrane at the labiomental sulcus. The **weather lines of the lip** are the distinct separation between the dry and wet portion of the lips. The **medial lobe** is the small, raised portion of the upper lip. The **angulus oris eminence** is the ridgeline that moves from the medial lobe to the corners of the mouth. The **frenulum** is a tissue fold on the interior of the mouth between the lips and the gums. The **mandibular suture** closes the mouth from the inside of the lips, septum, and mandible. The **musculature suture** closes the mouth from the inside of the lips, septum, and muscles of the lower jaw.

Techniques for Restoring the Mouth and Altering Expression

There are multiple techniques that can be used to restore the mouth. If sections of the mouth or teeth are incomplete due to trauma, restoration efforts begin prior to arterial injection (restore shape and form) or post-injection (fixation, dry tissue, sutures). Wax can be used to reconstruct the mouth or to correct features of the mouth.

Corrections include:

- **Lip line**: The mouth closure and lip line can be adjusted by filling the existing one with wax. Create a new groove and round the lips back into a natural shape.
- **Lip projection**: Increase the projection of the lip by adding wax and molding it with tools to meet the line of closure and reinstate natural curvatures. Reductions can be made by scraping or peeling a layer of wax off with a wired tool.
- **Corners of the mouth**: Wax can be used to fill in pulled, exaggerated lip corners or wrinkles that cause the appearance of a frown. Indentations and features can be etched into the wax with tools.

Cosmetic application steps are:

1. Apply natural lip color or selected lip color to lips or wax.
2. Feather out to apply natural shading.
3. Use tools to maintain natural features and the lip line.
4. Set with finishing powder.

Prognathism

Prognathism occurs when the mandible and/or maxilla extend beyond the typical symmetrical region, creating an improper alignment. There are various restorative arts techniques to address this, some of which require obtaining written permission from the family, such as extracting the teeth or realigning them if the family wants them to show. **Maxillary prognathism** occurs when the superior jaw (maxilla) protrudes. **Mandibular prognathism** occurs when the inferior jaw (mandible) protrudes. **Dental prognathism** occurs when the teeth are inserted at an angle or protrude. **Alveolar prognathism** occurs when tooth sockets are inclined or protrude. The most common procedures involve using wet cotton slings, mastic compounds, and suturing or gluing the lips before waxing. Other techniques include the use of a **mouth former**, which typically creates a more symmetrical mouth.

Anatomical Features of the Eye

The **orbit** (eye socket or orbital cavity) is the bone cavity in which the eye is located. The **supraorbital area** connects the supercilium and the superior palpebrae. **Eyelids** (palpebrae) are folds of skin that open and close to protect the eyeball from foreign material and to keep it moist. The **inner canthus** is the elevated region located at both inner edges of the closed eye. The **levator palpebrae superioris** is the facial muscle that opens the upper eyelid. **Cilia** (eyelashes) are the small hairs on the terminal point of the eyelids. **Supercilia** (eyebrows) are the hairs covering the superciliary arches. These are on the same transverse plane as the superior border of the ear. **Orbicularis oculi muscles** are responsible for closing the palpebrae, creating their line of closure. Closing this muscle compresses the **lacrimal gland**, which produces tears. **Occipitofrontalis muscles** are located on each side of the upper cranium. These muscles pull the forehead and eyebrows upward.

Significant Details of the Closed Eye

Compared to an open eye, the closed eye is slightly wider and lower laterally; the inner canthus is oval; and skin is smooth across the upper eyelid.

Eye profile features include:

- **Profile view**: The nose acts as a backdrop for the profile view of the eye. Proportions and curvatures between the supraorbital area (between the eyebrow and upper lid), superior and inferior palpebrae (upper and lower eyelid), and cheek can be compared with each other and the nose during restorations.
- **Supercilium**: This term refers to the eyebrow.
- **Supraorbital area**: The upper eyelid protrusion and its distance from the eyebrow affect the curvature of the supraorbital area.
- **Line of closure**: This arcs upwards laterally.
- **Superior and inferior palpebral sulci**: The superior palpebral sulci refers to the groove between the upper eyelid and supraorbital area, and the inferior refers to the groove below the lower eyelid and orbital pouch.
- **Line of closure**: This begins medially at the inner canthus and arcs to the outer canthus. The lateral side may be equal to or inferior to the medial side. Medial projection is greater than lateral projection. The line of closure is located two-thirds down the orbital cavity, while the lower eyelid makes up the inferior third.

The bilateral view shows the supercilium, inferior orbital margin, and line of closure.

Conditions of the Eye That Require Restoration

- **Sunken** or **enucleated eyes** can be built up by inserting cotton under the eyelids to restore shape and projection. Massage cream can protect against dehydration. After embalming, feature builder can be injected to increase protrusion.
- **Dehydration** causes separation between the upper and lower eyelid. Some cases can be restored simply by stretching and gluing the eye. Wax can be used to fill gaps along the line of closure or to restore the inner canthus to a natural depth. With extreme cases of dehydration, wax can be used within the ocular orbit to restore the entire shape and form of the eye.
- **Protrusions** can be reduced with external pressure (manual or water weights) during the embalming process or immediately after. In extreme or traumatic cases, incisions can be made to drain fluid, excise fat and tissue, or even remove the eye to reduce the form and rebuild natural contours.
- **Swollen orbital cavities** can be reduced with external pressure or by excision.
- **Ecchymoses** or **hematomas** within the orbital space may need to be treated with preservative fluids, bleaching agents, and reduction techniques.

Hair Restoration and Fingernail Preparation and Treatments

Decedents with natural or medically induced hair loss may wear wigs, toupees, scarves, wraps, or hats. Sudden hair loss (e.g., from a medical procedure, injury, or accident) requires restoration using synthetic hair or hair from the decedent's body.

- **Restoring facial or head hair**: Apply a layer of glue, wax, or rubber cement to the skin's surface. Starting at the inferior margin, push and roll the ends of the procured hair into the adhesive in layers. Cut and style the hair. Using an eyebrow pencil can make hair appear thicker.
- **Eyelashes**: Fake eyelashes can be trimmed and inserted under the upper eyelid to replace missing eyelashes. Alternatively, procure hair and insert it into wax to recreate lashes. Tape can also be used to create a lash set to insert under the upper eyelid. Lashes overlap and should be grafted using increments of overlapping hairs.
- **Eyebrows**: Hair is grafted into wax, angled upward and out from the inferior margin. An eyebrow pencil can be used to thicken or give the appearance of hair to the eyebrows.

Nail treatment involves the following steps:

1. Clean under fingernails.
2. Remove nail polish during or after the embalming process. Some embalmers obtain the family's permission first.
3. Cut and repaint fingernails as directed.

Cranial Restoration

Indiscernible cranial fractures may only be detected by nasal, oral, or ear leakage during injection. Visible **cranial restorations** begin by resetting fractures and normalizing facial features prior to arterial injection. Simple fractures are reset with exterior pressure and manual manipulations. Cranial autopsies are beneficial in facial and cranial trauma cases. Vascular disruptions from autopsies can reduce arterial pressure, which decreases some swelling risks. Interior access gives the embalmer the ability to internally restore fractures and features from within the cranium. After injection, the pieces can be glued or wired together to restore their shape and form. Sunken features or areas with missing bone and tissue can be filled internally with cotton or plaster of paris. Basket-weave sutures can be used to add support. Incisions are closed with sutures or glue depending on their depth and size. Visible areas should be sutured with an intradermal suture to reduce visibility. Hypodermic treatments, powders, hardening compounds, and cauterants are used as needed to ensure that tissues are preserved, firm, and dry in preparation for wax treatments. Non-visible areas can be glued with a liquid sealer, while visible areas are built up with plaster or wax. Hair restoration can be performed as needed.

PLANNING RESTORATIVE TREATMENTS

CATEGORIES OF CONDITIONS THAT REQUIRE RESTORATION

Classification of the case during the pre-embalming analysis establishes a treatment course to restore a natural appearance. In most cases, this involves restoring features (closing the eyes and mouth); addressing body conditions (such as edema, emaciation, and jaundice) with arterial chemicals and active arterial dyes; topically bleaching ecchymoses for later cosmetic application; and eliminating unwanted facial hair. The types of conditions necessitating restoration are:

- **Pathological**: disease (e.g., tumors, edema, jaundice, medication, or surgical procedures)
- **Trauma**: injuries resulting in death, immediate or prolonged (e.g., abrasions, lacerations, or fractures)
- **Postmortem**: autopsies, organ donation, or natural deterioration of the body (e.g., skin slip, gases, discoloration, compression/contact discolorations, indentations, and deformities)
- **Embalming**: caused by the process of embalming (e.g., swelling, dehydration, or discoloration)

Types of restorations include:

- **Non-wax**: Restoration is achieved without using wax. Cotton, mortuary mastics (putties), and tissue builder can restore deep or surface level features.
- **Wax**: Wax covers surface indentations, lacerations, and areas without skin to restore a lifelike appearance using smoothed, stippled, or contoured techniques.
- **Moist**: Areas that are wet, such as skin slip and open wounds, require post-injection treatment with chemical packs to dry the tissue.
- **Dry**: Internal tissue trauma, simple fractures, and missing hair are examples of dry conditions that need treatment with wax, glue, or cosmetics.

ORDER OF RESTORATION BEFORE ARTERIAL INJECTION

1. Sanitize the body and facial orifices. Remove medical devices that are near the face or in the way of the embalming processes.
2. Wash and rinse the body and hair with warm, soapy water to remove blood and foreign materials. Always wash with a sponge to avoid injury from compound fractures or foreign debris (such as glass, metals, needles, first aid equipment, or other sharps) that may be embedded in the body, caught in hair, or on the body's surface.
3. Position the body with bridges and blocks.
4. Shave and set features. Restore features as needed with eye caps, cotton, mastic compounds, and mouth formers. Stay creams can facilitate closures.
5. Suture lacerations and wounds with ligature or dental floss. Non-facial and non-cranial wounds can be sutured after arterial injection. Superficial and small lacerations can be glued rather than sutured. Preinjection sutures may need to be opened, drained, topically treated, and then re-sutured post injection.
6. Drain fluid pockets and remove lose skin and scabs.
7. Apply massage cream to the face and hands to prevent dehydration of intact tissues near areas of trauma.

8. Place weighted compresses on areas with swelling.
9. Bleaching compounds can be applied to hands and face prior to injection or after.

Order of Restoration Treatments During Arterial Injection

1. Arterial solutions should be prepared based on the condition of the body, using appropriate active dyes, arterial conditioners, and water treatment chemicals. For example, humectants can be used to treat emaciation; edema fluids for edema; and high indexes for traumatic injury, drowning, burn, or decomposition cases. Solution composition is altered based on how the injection progresses to ensure that adequate levels of preservation are established.
2. Inject arterial solution using selected arteries. Multiple injection sites may be needed to adequately distribute the solution throughout the body. Areas insufficiently reached with arterial injection can be hypodermically injected. Surface packs can be placed on tissue with open wounds or missing skin to begin dehydrating it.
3. While injecting arterial fluid, massaging helps distribute fluid, remove lividity, and push out coagulated materials. Raising and lowering the arms and legs allows gravity to help flush and flood tissue in the extremities.
4. Swelling of the eyes and neck can be reduced with weighted compresses. Cavity distension can be reduced during the aspiration process. Swelling within the neck can sometimes also be reduced during aspiration.
5. Reapplication of moisturizing massage creams throughout the embalming process and after injection prevents excessive dehydration of the face and hands.

Order of Restoration After Embalming

1. Following arterial injection and cavity treatment, the body needs to be given time to fixate and dry out, allowing compresses, cauterizing packs, bleaching agents, or hypodermically treated areas to soak into and treat tissues. Weighted compresses and gravity can reduce swelling over time.
2. Reaspirate as necessary.
3. Firm, dry tissue is needed for wax applications on the hands and face.
4. Glue sutures and dry areas of trauma.
5. Finalize setting the eyes and mouth, then glue them shut.
6. Use tissue builder to restore sunken features, smooth wrinkles, fill unnatural indentations, and rehydrate fingers. Use tissue-builder solvent to clean hypodermic needles and syringes.
7. Apply wraps, powders, and plastic garments as needed prior to dressing. Some embalmers choose to casket prior to beginning any significant restorations because moving the person can cause damage to previously applied wax and cosmetics.
8. Style hair.
9. Apply wax, cosmetics (e.g., tints, creams, sprays, and/or airbrush), and hair restorations (e.g., eyelashes, head hair, facial hair, and eyebrows). Recreate facial folds, wrinkles, and characteristics using wax and cosmetics for shadowing and proper pigmentations. Stippling re-creates natural pores. Cosmetics powders reduce shine, and cosmetic setting sprays can be used to protect against touch transfers.

Conditions Requiring Major Restorative Treatments

Decapitation

When the head is **severed** from the body, the trunk and head are embalmed separately. Fractures and lacerations are treated and sutured prior to arterial injection. Sutures may need to be redone after arterial injection to allow fluid to drain and to add powders. Post-injection, align and reattach the head to the body using wooden, plastic, or metal supports inserted into the foramen magnum and along the vertebrae; add additional supports within the deep tissues of the neck as needed.

Suture muscles together from the posterior neck, working toward the front in layers. Cotton soaked in plaster of paris can be wrapped around the sutured muscles. Splints provide additional support. Insert cotton to help restore the natural contours of the neck. Skin edges are treated and sutured, closing the severance. After the embalming restoration, additional surface treatment is performed as needed to preserve and curb leakage. Sutures are sealed with liquid sealer. The body is delicately dressed and casketed; wax and cosmetic restoration reconstruct the natural neck and facial structures and characteristics.

Severed extremities are treated similarly: they are injected separately and sutured back on. Gaping wounds left from missing extremities are treated and sutured closed post-injection.

Discolorations, Tumors, Fractures, and Lacerations

- **Discolorations**: During arterial injection, some intravascular discolorations and lividity can be removed as long as it has not settled into a postmortem stain. Most extravascular discolorations and ecchymoses cannot be removed; however, chemical bleaching agents can be used to help reduce the coloration boldness so less cosmetics may be needed to conceal the area and restore a natural coloration. Compresses applied topically provide a more uniform bleaching than hypodermic treatment does. Surface discolorations (e.g., blood, dirt, or betadine) can often be scrubbed off with soap; nonbroken skin discolorations (such as hematomas or postmortem staining) typically require a bleaching agent; and deep or superficial broken skin discolorations (e.g., desquamation/skin slip, abrasions, burns, or compound fractures) must be treated with drying chemicals and bleaching agents.
- **Tumors**: After arterial injection, tumors can be excised and the underlying tissue treated with preservative agents, cauterants, and bleaching chemicals as needed. Once the tissue dehydrates, restorative efforts (wax and cosmetics) can begin.
- **Fractures**: Internal fractures and compound fractures should be set prior to arterial injection. During arterial injection, the muscle around the fracture can fixate in a normal position.
- **Lacerations**: Visible lacerations should be preliminarily sutured prior to injection, while nonvisible ones can be sutured pre- or postinjection.

Treatment of Tissues

Hypodermic tissue building is a method of restoring tissue contour by injecting a liquid tissue builder into the tissue. It can be used anywhere that features need to be built out. The injection point is based on the area that needs treatment. For example, if the deceased has sunken tissues in the **supraorbital area**, the suggested injection point is between the supercilium and the superior palpebrae. Tissue building is often used at the line of closure for both ends of the mouth and at the points between the knuckles or on an abrasion.

Emaciation is a condition in which the tissue is thin and sunken due to loss of subcutaneous fatty tissue. Tissue builder is used to elevate these tissues to an ordinary height. A **scab** is a skin condition characterized by dried, crusted blood over a healing sore or wound that may also be oozing. A severely raised scab should be removed before embalming; petroleum jelly (Vaseline) is often applied first to soften it. **Desiccation** refers to the removal of water from tissues, typically by the use of chemical desiccators. **Searing** is the process of drying tissues by applying heat. A **cauterizing agent** is a chemical substance that sears tissue, shrinking and desiccating the tissue to dry it. The **electric spatula** is a temperature-controlled knife blade capable of extreme heat for searing tissue.

Sutures

Suturing is the process of stitching tissue together with surgical ligature. An **intradermal suture** (hidden suture) is a suturing method for closing incisions with the suture material hidden below the epidermis. A **bridge stitch** (simple interrupted suture) is a temporary piece of suture material that is used to properly align tissue and is later replaced with a permanent suture. A **worm suture** (inversion, draw stitch) does not enter the wound but instead extends down the edge of the tissue so the stitches are not raised and can be concealed in wax. A **basket-weave suture** (cross stitch) is a secure suturing method that crosses the edges of tissue tightly, holding them in position. This method is used for deep wounds or for closing cavities. A **baseball stitch** is a continuous line of stitches made from side to side across the incision, always from underneath, with a knot at each end of the row. A **whip stitch** (simple continuous) is similarly a running line of sutures across the incision with a knot at each end but consists of simple loops rather than the zigzag of the baseball stitch. A **purse-string suture** is a method of stitching around an incision and pulling it closed by tightening the suture.

Additional Products Used in Restoration

Hard restorative art wax may be softened by heat, petroleum jelly, or a **cream cosmetic**, which is a semi-solid product. **Massage cream** is an oily, soft material most often used to prevent dehydration, chemical burn, or razor burn. Applied to the face and hands, it can help to tack eyes or mouths closed. This is typically removed prior to cosmeticizing because otherwise the skin surface may be too oily for cosmetics to adhere evenly and naturally.

An **emollient** is a moisturizing agent that softens skin tissue. **Cake** is a cosmetic made of compressed powder used to even skin complexion. **Lanolin** is an oily, animal-based humectant applied topically to make and keep skin soft and supple.

Color and Pigmentation

Color is the brain's interpretation of light as it reflects off an object in various wavelengths. Color **conversion** is the color-changing phenomenon that occurs when one color overtakes another, resulting in a new and different color. **Overtone** is the colorant effect achieved by the addition of an overlying color to dominate the overall effect and create a more general coloring. A color's **undertone** is its underlying color that determines its "temperature," typically warm (red, orange, or yellow) or cool (green, blue, or purple). An **opaque** object is one that does not allow light to pass through it. In art restoration, this is achieved by using a liquid or cream cosmetic to conceal underlying discoloration. A **translucent** object allows light to pass through but with diffusion, so clear visibility and perception of dissimilar objects are hampered by a slightly cloudy appearance. A **transparent** object allows light to pass through clearly so that the objects behind it are clearly distinguishable. A **colored light** is a bulb illuminating a particular hue. A **colored filter** is a piece of material applied over a white light to transmit the light of certain wavelengths while absorbing others.

Color and Hue Terminology

A **hue** is a property that describes the color of an object and represents a variation in wavelength of the primary colors. A **cool hue** is a variation of blue, green, or purple, characterized by short wavelengths that create the illusion that an object is farther away. A **warm hue** is a variation of red, orange, yellow, and other colors with longer wavelengths, creating the illusion that an object is closer. The **color wheel** is a circle in which all the hues are arranged in orderly intervals. **Complements** are hues that are directly opposite one another on the color wheel. Mixing two complements in equal quantities will produce gray. **Chroma (intensity)** is the brightness or dullness of a hue. **Value** refers to the visible lightness or darkness of a particular hue. A **tint** is a variation of a hue achieved by mixing it with white. A **subdued** hue is dulled or muted. **Color harmony** describes an aesthetically pleasing combination of colors.

COLOR THEORY

Color theory, or pigment theory, is the science of how to coordinate, mix, and blend colors to achieve a specific aesthetic. Understanding color theory aids in cosmetic selection for matching skin tone, covering imperfections, and restoring the natural, lifelike aesthetics of the decedent. In the Prang system, colors are separated into **primary colors** (red, yellow, and blue); **secondary colors** (orange, green, and violet), which are two primary colors combined; and **tertiary colors** (indigo, red-violet, vermilion, amber, chartreuse, and aqua), which are one primary and one secondary color combined. Color wheels show the relationships among these three categories. Colors next to each other blend into one another, while colors opposite are complementary. Complementary colors act as concealers. Green conceals unwanted red patches and imperfections. Orange conceals bruising. Purple conceals yellows or jaundice.

Neutral colors are black, white, and gray. Tints have white mixed in, shades have black mixed in, and tones have gray mixed in. Mixing and blending neutrals with other colors alters the color intensity (bright or dull) and value (lightness or darkness). The application of lighter and darker cosmetics can be used to construct depth and accentuate, highlight, contrast, or conceal features.

COSMETOLOGY

Cosmetology is the study of the various techniques and products for improving or changing the appearance of skin, hair, and nails. A **cosmetologist** is a professional trained in the application of the cosmetic material called **makeup** and the styling of hair. A **cosmetic** is a manufactured product that can create an altered appearance. A **cosmetic compound** is a mixture of pigments in a product that can be applied to a surface. A **cosmetic base** is the foundation that is applied to the skin before another product is applied on top of it. A **colorant** is a dye, pigment, or cosmetic substance that adds color to an object. **Corrective shaping** is a method of cosmetic application that uses highlighting on certain facial features to make them appear larger or smaller by use of shadowing.

SKIN COSMETIC TREATMENT

The **pores** of the skin are very small orifices for sweat glands. **Complexion** describes the overall appearance of the skin tissue, particularly its surface quality and color. A darker complexion is due to more melanin being present in the skin tissue. **Powder** is a finely crushed substance in a variety of colors, capable of being distributed across a surface to cover blemishes or adjust skin tone. A **powder puff** is a pad used to apply powder to the skin. A **powder brush** is a small brush used to apply and distribute powder. A **powder atomizer** utilizes forced air to distribute powder. An **eyebrow pencil** colors the brow hairs and can create the effect of an eyebrow if hair is missing. **Eye shadow** is a powder, cream, or liquid colorant used to shade the upper eyelid.

TYPES OF MORTUARY COSMETICS

Cosmetics can be selected based on the decedent's natural appearance as seen in photographs, along with their postmortem and post-embalming surface imperfections.

- **Tints**: Transparent liquids and tinted massage cream deposit faint and translucent coloration to the skin, restoring a lifelike hue.
- **Semi-opaque emollient cream**: This is similar to tinted massage cream but covers grayed-out skin or minor imperfections discreetly.

- **Opaque cream cosmetics**: Oil-based cosmetics, with soft or firm consistency, can be applied to cover discolorations. Stippled lightly into the pores, these creams can create a natural looking undertone.
- **Liquid opaque cosmetics**: Often resin-based, these are applied using brushes, fingers, aerosol cans, or airbrushes.
- **Additional cosmetics**: Other cosmetics include lip color, lip liner, rouge, eye shadow, eye liner, mascara, eyebrow pencil, and nail polish.

Cosmetic remover, mortuary solvent, or dry wash can be used to clean cosmetics out of hair using a comb and toothbrush or cotton swab. Cream cosmetics that are the same color as the hair, thinned with mortuary solvents, can be brushed onto affected hair to restore the natural color. Cosmetics can be applied to unembalmed decedents using the same cosmetics and similar techniques as embalmed people. Cosmetic sponges work well to apply, absorb excess, and blend cosmetics on unfirm skin surfaces.

Mortuary Cosmetic Application

Cosmetics can be applied with numerous tools, including brushes of varying function, size, length, and stiffness; sponges; applicators; and by hand.

- Apply liquid or cream tints to the skin to distribute an even, tinted undertone.
- Smooth skin variances and cover blemishes with a base cosmetic. Mixing hues aids matching.
- Use warm color (pinks, reds, deeper tones) highlights above the eyebrows, down the bridge of the nose, and along the cheeks, earlobes, and chin.
- Apply cosmetics to the eyes for a natural appearance or following the person's cosmetic preferences.
- Natural lip color is typically the same color as the cheeks (warm coloration) and applied thicker using vertical brush strokes. The mouth can be shaped wider with cosmetics or narrowed using wax. Blend lip color and base cosmetic along the exterior margins of the upper and lower lips.
- Apply a brown toner to smooth out and blend cosmetic variations (warm coloration deposits and lip margins) to emulate a natural appearance.
- Finishing powders, which set and dry cosmetics, can be dusted over the skin surfaces using a brush, powder blower, or powder puff. Matte powders reduce cosmetic shine, while a sheen finish mimics the natural facial oils.

Color Considerations in Cosmetic Application

Selecting Cosmetics to Match Skin Tone and to Cover Discolorations

Melanin is the pigmentation present in the epidermis that affects complexions. The more **melanin**, the darker pigmentation a person has. Freckles and moles are areas with high amounts of melanin. These features need to be re-created on facial features when thick, opaque cosmetic applications are necessary. Another impactful factor of complexion comes from the hemoglobin within superficial capillaries. Tints or base colors can be applied directly to the skin of the hands and face to emulate hemoglobin coloration. Cosmetics and powders can be used to alter and correct a decedent's complexion and skin tone to their lifelike state. Individuals who wore makeup require an even cosmetic application to smooth out skin tones, whereas those who did not should have a more natural variance. Shades of cosmetics can be blended to match each individual's complexion. In cases of extensive discoloration, a complementary color can be applied to conceal the discoloration. Opaque cosmetics can be applied and stippled into the skin. Finishing powder helps dry and set the cosmetics. Finishing spray can also be used as a barrier.

Effects of Lighting on a Decedent

Lighting can aid in restoring the exposed skin of decedents to its natural coloration. The color of the lights can be changed to cast a white, yellow, red, or pink hue upon the viewing area. Red and pink lights cast a tint over the entire face and emulate the red hemoglobin undertone. These colors wash out the warm, red areas of the face, requiring more warm coloration to be applied to strengthen these highlights. Magenta accents red colorations on the decedent's skin and also benefits jaundice. Tinted light shades can cast additional color upon the decedent. Ivory, eggshell, or pink **light shades** all enhance appearances by tinting light from the bulb as it filters through the shade. Altering the light intensity by dimming or brightening can also be helpful in obtaining a realistic appearance. Cosmetics that look natural in bright light will look duller in dimmer light. Uneven lighting creates atypical shadows on the face. Installing consistent lighting between the viewing room and preparation room improves cosmetic outcomes. Some funeral homes take their own lighting for viewings at other locations. Taking cosmetics along in case the lighting is completely different allows for cosmetics to be adjusted as needed.

Other Preparation of the Deceased

Types of Medical Devices in or on Decedents

- **Pacemaker**: Remove if final disposition is cremation.
- **Intravenous lines (IVs) and arterial lines** (peripheral IVs; midlines, PICC, and internal jugular central lines; tunneled central lines; or ECMO tubes):
    - Removing after injection increases resistance, which reduces leaking.
    - Waiting to remove jugular lines until after the jugular is raised reduces leaking and improves visibility.
    - Any lines impeding injection or drainage should be removed.
- **Urinary catheters**: Deflate the balloon (release valve or cut the tube) and remove prior to injection.
- **Chest tubes, drains, and colostomy/ostomy bags**: Remove after cavity embalming to reduce drainage and odor.
- **Endotracheal tubes**: Remove before beginning facial sanitary care.
- **Port**: The port doesn't need to be removed. Internally cut and remove the line into the jugular to prevent interference with drainage instruments (angular forceps or drain tubes).
- **Intraosseous (IO)**: Twist and pull out.
- **Staples**: Remove with forceps or a staple remover if they are in the way or an incision needs to be treated.

Caution should be taken when removing medical devices. When a tube is cut, fluid can quickly exit the tube. Always cut while holding an absorptive cloth between you and the tube. Sharps are disposed of in a sharps container; everything else is placed in biohazard garbage. Notate all removed devices on the embalming report.

Special Ceremonial Preparations

Preparing a Decedent in the Jewish Rite

In the **Orthodox Jewish** tradition, burial should take place within 24 hours of death according to the Torah. In the modern world, this is often not feasible between securing legal documentation and coordinating with family members, the **Rabbi,** and the cemetery; however, burials do take place as quickly as possible. Most Jewish families elect not to embalm; rather, the **Chevra Kadisha** perform the **tahara**, a washing and prayer ceremony**.** Women prepare women and men prepare men. Warm water is used to wash the body from head to toe, and all orifices are cleaned. The body is dried and dressed in a **tachrichim**, a simple white burial shroud used to equalize the rich and the poor. Men are buried with a **tallit**, a prayer shawl. The body is placed into an **aron**, a casket constructed only of wood, with a small amount of dirt from Israel. **Conservative** and **Reform** Jewish families do not adhere strictly to traditions. They may have the funeral director wash, dress, and casket their loved one; use clothing other than a shroud; or have embalming done.

Preparing a Decedent Following the Tradition for an Islamic Funeral

A person practicing Islam identifies as Muslim, worships Allah, follows the Quran, and attends a mosque. According to Islamic religious law, the burial should take place within 24 hours, but within 3 days is acceptable. Immediately after death, family members of the same gender **wash the body** three times (this can be done more but must be done an odd number of times) in a specific order. The spouse is allowed to participate in this ritual. The deceased is **shrouded**, and hands are placed on the chest in a position of prayer. The body is covered with a white sheet. Men are placed on three white sheets and women on five. The body is wrapped in one sheet at a time and secured with strips of cloth or rope. Traditionally, the body is not placed in the casket but is buried wrapped in cloth. Some sects will allow a casket or carrying tray for ease of transportation. There are no viewings in the Islamic faith. Organ donation is acceptable, but embalming and autopsies are strongly discouraged as they are considered desecration of the body. Cremation is prohibited because of a belief in a physical resurrection.

Preparing a Body for Viewing Without Embalming

Viewings without embalming can be requested by families for religious or other reasons.

- Refrigerate the body until the viewing. Regulations and specifications are dictated by state law.
- Complete topical sanitary care. Wash the entire body, including hair; shave facial hair if applicable.
- Sanitize all facial orifices, including the eyes, nose, mouth, and ears.
- Set the features. Close eyes with eye caps or cotton and mouth with dental ties or sutures.
- Aspirate if allowed, but the presence of purge necessitates aspiration.
- Dress and repose the body.
- Comb and style hair.
- Apply cosmetics. Cream-based cosmetics help retain moisture. Massage cream helps prevent the lips, eyelids and canthi, and fingers from dehydrating.

Decedent Care When Receiving from Another Funeral Home

When the body is embalmed, but not dressed and casketed:

- Review documentation such as the death certificate, cause of death, embalming report, and personal effects inventory records to familiarize yourself with the case.
- Discuss details with the family, including roles, needs, plans, service arrangements, and requests.
- Conduct a case analysis by inspecting the body to ensure that it is well preserved. Identify and treat any problem areas such as leaks, skin slip, blebs, discolorations, and areas that received insufficient distribution.
- Reaspirate.
- Apply plastics as needed and dress the body.
- Casket, style hair, perform restoration as needed, and cosmeticize (order can vary based on the director's or embalmer's preference).

When the body is embalmed, dressed, and casketed:

- Review documentation.
- Coordinate details with the family and other parties as needed.
- Inspect the body and the interior of the casket to ensure problems did not arise during transportation. Make sure the oral and nasal cavities are still clean and dry (no sign of purge). Check for abdominal distention or pressure; if present, the body will need to be reaspirated.
- Touch up restoration work and cosmetics as needed.

When the body is not embalmed:

- Review documentation and personal effects.
- Prepare for services requested. Embalm the body if requested; sanitize, set features, and prepare for identification viewing if a cremation is requested; or, for direct burials, dress and casket.

Body Positioning in a Casket or Alternative Container

Altering the position of the body post-embalming (after fixation) is challenging; positioning prior to injection prepares the body to be reposed.

Typical positioning is as follows:

- Position the head above the chest, and chest above the abdomen. Utilize blocks and table slope during embalming; in the casket, the bed should be sloped in a similar fashion, with the head higher than the feet.
- Position the head straight or turned 15° to the right.
- The arms should be bent at the elbow so the hands can rest naturally atop the lower abdomen. Postinjection, the hands can be positioned in a relaxed manner or propped atop one another.
- Some casket beds tilt, which is helpful in cases of spinal curvatures, malformations, or osteoporosis. Pillows, foam blocks, and towels can be discreetly used—hidden under the interior linings and blankets of the casket—to prop the person in a straight, comfortable manner for viewing.
- For cases of trauma, the body is typically placed in the casket with the head to the left, but it can be turned (placed backwards) to hide trauma to the right side of the face. If the family has selected a half-couch casket, a reverse half-couch will be needed. The head can be tilted, along with the bed of the casket, to help conceal trauma.

Reaspiration, Reinjection, and Delayed Aspiration

Problem areas can arise between embalming and services. **Reaspiration** is when the body is aspirated again post-embalming. Reaspirating cases prior to dressing and casketing is a standard procedure in many funeral homes, and it may also be necessary in other cases. Reaspiration is used to eliminate existing oral or nasal purge, reduce the risk of developing further oral or nasal purge, reduce the buildup of gas and fluid within the cavity, and reduce fluid and gas accumulation prior to transporting the body to another funeral home or location. **Reinjection** of additional cavity fluid may be needed after reaspiration if gas develops or tissue appears unpreserved. **Delayed aspiration** is when aspiration is delayed to allow arterial fluid to more effectively saturate tissues rather than performed immediately following arterial injection.

Scenarios in Which Reaspiration Is Required

Reaspiration of a body is necessary in the following cases:

- Remains received from another funeral home (by air or vehicle transportation), to ensure that the body was aspirated properly and did not develop fluid or gas accumulations during transportation or over time
- Extended holds between embalming and time of services
- Cause of death involving infections like sepsis and pneumonia
- Death following an abdominal surgery
- Death due to drowning

- Ascites or other serous cavity edema
- Vein distention caused by a buildup of gas throughout the body
- Obese cases to prevent fluid and gas accumulation; reaspiration reduces the risk of purge

Using Protective Plastic Garments on Decedents

Plastic garments are used on the decedent (embalmed or not) prior to dressing to shield the clothing and casket, alternative container, or viewing table from problem areas that may leak. They can also be used as a cautionary measure. For example, some funeral homes require that bodies are put in **coveralls** or **pants** to protect from potential anal, bladder, or vaginal leakage.

For problem areas:

- Treat the area using chemicals or glue, wraps, and packs as needed.
- Put plastics on.
- Add powders with absorptive, odor, or preservative properties. Many also prevent mold growth.
- Secure loose ends that could leak. Tape around the elastic band(s) on sleeves, stockings, coveralls, and pants to help prevent leaking.
- **Unionalls** are recommended for cases with multiple leaking extremities, many problem areas, trauma, burns, drownings/water deaths, decomposition, autopsies, organ donation, and long-bone donations.

After the plastic garment is secured, the person can be dressed and casketed.

Funeral Service Sciences

Anatomy

Anatomy is the division of science that studies the organization of the human body. **Gross anatomy** is the study of the body with the unaided eye. **Histology** (microscopic anatomy) is the study of the body with the use of a microscope. **Pathological anatomy**, also called human pathology, is the study of how disease affects both the structure and function of the body. **Regional anatomy** is the study of a particular body region. **Systemic anatomy** is the study of body systems and organs. **Topographical anatomy** is the study of the surface shape or form of the body. **Physiology** is the study of how the body functions. Like anatomy, physiology exists on several levels, from molecular processes within cells to the whole body interacting with the environment.

Cytology

Cytology is the study or examination of cells within the tissues of the human body. Cells vary in shape, size, and function. When similar cells group together, they form **tissues**.

Four common classifications are:

- **Epithelial tissue** is a dense layer of cells that acts as a protective shield and is found in surface layers of the skin, blood vessels, mouth, stomach, respiratory tract, etc. It is categorized based on the shape (squamous, cuboidal, columnar, or transitional) and organization (simple, solitary layers or stratified, multiple layers) of the cells within the tissue.
- **Connective tissue** cells vary immensely in structure, form, and function and are found in bones, ligaments, tendons, organs, adipose, cartilage, blood, etc. Connective tissues have an intercellular **matrix** that varies in composition and density.
- **Muscle tissue** contains flexible cells that allow the tissue to relax and contract, supporting movement.
    - **Skeletal**: voluntary, attach to bone, cross-striated fibers
    - **Cardiac**: involuntary, control heart contractions, slightly crossed and striated fibers
    - **Smooth**: involuntary, within blood vessels and organs with cavities or structures with ducts, narrow and smooth fibers
- **Nervous tissue** is responsible for sending messages and regulating function throughout the body. Cells are either neurons or glia and are present in the brain, spine, and nerves.

Human Anatomy Terms

The **anatomical position** is a standing position with feet and palms facing forward and thumbs angled away from the body. A body in a **supine** position is lying face up with palms up, whereas a **prone** position is face down. The view of the body when it is cut from side to side, resulting in a front and back division, is called the **frontal plane** or **coronal plane**. The **midsagittal (medial) plane** divides the body down the center from top to bottom into left and right halves. These halves are considered to have **bilateral symmetry** externally. Other planes parallel with the midsagittal are called sagittal planes. The **transverse (axial) plane** divides the body into upper and lower halves. **Curvature** means bending away or toward something. An **accessory** is something that serves in an auxiliary fashion or assists a structure or function.

Human Anatomy Directional Terms

Anterior (ventral) refers to the frontal part of the body or a part that is in front of another. **Posterior** (dorsal) refers to the rear part of the body or a part that is behind another. **Superior**

positioning means that one part of the body is located above another part. **Inferior** positioning means that one part of the body is located below another. **Medial** refers to the middle or median plane of the body. **Lateral** refers to the side of the body.

Proximal refers to the portion of the body closest to a reference point. **Distal** refers to the portion of the body farthest from a reference point. **Peripheral** describes the outermost regions or perimeter of part of the body, farthest from the center. **Superficial** describes a region at or near the uppermost surface. **Deep** refers to the region of a body located farthest below the surface. **Pectoral** refers to the frontal portion of the chest. **Suprarenal** is the part of the body above the kidney.

Anatomical Body Cavity and Organ Terms

The human form has two major cavities: dorsal and ventral. The **dorsal cavity** is in the back of the body and is divided into the cranial cavity and the spinal cavity. The **ventral cavity** is in the front of the body and is divided into the thoracic cavity and abdominopelvic cavity. The **thoracic cavity** is further divided into the pleural cavities and the mediastinum, which contains the pericardial cavity. The **abdominopelvic cavity** is divided into the abdominal cavity and the pelvic cavity. The **viscera** are the internal organs confined within a cavity. A **capsule** is an uninterrupted casing surrounding a cell, organ, or structure. The **cortex** is the outermost layer of an organ.

Cells

Biology defines **cells** as structures that are the basis of all living things. Cells can function individually in single-celled organisms or together in complex organisms. The human body is composed of trillions of cells. Their size, shape, structure, and function vary.

Components of animal cells:

- The **plasma membrane** is the exterior margin of the cell, contains the cell's cytoplasm and structures; allows fluid to enter and exit the cell; and aids in cell identification. It is composed of fat molecules (phospholipids and cholesterol) and protein molecules that act as chemical/hormone receptors.
- **Cytoplasm** is matter within the cell containing **organelles**, internal structures contributing to cell function.
    - **Ribosomes** produce enzymes and proteins.
    - The **endoplasmic reticulum** produces fats, carbohydrates, and proteins of the plasma membrane and transports proteins from the ribosomes to other areas of the cell.
    - The **Golgi apparatus** receives molecules and chemically processes them before releasing them to exit the cell by merging through the plasma membrane.
    - **Mitochondria** produces energy for the cell through chemical reactions.
    - **Lysosomes** break down and process foods and substances.
    - **Centrioles** aid in cell division.
    - **Cilia** assist with movement.
- The **nucleus** controls organelles and is responsible for cellular reproduction.

Layers of the Integumentary System

The primary function of the **integumentary system** is to provide a protective barrier for the internal body. The system consists of skin, hair, nails, and glands associated with skin, hair, and nails. There are three layers of skin: epidermis, dermis, and hypodermis. The **epidermis** is the outer layer. It provides protection, produces keratin to thicken skin, and produces pigment to protect the body from the sun. The **dermis** is a thicker layer that contains connective tissue, hair follicles, and sebaceous glands. The **hypodermis** is the innermost layer. It contains fat cells and connective tissues that protect, regulate warmth, and cushion the body. Hair can provide some protection from the elements and insulation from heat and cold, as well as sensory input such as the presence of parasites. Fingernails and toenails are sheets of hard keratin that protect the extremities.

Bone Markings

Osteology is the division of science that studies bones. An **articulation** is the point where two bones meet. Bones have many parts that stick out or are recessed from the rest of the bone. A **protuberance** is an outward growth of bone. A **condyle** is an arched protuberance at the end of a bone, creating an articulation. An **epicondyle** is a protuberance on top of a condyle. A **tubercle** is a small, round protuberance. A **tuberosity** is a rough protuberance where muscles or ligaments attach. A **process** is a large or sharp protuberance. A **crest** is a ridge along the edge of a bone. A **facet** is a flat surface. A **fossa** is a depression or shallow area in bone. A **fovea** is a smaller depression. A **foramen** is a natural opening in a bone. A **canal**, **fissure**, or **meatus** is a smaller opening in a bone. A **sinus** is a space within a bone.

Bones

The axial skeleton is made up of the 80 bones of the head, spine, and chest.

- **Head**: The cranium includes frontal (forehead), parietal (back), temporal (side), mandibular (lower jaw), maxillary (upper jaw), nasal conchae and septum (nose), and zygomatic (cheek) bones. The ear includes the malleus (hammer), incus (anvil), and stapes (stirrup) bones. The hyoid is not connected to any other bone.
- **Spine**: The spine includes seven cervical (neck), twelve thoracic (upper back), and five lumbar (lower back) vertebrae, the sacrum, and the coccyx (tail bone).
- **Chest**: The chest contains the ribs, scapula (shoulder blade), and clavicle (collar bone).

The appendicular skeleton is made up of the 126 bones of the pelvis, upper appendages (arms), and lower appendages (legs).

- **Pelvis**: The pelvis includes the ilium (upper), ischium (lower), and pubis (front).
- **Arms**: Arm bones include the humerus (upper), radius and ulna (forearm), carpals (wrist), metacarpals (hand), and phalanges (fingers).
- **Legs**: Bones of the leg include the femur (thigh), patella (knee), tibia and fibula (calf), tarsals (ankle), metatarsals (front foot), calcaneus (heel), and phalanges (toes).

Review Video: Skeletal System
Visit mometrix.com/academy and enter code: 256447

Arthrology

Arthrology is the study of joints and articulations. A **joint** is the site at which an articulation (connection) occurs. **Diarthrotic articulations** are moveable joints with synovial fluid and cartilage cushions that are held together by ligaments, like the limbs. **Amphiarthrotic articulations** are slightly moveable and are sutural or fibrous in nature. **Synarthrotic articulations** are immovable joints, such as the spine and skull. **Cartilage** is a dense connective tissue composed of collagen and/or elastin fibers on the end of bones, which provides a smooth surface for articulation by reducing friction. **Hyaline cartilage** is found in the nose, larynx, trachea, ribs, and sternum, and the entire skeleton of an embryo. **Elastic cartilage** is found in the outer ear (pinna) and epiglottis. **Fibrocartilage** is found in the knee, in the pubic bones in the pelvic region, and between the vertebrae in the spine. A **ligament** is a fibrous band of connective tissue stretching from one bone to another in a joint to provide lateral stability. Ligaments also connect cartilages and other structures. A **tendon** is also called a **sinew** and connects muscle to bone. Tendons grow into the bone and make mineralized connections with the bone. **Symphysis** refers to bones that have grown together and fused, such as the pelvis.

Digestive System

The gastrointestinal tract (GI tract) is a system of organs in the abdomen. It is responsible for the ingestion and digestion of food, absorption of nutrients and medications, and elimination of waste products. The GI tract is divided into two sections. The **upper GI tract** consists of the mouth (buccal mucosa, tongue, and teeth), pharynx, esophagus, and stomach. The **lower GI tract** comprises the small intestine (duodenum, jejunum, ileum, and ileocecal valve) and the large intestine (ascending, transverse, and descending colon; sigmoid flexure; rectum; and anus). The accessory organs of digestion include the liver, the gallbladder, and the pancreas. The liver produces bile as a byproduct of breaking down old red blood cells. The liver excretes bile into the small intestine to break up fatty foods by way of the biliary system. The gallbladder's only function is to store and concentrate bile, so if painful stones form in it, the gallbladder can be safely removed. The pancreas secretes hormones and excretes digestive enzymes.

Review Video: Gastrointestinal System
Visit mometrix.com/academy and enter code: 378740

Urinary System

The urinary system starts with two bean-shaped **kidneys** (located in the lower abdomen on either side of the spine), which filter toxins and excess fluid from the blood, creating urine. The kidneys produce 2–3 liters of urine daily. The kidneys also maintain the acid-base balance, regulate electrolyte concentrations, control the volume of blood, and govern blood pressure.

The concave side of the kidney contains an opening called the hilum, which is the point of entrance for the renal artery, renal vein, nerves, and ureter. The kidney is surrounded by a capsule of fibrous and connective tissue. The renal cortex is the outer part of the kidney. Inside the cortex is the renal medulla, split into 10–20 renal pyramids. The tip of a renal pyramid is called a papilla. Each papilla drains into a minor calyx. Several minor calyces act together to drain into a major calyx. The major calyces drain into the renal pelvis, from which urine then drains to the ureter.

Ureters carry the urine to the bladder, and a **urethra** carries the urine to the **external meatus** (opening) during urination. The urethra of the female is about 0.5–1.5 cm long, and the male urethra is about 15–29 cm long.

Review Video: Urinary System
Visit mometrix.com/academy and enter code: 601053

Male Reproductive System

The functions of the male reproductive system are to produce, maintain, and transfer **sperm** and **semen** into the female reproductive tract and to produce and secrete **male hormones**. The external structure includes the penis, scrotum, and testes. The **penis**, which contains the **urethra**, can fill with blood and become erect, enabling the deposition of semen and sperm into the female reproductive tract during sexual intercourse. The **scrotum** is a sack of skin and smooth muscle that houses the testes and keeps the testes outside the body wall at a cooler, proper temperature for **spermatogenesis**. The **testes**, or testicles, are the male gonads, which produce sperm and testosterone. The internal structure starts with the **epididymis**, which stores the sperm as it matures. Mature sperm moves from the epididymis through the **spermatic duct** to the **ejaculatory duct**. The **seminal vesicles** secrete alkaline fluids with proteins and mucus into the ejaculatory duct also. The **prostate gland** secretes a milky white fluid with proteins and enzymes as part of the semen. The **bulbourethral**, or Cowper's, glands secrete a fluid into the urethra to neutralize the acidity in the urethra, which would damage sperm.

Female Reproductive System

The female reproductive system produces **ova** (oocytes or egg cells), transfers the ova to the **fallopian tubes** for fertilization, receives the sperm from the male, and provides an environment for the developing **embryo**. The external portion of the female reproductive system includes the labia majora, labia minora, Bartholin's glands, and clitoris. The **labia majora** and the **labia minora** enclose and protect the vagina. The **Bartholin's glands** secrete a lubricating fluid. The **clitoris** contains erectile tissue and nerve endings for sensual pleasure.

The internal portion of the female reproductive system includes the ovaries, fallopian tubes, uterus, and vagina. The **ovaries**, which are the female gonads, produce the ova. Fertilization typically occurs in the fallopian tubes. If fertilized, the egg travels to the **uterus**, where it implants in the uterine wall. The uterus protects and nourishes the developing embryo until birth. The **vagina** is a muscular tube that extends from the **cervix** of the uterus to the outside of the body. The vagina receives the semen and sperm during sexual intercourse and provides a birth canal when needed.

The female reproductive system also includes **mammary glands** (breasts), which are modified sweat glands that produce milk after childbirth.

> **Review Video: Reproductive Systems**
> Visit mometrix.com/academy and enter code: 505450

Respiratory System

The respiratory system has two divisions. The **upper respiratory tract** consists of the nasal cavity and pharynx and their associated structures. The **lower respiratory tract** consists of the larynx, trachea, bronchi, and lungs. **Internal respiration** is the exchange of oxygen, carbon dioxide, and trace gases at the cellular level. **External respiration** is the exchange of oxygen, carbon dioxide, and other gases between the lungs and blood, commonly known as breathing. The passage of gases through the respiratory system is:

1. Air is inhaled through the **nostrils** and **mouth**.
2. Air passes through the **pharynx** to the **larynx** (voice box).
3. The **epiglottis** flips to cover the esophagus.
4. Air passes into the **trachea** (windpipe).
5. The **diaphragm** contracts and flattens to raise the ribs as breathing occurs.
6. **Intercostal muscles** between the ribs pull the ribs up, enabling the chest to expand and air to pull inward.
7. The trachea splits into the left and right **bronchi** that connect to the **lungs**. The bronchi split into fine branches called **bronchioles**.
8. The bronchioles end in **alveoli** where the red blood cells absorb oxygen (O_2) from the inhaled air and give off carbon dioxide (CO_2).

> **Review Video: Respiratory System**
> Visit mometrix.com/academy and enter code: 783075

Cardiovascular System

The cardiovascular system controls blood flow throughout the body and to the tissues, controls gas exchange (carbon dioxide and oxygen) by transporting oxygenated blood from the lungs, serves as a reservoir for blood, maintains blood pH through a buffer system, responds to infections, and facilitates coagulation (blood clotting). The cardiovascular system is made up of the heart, the venous system (vessels), and blood. It is responsible for oxygenation of cells, perfusion (carrying of blood with oxygen, glucose, and nutrients to cells), and removing waste products such as carbon dioxide. The **lymphatic system** is composed of ducts that help remove fluid, or **lymph**, from tissues and disperse it back into the vessels of the circulatory system. **Lymph nodes** function to filter out pathogenic materials and foreign substances. **Lymphocytes**, a type of white blood cell, originate in lymph nodes and are streamed into the circulatory system to aid in fighting infection and disease.

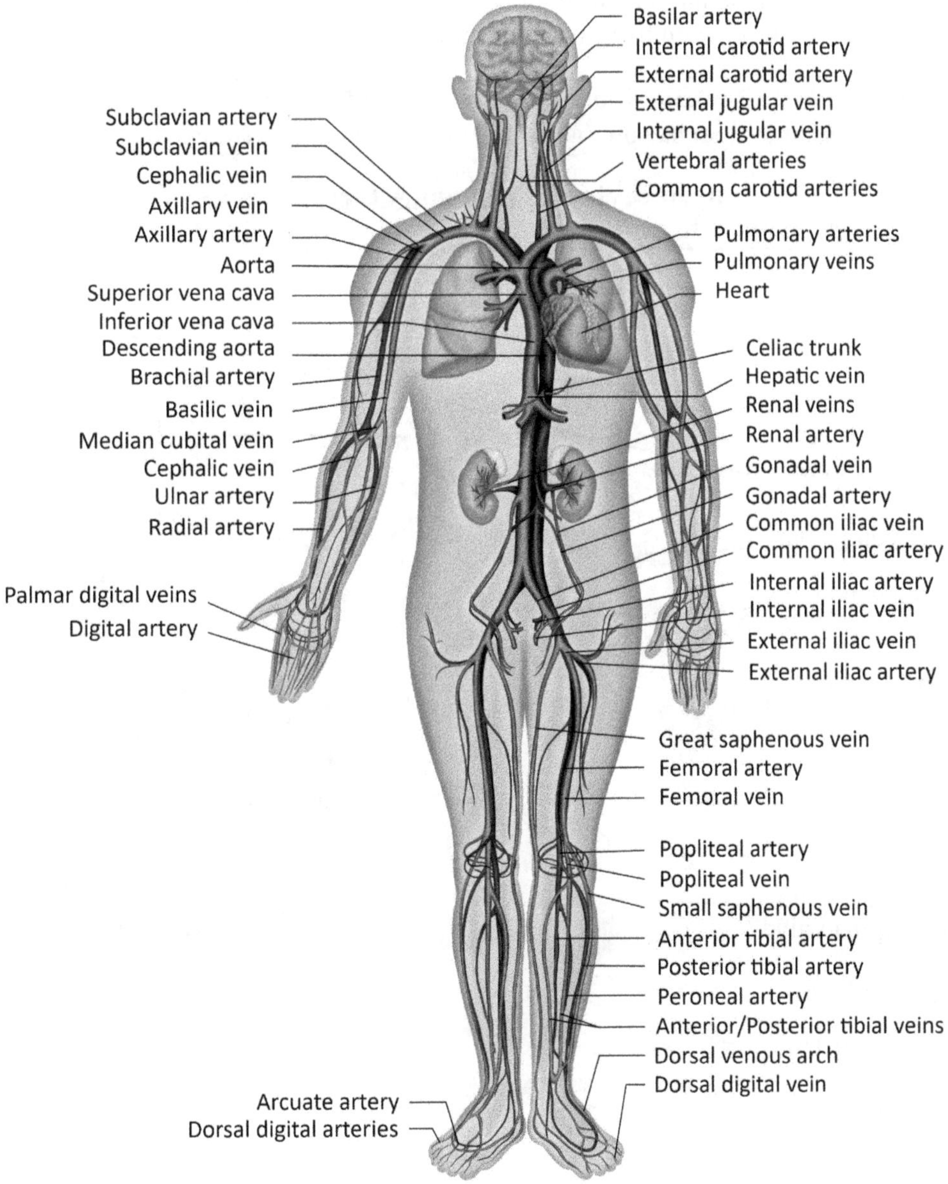

Cardiovascular System Components

The cardiovascular system has the following components:

- **Heart**: The heart has four chambers—two upper (right atrium and left atrium) and two lower (right ventricle and left ventricle). The heart muscle receives blood from four major coronary arteries (right, left main, left anterior descending, and left circumflex) and their branches and then distributes blood via the aorta and pulmonary arteries.
- **Vessels**: The venous system includes veins, venules, and venous capillaries and returns blood back to the heart via the inferior and superior vena cava. The arterial system (including the coronary arteries) branches from the aorta after it leaves the heart and includes arteries, arterioles, and arterial capillaries.
- **Blood**: Blood consists of red blood cells (erythrocytes), white blood cells (leukocytes including monocytes, lymphocytes, basophils, neutrophils, and eosinophils), platelets (thrombocytes), and plasma, the liquid portion of the blood (which contains clotting factors). Blood carries oxygen from the lungs and distributes it to the rest of the body.

Review Video: Cardiovascular System
Visit mometrix.com/academy and enter code: 376581

Review Video: Pulmonary Circuit
Visit mometrix.com/academy and enter code: 955608

The Heart

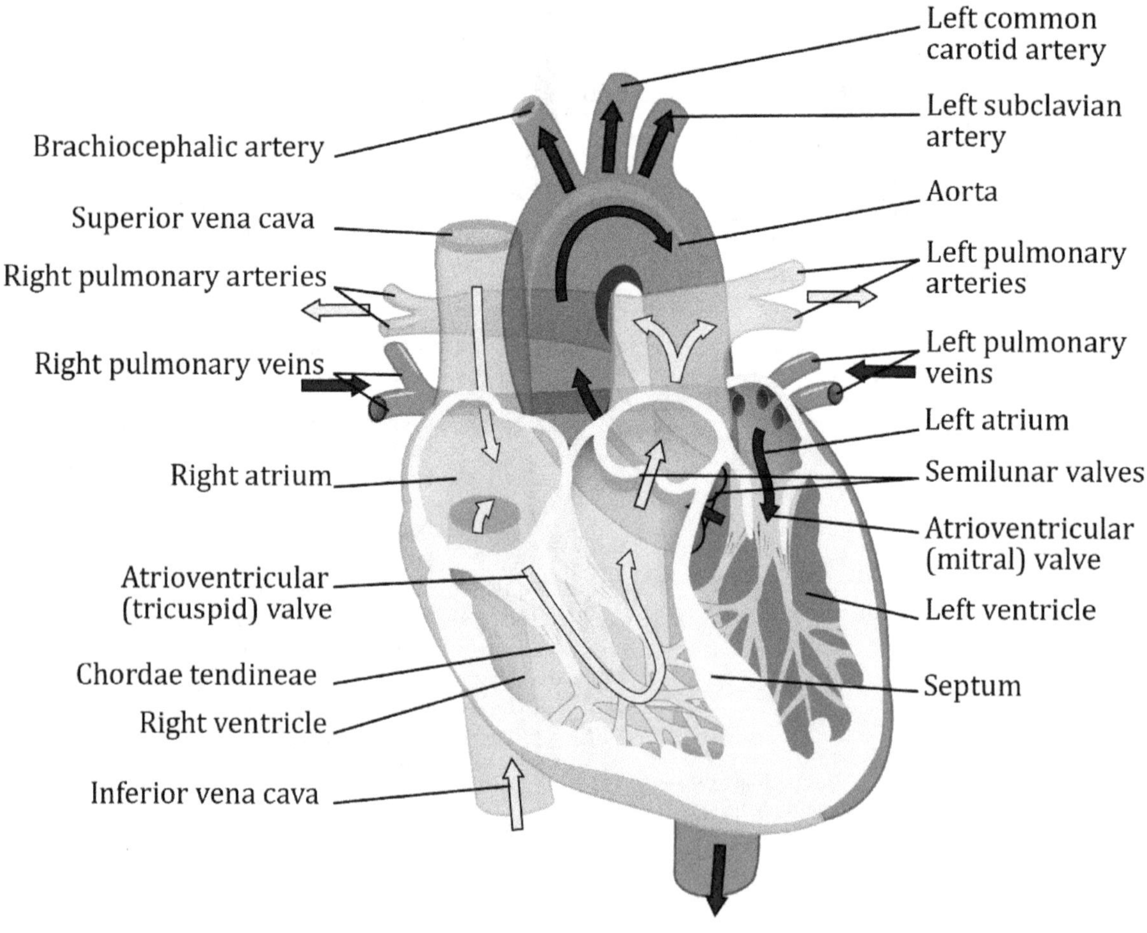

The heart is about the size of a fist. It is located in the middle of the chest, behind the sternum, and leans slightly left. The heart is covered by a double-layered membrane called the **pericardium**. The heart itself has **four chambers**. The two upper chambers are the **right atria** and **left atria**; the lower chambers are the **left ventricle** and **right ventricle**. The left and right atria and the left and right ventricle are separated by a muscular structure called the septum. The **tricuspid valve** controls the flow of deoxygenated blood from the right atrium to the right ventricle. The **pulmonary semilunar valve** controls the flow of blood from the right ventricle to the pulmonary artery, which carries the blood into the lungs, where it is oxygenated. The blood then flows through the pulmonary vein back to the heart, where the **mitral valve** controls the flow of the blood from the left atrium to the left ventricle. The **aortic semilunar valve** regulates blood flow from the left ventricle to the aorta. From the aorta, the oxygenated blood is conducted to the rest of the body, becomes deoxygenated, then travels back to the right atrium.

Review Video: How the Heart Functions
Visit mometrix.com/academy and enter code: 569724

Review Video: Heart Blood Flow and Heart Anatomy
Visit mometrix.com/academy and enter code: 783139

Arteries and Veins

Arteries (other than the pulmonary and umbilical arteries) carry oxygenated blood away from the heart throughout a living body; postmortem, they are used to inject arterial solution. Arteries split into arterioles, which connect to capillaries. They are thicker than veins and have a rubbery, noodle-like consistency needed to withstand high pressure.

Both arteries and veins have three layers:

- **Adventitia**: outer layer composed of connective tissue
- **Media**: middle layer of muscle and elastic tissues (thicker in arteries)
- **Intima**: inner layer composed of epithelial cells

The inside of the vessels is called the **lumen**. When incising the vessels, it is important to cut through all the layers, exposing the hollow center in which to insert instruments.

Veins (other than the pulmonary and umbilical veins) carry unoxygenated blood from the body tissues back towards the heart. Capillaries connect to venules, which join into larger veins. Veins can stretch or constrict to increase or decrease blood volume because they function under lower pressure than arteries. They collapse postmortem when blood flow stops. Veins have valves. As the heart pumps blood, these valves open and close to prevent blood from being pulled backwards by gravity.

Path of Embalming Fluid Through Arteries, Veins, Collateral Circulation, and Anastomosis

Arteries are used to inject embalming fluid. Fluid travels through the vascular system just like in life. Arteries branch into **arterioles,** smaller arteries, which connect to capillaries. **Capillaries** connect arterioles and **venules**, small veins. Capillaries allow fluid to leave the vascular system and enter tissues. There it interacts with muscles, tissues, and cells. Embalming fluid enters the interstitial space and can push other fluid back into the capillaries. Fluid that reenters the capillaries flows into venules. Venules connect back to veins, leading back to the superior and inferior vena cavae to the right atrium.

A circulatory anastomosis is when two vessels conjoin. The **circle of Willis** is an anastomosis of arteries to supply the anterior and posterior brain with blood. Blood can flow either direction through the circle depending on bodily needs. This allows for **collateral circulation**, which is when blood reaches an area by another vascular path. Change in pressure from a blockage allows directional flow changes to ensure that the brain still receives proper blood flow. Collateral circulation typically consists of small vessels that can reach an area of the body by an indirect or alternative route. This is resourceful in life and helpful postmortem during embalming.

Fetal Circulation

In utero, a fetus receives nutrients and oxygen from the mother through the **placenta**. The placenta forms and attaches to the uterine wall, forming a connection between the mother's and baby's blood. Blood and nutrients are carried to and from the placenta's vascular system by the **umbilical cord**, which consists of two arteries and one vein. The arteries carry deoxygenated blood while the vein carries oxygenated blood. The vein carries blood directly to the inferior vena cava. The lungs and liver are bypassed by most of the blood as they are not fully functioning in utero. This specialized vascular system ceases to function following birth. As the baby inflates its lungs, pressure collapses the umbilical vessels and closes the bypasses in the heart.

Spontaneous abortion, or **miscarriage**, is most likely to occur during the first 10–13 weeks; however, early pregnancy loss can occur in the first 20 weeks. After 20 weeks, the loss is classified as **stillborn**. Preservation of fetal loss is difficult. Gestational age, vascular fragility, birth scenario, potential malformation, and postmortem exams all contribute to embalming challenges. Topical embalming, rather than vascular, may be necessary if preservation is requested by the family.

Endocrine System

A **gland** is an organ, group of cells, or single-celled body structure with the function of manufacturing a secretion. The **endocrine** system is a glandular system that has no specific ducts or passageways but is capable of secreting chemicals directly into the blood. The major glands that comprise the endocrine system, the hormones they secrete, and diseases resulting from their dysfunction include the following:

Gland	Hormones	Disease
Adrenal Cortex	Aldosterone Cortisol Androgens	Addison's disease Cushing's disease
Adrenal Medulla	Epinephrine Norepinephrine	Anxiety attacks Depression
Anterior Pituitary	Adrenocorticotropic hormone (ACTH) Follicle-stimulating hormone (FSH) Gonadotropic hormones Growth hormone (GH) Luteinizing hormone (LH) Prolactin Thyroid-stimulating hormone (TSH)	Dwarfism Gigantism
Hypothalamus/ Posterior Pituitary	Inhibiting hormones (stop the release of other hormones) Antidiuretic hormone (ADH) Oxytocin Releasing hormones (trigger the release of other hormones)	Diabetes insipidus

Gland	Hormones	Disease
Kidneys	Calcitriol Erythropoietin	Hypertension
Ovaries	Estrogen Progesterone	Endometriosis Menometrorrhagia
Pancreas	Insulin Glucagon	Diabetes mellitus
Parathyroid	Parathyroid hormone	Tetany Renal calculi
Pineal	Melatonin	Alzheimer's disease
Testes	Testosterone	Gynecomastia Klinefelter syndrome
Thymus	Thymic factor (TF) Thymosin Thymic humoral factor (THF) Thymopoietin	DiGeorge syndrome
Thyroid	Calcitonin Thyroxine (T4) Triiodothyronine (T3)	Cretinism Hypo/Hyperthyroidism Goiter Myxedema
Digestive tract	Gastrin Cholecystokinin Secretin Ghrelin Motilin	Gastritis Gastroesophageal reflux

Review Video: Endocrine System
Visit mometrix.com/academy and enter code: 678939

Nervous System

The human nervous system is divided into the central nervous system (CNS) and the peripheral nervous system (PNS). The **CNS** is composed of the brain and spinal cord. The brain controls bodily processes consciously (e.g., higher thinking/mental faculties, voluntary muscle action, memory, etc.) and unconsciously (e.g., heart rate, blood pressure, breathing, digesting food, etc.). The spinal cord has nerves that innervate major organs and muscles and initiate muscle movement or organ function at the command of the brain.

The **PNS** is made up of the nerves. The PNS is divided into the somatic nervous system and the autonomic nervous system. The autonomic nervous system is further divided into the sympathetic nervous system and the parasympathetic nervous system. The meninges are membranes that protect the brain and spinal cord. Ventricles are spaces within the brain. The ventricles are filled with cerebrospinal fluid.

Review Video: What is the Function of the Nervous System?
Visit mometrix.com/academy and enter code: 708428

Nervous System Structure and Function

The nervous system is composed of the central and peripheral nervous systems. The **central nervous system** includes the main organs of the nervous system: the brain and the spinal column. The **peripheral nervous system** includes all parts of the nervous system that branch off from the central nervous system, such as cranial and spinal nerves.

The nervous system consists of billions of **neurons**—special cells made up of a cell body, axon, and dendrite. Function determines neuron nomenclature:

- **Afferent neurons** transmit information from muscles and organs to the central nervous system.
- **Interneurons** transmit information from neuron to neuron.
- **Efferent neurons** transmit information from the central nervous system to muscles or glands.

The nervous system has three main functions:

- **Sensing**: The nervous system perceives internal and external alterations to the body.
- **Integrating:** The nervous system computes sensory information to communicate to the body the correct action to take.
- **Motor**: The nervous system transmits information to the muscles of the body when it is time to initiate movement and control this movement.

The human body uses sensory inputs to gather information about itself and the surrounding world. This information travels to the central nervous system, where the information is processed and acted upon through a process called **integration**. The brain makes decisions based on the information gathered or rejects the information if necessary. If the brain decides to act on the information gathered, it initiates movement through motor pathways. Because the nervous system controls all human movement, it is important to train it to ingrain correct movement and improve reaction time.

Myology, Muscle Characteristics, and Muscle Components

Myology is the study of the purpose, composition, movement, and pathologies of muscles. There are three types of muscles: skeletal muscles (involuntary and striated), smooth muscles (involuntary and smooth), and cardiac muscles (involuntary and cardiac tissue). Involuntary muscles use low-energy movements regulated without conscious thought or control. Humans do not tell their heart muscles to contract; they do so involuntarily. Voluntary muscles are controlled; these movements require more energy. The conscious movement of facial muscles to create a smile is voluntary. Muscles are composed of groupings of contractible and structurally similar cells, called **muscle fibers**.

Skeletal muscles support movement, posture, and heat generation. They typically connect one bone to another and pass over a joint. The **origin** is where muscle attaches to the less mobile bone, while the **insertion** of the muscle connects to the more mobile bone. When the muscle body contracts, the more mobile bone moves toward the more stationary bone. **Tendons** attach muscles to the bones at the muscle's origin and insertion points. **Synovial fluid** from the synovial membrane of either bursae or tendon sheaths lubricates muscles and joints, aiding in movement. Muscles are composed of water, protein, fat, and glycogen.

Review Video: Muscular System
Visit mometrix.com/academy and enter code: 967216

Muscles of the Head and Neck

The muscles of the head and neck include:

- **Frontalis**: extends from the occipital bone to the integument of the eyebrow; lifts eyebrows
- **Temporalis**: extends from the temporal bone to the mandible; raises jaw to close mouth
- **Orbicularis oculi**: circular muscle around the eye attaching to both the maxilla and frontal bone; shuts eye
- **Orbicularis oris**: circular muscle around the mouth; closes mouth, abutting the top and bottom lips
- **Levator anguli oris**: raises the position of the mouth
- **Levator labii superioris alaeque nasi**: simultaneously elevates and extends the upper integumentary lip and flares the nostrils
- **Levator labii superioris**: raises and stretches the upper lip
- **Zygomaticus major**: extends from the zygomatic bone to the upper lip and corner of the mouth; raises the corner of the mouth and lips
- **Masseter**: zygomatic arch to the mandible; lifts jaw
- **Sternocleidomastoid**: extends from clavicle and sternum to the mastoid process; raises jaw, turns head and neck
- **Trapezius**: extends from the skull and vertebra to the scapula; rotates neck and mobilizes scapula

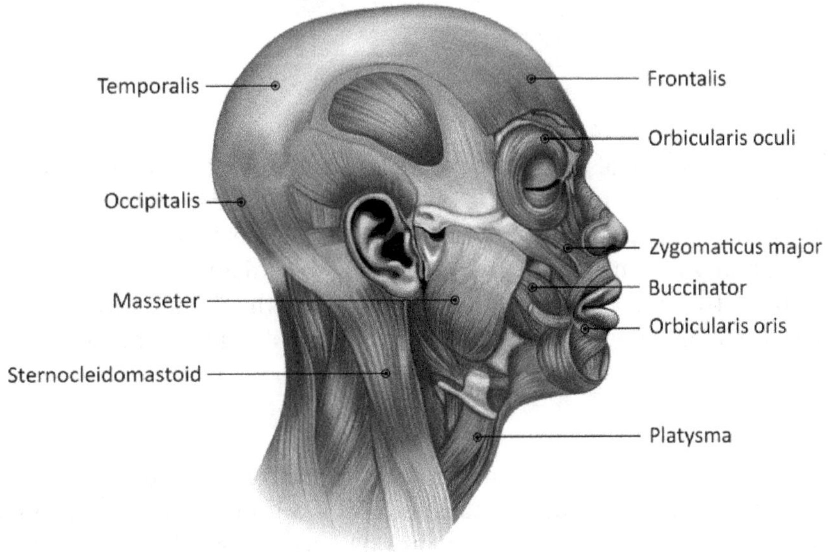

Muscles of the Chest and Trunk

The primary muscles of the chest and trunk are:

- **Pectoralis major**: extends from the sternum, clavicle, and ribs to the humerus; flexes and moves the arm toward the body (adduct)
- **External oblique**: abdominal midline to thoracic ribs; flexes the abdomen, twists and bends the trunk
- **Internal oblique**: abdominal midline (linea alba) to pelvis; flexes the abdomen, turns the trunk

- **Transverse abdominis**: extends from the midline to ribs, vertebrae, and pelvis; flexes the abdomen and reinforces the trunk, spine, and pelvis
- **Rectus abdominis**: central abdominal muscles extending from the ribs to the pubis; tightens the core to support movement

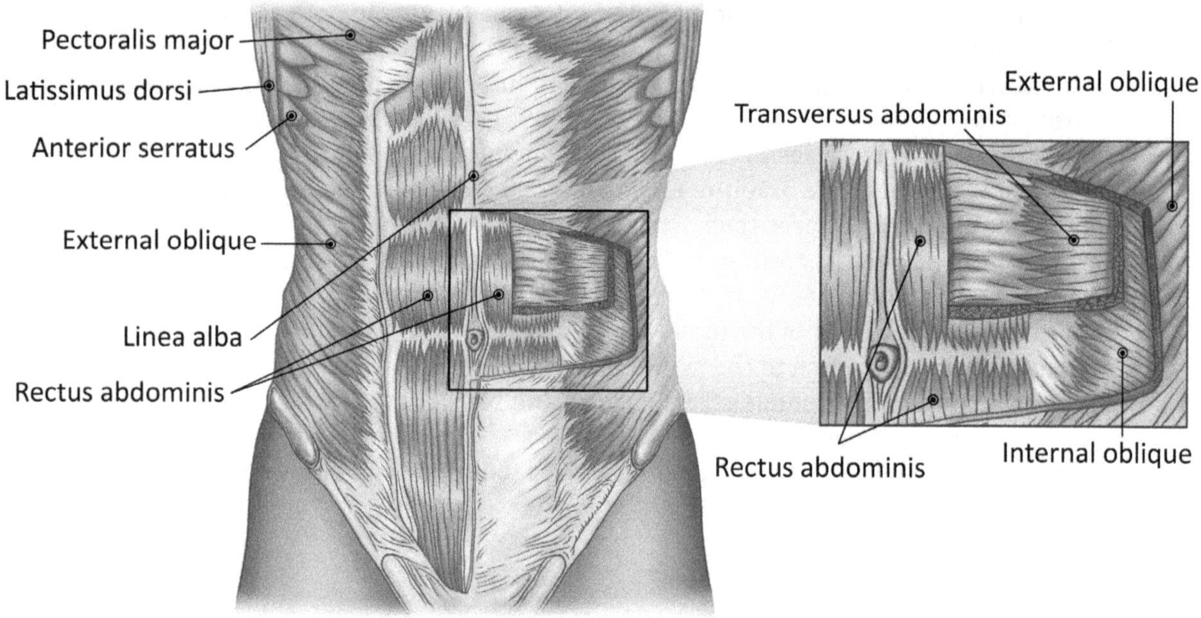

Chemistry

Chemistry is the scientific study of the nature of matter and how it changes. **Inorganic chemistry** is the study of the characteristics and properties of compounds that contain little, if any, carbon. **Organic chemistry** is the study of the characteristics and properties of certain carbon compounds. **Biochemistry** is the study of compounds found in living organisms. **Embalming chemistry** is the study of the types of matter and changes in matter following the disinfection and preservation of human remains. All the major divisions of chemistry are involved to some degree during embalming.

Chemistry Terms

The **atom** is the smallest particle of an element that is consistent with the properties of the element. A **molecule** is a group of atoms; it is the smallest unit of a compound held by a chemical bond. An **element** is an uncomplicated substance that cannot be decomposed by normal chemical resources. An atom's **valence** is an indication of its ability to form bonds with other atoms. A **formula** is a combination of symbols used to express the chemical composition of a substance; for instance, the formula for water is H_2O. **Ionization** is the disassociation of a substance in solution into ions. An **ion** is an atom that has lost or gained an electron, becoming a charged particle. **Acids** are substances that yield a hydrogen or hydronium ion in water. **Bases** are substances that yield hydroxide ions in water. An **amphoteric compound** can chemically behave as either an acid or a base. **Salts** form by neutralizing an acid and a base together.

Measurements in Chemistry

Measurement and calculations in chemistry, like all sciences, use the **metric system**, which is based on meters for distance, grams for weight, and liters for volume. **Parts per million (ppm)** is a mathematical value identifying dilution amounts. For example, 1 ppm equals 1 milligram per liter.

This is used to measure the amount of formaldehyde gas per million parts of air by volume in a given space. It is also used to measure the amount of a chemical per million parts of solution. The **pH** measures the hydrogen ion concentration of a solution, mathematically representing its acidity or alkalinity. A pH of 7 is **neutral**. A solution with a pH below 7 is considered **acidic**; the lowest pH is 0. A solution with a pH above 7 is considered **basic**, or **alkaline**. The pH scale goes up to 14, though some very strong bases actually have a higher pH.

PHYSICAL AND CHEMICAL STATES OF MATTER

All objects are composed of **matter**. It is characterized by both physical and chemical properties. A **liquid** is made up of molecules that demonstrate unrestricted movement. A **physical change** is one that does not cause a change in the chemical composition of matter, including **physical properties** like odor, hardness, color, and density. A **chemical change** results in the formation of a new substance, including a change in the **chemical properties**. This indicates that the characteristics of its chemical structure have changed. **Osmosis** is the movement of a solvent through a membrane, most often from a solution of lower solute concentration to one of greater solute concentration. The process of osmosis and the factors that influence it are important for the embalmer to understand so he or she can attain the proper balance of extracellular and intracellular fluids.

SOLUTIONS, MIXTURES, AND COMPOUNDS

A **solution** is a liquid mixture consisting of substances that have been dissolved. A **solvent** is the agent that causes the dissolving and is the main ingredient in the solution. A **solute** is the substance that is dissolved in the solution. **Solvation** is the act of dissolving. **Solubility** is a measure of how well two substances mix. **Diffusion** describes the progression of fluids from a more concentrated area to a lesser one, as in the case of embalming chemicals moving from intravascular arteries and veins to extravascular capillaries. A **mixture** consists of two or more materials that are together but are not chemically combined; the relative amounts of these materials can vary. **Compounds** are substances that consist of two or more atoms combined chemically in definite proportions by mass.

SPECIFIC SOLUTION TYPES

A **hypotonic solution** has a lower concentration of solutes than a comparable solution or a cell. A **hypertonic solution** has a greater concentration of solutes than a comparable solution or a cell. An **isotonic solution** has an equivalent concentration of solutes as a comparable solution or a cell. A **dilute solution** has a small concentration of solute. **Vehicles** or carriers are liquid solvents to mix various ingredients into embalming fluids. **Hardness of water** describes a concentrated mineral and salt presence in water. This chemical state often requires supplemental fluids that remove or separate the minerals out of the solution to reduce their effect on vascular embalming.

CARBOHYDRATES, HEXOSES, LIPIDS, AND ENZYMES

Biochemistry is the study of the chemical characteristics, interaction, and systems that occur within living things, relating to both normal function and pathologies. **Carbohydrates** are biomolecules containing aldehydes (aldoses) or ketones (ketoses), typically classified as sugars, starches, glycogen, or cellulose. **Hexoses** are simple sugar carbohydrates with six carbons such as glucose (blood), galactose (brain and nerves), and fructose (fruits; two times sweeter than glucose).

Lipids must contain carbon, oxygen, and hydrogen but, unlike carbohydrates, can have additional components like phosphorous or nitrogen. Lipids (fat) are the result of a chemical reaction of an aldehyde with fatty acids. Fats are solids at room temperature, while **oils** are liquids at room temperature. When soap is introduced to oils or fats, it acts as an **emulsifier**, allowing substances that do not normally mix to mix. Lanolin, an oily wax, is in some embalming chemicals, creams, and cosmetics.

Enzymes are colloidal compounds that enable quicker chemical reactions within the body. An enzyme only reacts with specific substances, at the correct temperature, within a particular pH range. Postmortem, enzymes will begin to break down the body's own tissues (autolysis). Enzymes need to be treated during the embalming process to prevent bodily deterioration.

PROTEINS

Proteins are formed when amino acids link, forming a polymer. Formaldehyde is used to preserve and coagulate proteins for preservation. **Albumin** is the primary protein in blood plasma and serves to grow and repair tissues. **Proteolysis** is the process of protein decomposition. **Preservative demand** (formaldehyde demand) is the amount of preservative required to effectively preserve remains, depending on the tissue condition as determined in the embalming analysis. **Denaturation** is the process by which a protein's molecules change due to addition of heat or chemicals. The **denatured protein** structure has been changed by physical or chemical agents. An **enzyme** is a protein that, when present, serves as a catalyst for the ensuing chemical reaction.

CARBONS, HYDROCARBONS, HALIDES, ETHERS, AND CARBOXYLIC ACIDS

Organic compounds include alcohols, ketones, ethers, esters, and acids, which are composed of carbon, oxygen, and hydrogen, often with other elements. **Hydrocarbons** contain only carbon and hydrogen elements. They bond in chains (aliphatic or acyclic) or rings (aromatic or cyclic). These are commonly known as alkanes, alkenes, alkynes, etc. **Alkyl halides** are alkanes that have one or more halogen elements replacing hydrogens. Chloroform is an example of this type of compound.

Carboxylic acids have a carbon double-bonded to oxygen (COOH) on the end of the molecule. Formic acid (HCOOH) is a carboxylic acid created when formaldehyde is oxidized. **Ethers** are created when water is removed from alcohols (dehydration). Oxygen must be in the middle of the carbon chain for this reaction to occur.

ORGANIC PRESERVATIVES IN VASCULAR EMBALMING

An embalmer prepares **arterial fluid**, a mixture of liquids for vascular injection into a body. It includes preservatives, water or alcohol, and sometimes supplemental chemicals. The translocation of this fluid though the body inactivates saprophytic bacteria and renders the body tissues less susceptible to decomposition. The three chemical preservatives are alcohols, aldehydes, and phenolic compounds. **Alcohols** are colorless, liquid, organic compounds with one or more hydroxyl (-OH) groups. The general formula is R-OH (R is a hydrocarbon group). Alcohol is required to prevent the polymerization of formaldehyde (HCHO) into paraformaldehyde (solid form of formaldehyde). **Aldehydes** are organic compounds with one or more -CHO groups. The general formula is R-CHO (R is a hydrocarbon group or hydrogen). **Phenolic compounds** are triple-based arterial fluids containing alcohols, aldehydes, and phenol (carbolic acid). Phenolic compounds are drying agents that are derivatives of benzene containing one or more -OH groups, used principally with jaundice to prevent the skin from turning yellow or orange.

ORGANIC CHEMICALS IN EMBALMING

Iodophors are disinfecting solutions that contain iodine. **Hypochlorites** are compounds that contain chlorine. **Ketones** (R-CO-R) are any class of simple organic compounds that include the carbonyl group inside the carbon chain so that the carbon atom is joined with two other carbon atoms. An example is acetone. An **ester** (RCOOR) is created when an alcohol and an organic or carboxylic acid come together through the elimination of water. Esters serve as perfuming or masking agents in embalming. **Amines** ($R\text{-}NH_2$) are organic derivatives of ammonia. They are the transitional products of decomposition and are characterized by a strong, fishlike odor.

Chemical Properties of Formaldehyde

Formaldehyde, or **methanal** (HCHO), is the simplest aldehyde. It is a colorless gas with a pungent odor and is dehydrating to mucous membranes. This dehydration affects the skin to a lesser degree and is readily soluble in water to a saturation level of 37%. At this saturation level it is called **formalin**. Silver, iron oxide, molybdenum, and vanadium act as catalysts to produce the oxidation processes needed to convert methanol for formaldehyde. A **polymer** is a substance formed by bonding several monomers or basic chemical units through a process called polymerization. Once polymerized, formaldehyde dries to a state called **paraformaldehyde**. Formaldehyde is unstable in alkaline solution and will decompose. It will polymerize if the medium becomes too acidic. Formaldehyde will react with ammonia to form **urotropine**, an antiseptic used to treat urinary tract infections. A body in advanced decomposition requires much higher concentrations of formaldehyde than a non-decomposed body. This occurs because HCHO has an affinity for nitrogen, a crucial element found in protein. **Hydrolyzation** occurs when water breaks down a compound to form an acid and a base composition. When protein hydrolyzes, more nitrogen is out in the open. This causes the formaldehyde to react with the nitrogen.

Modifying Agents

Supplemental fluids are added to arterial fluids for reasons other than preservation or disinfection. They include preinjection, co-injection, and humectants. **Modifying agents** are added to a mixture or solution for embalming based on the type of embalming, the environment, and the arterial fluid to be used. Their purpose is to influence the chemical reactions produced by the preservative solution and to control the action of the main preservative agents. Four typical ingredients are added to arterial fluids in embalming. **Anticoagulants** are supplemental chemical agents mixed with the arterial fluid to thin the blood in the dead body and facilitate fluid translocation, counteracting the normal postmortem increase in blood viscosity. **Humectants** are chemicals that help embalmed tissue to retain moisture. **Buffers** help to maintain pH by affecting the stabilization of the acid-base (pH) balance within embalming solutions and in the embalmed tissues. **Surfactants** are chemical wetting agents that improve the movement of a substance (surface tension) by reducing the molecular cohesion of a liquid so it flows freely through smaller apertures.

Poisons vs. Toxins

There are many potentially hazardous chemicals used to sanitize and preserve decedents in preparation for their funeral rites. **Poisons** are chemicals that have a detrimental impact on a living species. Chemicals used in the embalming process act as poisons on pathological organisms within a decedent. Inorganic poisons are products of non-living things (e.g., lead). Organic poisons, produced by plants and animals, are considered **toxins**. **Detoxification** is the process of reducing the concentration of a toxic poison.

Hazardous chemicals used in the preparation of human remains can be toxic, flammable, or explosive or cause bodily harm to humans or the environment. Never mix chemicals unless the label specifically states that it is acceptable as reactions may create products that are even more hazardous. For example, household bleach (sodium hypochlorite) and ammonia are individually hazardous but can be used with proper precautions, including personal protective equipment such as gloves, eye protection, and respirators. Mixing the two produces chloramine gases, which are highly toxic and can be fatal.

Examples of Hazardous Chemicals Used in the Preparation Room

Hazardous chemicals used in the preparation room include:

- **Acetone**: clear, unstable (flammable), and mildly toxic liquid used in embalming fluid, nail polish remover, and everyday items like furniture and shoe polish
- **Ammonia**: clear gas with an intense odor; toxic in high concentrations, causing burns, irritations, and lung damage; used in cleaning chemicals
- **Formaldehyde**: clear gas with a strong odor, flammable, highly toxic; used in embalming chemicals, powders, and gels for preservation; also used in the production of everyday items like furniture, paper, and medicines
- **Glutaraldehyde**: a more stable liquid, considered moderately toxic; used in embalming chemicals as a preservative and germicidal agent
- **Paraformaldehyde**: formaldehyde in a solid state; extremely toxic; used in embalming powders and compounds to aid in preservation

Impact of Medicinal Treatments and Chemical Drugs

People are commonly treated with multiple drugs prior to their death due to disease, pain, and other medical conditions. All drugs affect and alter cells and tissue throughout the entire body. These chemical agents decrease the effectiveness of arterial embalming chemicals primarily due to the physiological changes they impart upon the decedent's organs, tissues, and cells. The drugs do not affect the arterial chemicals themselves. Drugs can reduce the ability of fluid to move in and out of the cell membranes, reducing intracellular preservation. Liver failure from drug use can cause jaundice. Kidney failure from drugs results in increased nitrogenous waste, which reduces the effectiveness of preservatives.

Chemical impacts on the body and the embalming process include:

- **Antibiotics**: circulatory obstructions, jaundice; reduced distribution and preservation
- **Corticosteroids**: dilution of arterial fluid from edema; difficulty neutralizing intracellular autolytic enzymes due to reduced cell permeability
- **Cancer chemotherapy**: weight loss, increased nitrogenous waste, edema, jaundice, fragile bones, purpura; preservation approach must treat the presenting conditions without further dehydrating the body
- **Tranquilizers, sedatives, and stimulants**: weight loss, dehydration, protein insufficiency; difficult to fixate with excess nitrogenous waste
- **Cardiovascular drugs**: coagulation problems, increased nitrogenous waste from less-effective circulatory system; reduced distribution

Decomposition Caused by Physical and Chemical Changes

Following death, the body is subject to physical and chemical changes. Physical changes, in which the environment impacts the state of the body, include algor mortis, hypostasis, dehydration, and livor mortis. Chemical changes, in which internal chemical reactions alter the state of the body, include postmortem caloricity, body pH, rigor mortis, and decomposition. Many chemical changes begin with **autolytic enzymes**, which are naturally occurring proteins that do not cease functioning when the body dies. Postmortem, they begin to break down tissues by causing chemical interactions that create new substances within the tissue.

Postmortem caloricity is an increase in body temperature following death. It is caused by the chemical reaction responsible for metabolism. Oxygen within the body postmortem continues to fuel metabolic reaction. **Anabolism** takes body energy to join molecules together. **Catabolism** is the metabolic phase that breaks these complex molecules apart to produce heat and energy for the body to use. Postmortem, this heat and energy release causes rigor mortis and decomposition to occur at a faster rate.

Effects of Body pH and Rigor Mortis in Embalming

During life, the **pH** of the body typically is around 7.4. Postmortem, the acidity of the body increases (lower pH) as rigor mortis advances. Rigor mortis is caused by a buildup of lactic acid. As acid levels increase, soft proteins of the tissues begin to deteriorate. This begins to shift the pH of the body back into the alkaline (basic) range. Protein decay releases nitrogen into the tissues in the form of ammonia and amines. This altered pH can interfere with arterial distribution and cause splotching.

During rigor mortis, the muscles of the body stiffen as their proteins bind together. Embalming while the body is in rigor mortis is problematic because it increases intravascular resistance, increases the amount of preservatives that must be used (formaldehyde is unable to bond with proteins), causes splotchy distribution, and can deceivingly present as fixation from arterial chemicals.

Decomposition

Decomposition involves the chemical breakdown of proteins, carbohydrates, and lipids within the body.

- **Proteins**: Postmortem, protein chains begin to be broken down by catalytic enzymes. Autolysis is caused when the pH of the body becomes acidic, collapsing the cell membrane and releasing digestive enzymes that begin digesting the cell components. Hydrolysis is when a compound and water react with one another, separating the compound into multiple smaller molecules. The decomposition of proteins is called putrefaction and can be caused by anaerobic or aerobic bacteria.
- **Carbohydrates**: Fermentation is the deterioration of carbohydrates caused by bacteria. As carbohydrates decompose, they release organic acids that do not have an odor or affect the embalming process.
- **Lipids**: Body fat is subject to hydrolysis and is broken down into fatty acids and glycerol. There is no substantial impact on embalming, nor does this deterioration have an odor.

The typical order of decomposition is cells, tissues, and then organs. Tissue decomposition typically progresses as soft tissues, firm tissues, and then hard tissues. Signs of decomposition are color, odor, skin slip, gas, and purge.

Embalming impacts include reduced distribution, unwanted tissue distention, and requiring more arterial fluid. The signs of decomposition require treatment during embalming and post-embalming care.

Pathology

Pathology is the study of diseases, symptoms, and progression. Antemortem, pathologists examine and test biopsied or removed blood, tissues, organs, growths, and tumors to aid in medical diagnoses. Postmortem pathology involves autopsies to determine cause of death and influencing factors. **Gross pathology** uses the unaided eye to study the structural changes that disease causes in the human body. **Physiological pathology** studies the types of alterations a particular disease makes to a normally functioning body. **Clinical pathology** studies disease by testing body fluids, secretions, and excretions. **General pathology** studies the broadly observed effect of disease, while **special pathology** is a specialty within pathology, such as focusing on one system or diagnostic method. **Etiology** is the cause of a disease or the study of the causes of diseases. **Pathogenesis** refers to the way a disease develops over the course of time. A **pathogenicity** occurs when a disease causes pathological changes. A **prognosis** is a medical expectation of the body's condition at the conclusion of a disease.

Reversible Cell Injury, Cellular Adaptation, and Irreversible Cell Injury

Following chemical, biological, or physical injury, a cell can adapt, reverse injury through healing, or die. **Reversible cell injury** can be a result of stimulation or environmental impacts (low levels of toxins, temporary hypoxia, or brief anoxia). Cellular homeostasis can be altered when the demands exceed or reduce their required function; for example, cell metabolism can increase or decrease slightly without straining the cell irreparably. **Adaption** occurs if demands aren't too extreme and the cell "learns" to function in adverse conditions. Most cells return to normal function when standard stimulation returns. Adaptation that occurs in cases of cell loss (death) typically are not reversible (osteoporosis, atrophy, aging). **Irreversible cell injury** occurs when too much strain is placed on the cell and it is unable to maintain homeostasis. Toxins, hypoxia, anoxia, and injury can cause alterations to the nucleus or cell destruction. Enzymes are released when a cell dies.

Autopsies

An **autopsy** is an examination of the body following death to determine cause and manner of death. It is completed by a pathologist, forensic pathologist (medical specialty), or medical examiner (job title). A coroner or medical examiner orders a **forensic autopsy** when the cause of death is not clear for unattended deaths or when further postmortem examination of the body is required to identify the body or due to death of a suspicious nature, violence, trauma, or accident. **Hospital autopsies** are ordered when the medical diagnosis is unclear, when unexpected complications occurred, when experimental medical treatments were used, following unsuccessful diagnostic surgeries, in cases of death during childbirth, in cases of contagious disease, or when other undeterminable and questionable circumstances lead to death. The family must give permission for hospital autopsies, whereas forensic autopsies can be required. It is important that the embalmer complete an accurate embalming report for every embalming, but it is essential to have a detailed report for autopsy cases. Record the type of autopsy that was performed (partial, cranial, spinal, or full). Notate whether all of the viscera were returned with the body. The embalmer may not be able to determine whether all of the viscera were returned.

Attitude toward Autopsies, Postmortem Examinations, and Organ Donation

Funeral professionals sometimes view autopsies, postmortem examinations, and organ donation as adding to their workload and an unwanted challenge of their skills. Embalmers are trained to handle these cases and should do so with professionalism, tact, and poise. On a technical level, autopsies can often aid in arterial distribution and restoration of traumatic or accidental death cases. They can also provide the family with closure, answers, peace of mind, and an opportunity to seek justice in criminal or accidental deaths. Organ donation provides the therapeutic effect of seeing their loved one helping someone else live a better life. Some people find it cathartic to know that parts of their loved one live on.

Funeral professionals should never make negative comments to the family or public about these procedures and examinations. They should never use their professional status to sway a family in their decision-making. An exception to this falls under the scope of **professional reporting**, when a funeral director makes observations of a decedent that are conflicting and inconsistent with family, caregiver, or medical reports. Suspected abuse should be reported to the appropriate authorities according to state law so that a proper investigation can ensue.

Manner of Death and Cause of Death

Autopsies are conducted to determine the cause and manner of death. **Cause of death** can be divided into primary, secondary, and additional contributing causes. **Manner of death** is how the death is classified: natural, accidental, suicide, homicide, undeterminable, or pending. **Pending** death determinations are awaiting results from continued investigations, toxicology panels, or other laboratory testing.

During the postmortem examination, the pathologist examines the surface of the body and internal organs, notating normal, abnormal, and trauma areas. Removing, weighing, examining, and sectioning organs and tissue, they determine what pathologies and diseases are present in the body and which ones likely caused or contributed to death. Tumors, aneurysms, vascular blockages, and cardiac conditions are some examples.

People can have antemortem symptoms that are used to diagnose and determine a cause of death during a medical evaluation or postmortem exam. **Syndromes** are a set of specific symptoms that present together and are used to define a condition. **Disorders** are classified by symptoms that alter or impair natural function and may not have a determined cause. **Disease** is a medical ailment with a definite cause. **Abnormalities** within the human body are atypical ailments, structural irregularities, or uncharacteristic functions resulting from pathologies, genetics, or traumas.

Human Body Conditional Change and Injury

A **chronic** condition refers to a disease or condition that is ongoing, whereas an **acute** condition is one that appears suddenly. **Dehydration** is the natural reduction of fluids or moisture from the body tissues occurring antemortem or postmortem. **Emaciation** is extreme thinness. **Cyanosis** is an observed superficial condition characterized by a bluish color of the skin or mucous membrane, caused by a lack of oxygen. **Jaundice** is a yellowed appearance of the skin or mucous membranes usually caused by liver disease. A **contusion** is a superficial condition in which blood vessels are damaged by trauma and exhibit a bruising hematoma and swelling. A **concussion** is an impairment to the brain as a result of blunt trauma to the head. An **aneurysm** is a condition in which a bulging sac forms on an artery. **Degeneration** is the decline of tissue health and function due to a disease or injury. **Pus** is a whitish-brown liquid composed of bacteria and white blood cells that forms around the site of tissue inflammation. A **pustule lesion** is a raised, inflamed area containing pus.

Abnormal Tissues

Dysplasia is tissue that develops and grows in an abnormal manner. **Dilated** refers to an abnormally enlarged size. **Aplasia** is an abnormal or incomplete growth of an organ or other body part. A **polyp** is an unusual tissue growth on a mucous membrane. **Ectopic** describes a condition in which tissue is not in its normal place, such as an extrauterine pregnancy. **Edema** is the accumulation of excess fluids among tissue cells. This fluid dilutes the potency of the embalming fluid as it reaches the tissues. **Hydrocephaly** is a buildup of cerebrospinal fluid in the brain. A **hydrocele** is a buildup of fluid in the scrotal sac. A **hernia** is an atypical bulge of tissues or an organ pressing against the normal limits of the cavity. An **islet** is a small, aggregated group of one kind of tissue within another type of tissue. A **lesion** is abnormal tissue structure caused by a disease or injury. A **furuncle** is an infection that exists in a sweat gland or hair follicle. A **carbuncle** is a cluster of boils in the skin emanating from subcutaneous tissue that releases pus and is surrounded by dead tissue.

Inflammation and Inflammatory Process

Inflammation is the body's response to an injury caused by chemicals, microbes, disease, or physical trauma involving nerves, vasculature, and blood cells. Inflammatory responses can only happen in living tissue. Signs of an inflammatory response discovered during an autopsy indicate that the injury occurred prior to death. The purpose of inflammation is to protect the body and promote healing.

Stages of inflammatory response:

- Vascular changes following a damaging stimulus allow nerves to send messages to the capillaries to briefly constrict and then immediately dilate arterioles to increase blood flow into the capillaries of the affected area. Venules also dilate to accommodate the influx of blood to the area. The increase in blood flow causes redness, swelling, and warmth.
- Increased vessel permeability allows fluid and cells to easily enter the area and increases the capillary pressure. Leukocytes and platelets stick to the endothelial cells of the vascular wall. This permeability allows fluid known as an **exudate** to enter the surrounding space, causing edema.
- Phagocytosis of bacteria and other debris helps clean the injured area.

Inflammation is classified by duration (acute or chronic), etiology (cause), location (localized or systemic), and pathology (examination of affected area). Common symptoms associated with inflammation are redness, swelling, heat, pain, and fever.

Neoplasms

Neoplasms form from uncontrollable new cell growth. Neoplastic cells are autonomous (independent growth), unaffected by normal cell regulators, and do not follow typical growth standards. Neoplasms form masses of cells (tumors) but can also present as abnormal cells found throughout the body. Histological analysis determines cell type and clinical classification (benign or malignant). **Benign neoplasms** have a slow expansion rate, do not metastasize, are superficially smooth, are similar to surrounding tissue, and have distinguishable cells with a standard nucleus. **Malignant** neoplasms grow rapidly, metastasize, are atypically shaped, can become necrotic or bleed, and are not similar to surrounding cells; cells are not clearly differentiated in malignant neoplasms, making them hard to remove. A **cyst** is an encapsulated sac under or on top of the body surface composed of air, pus, fluid, or some combination of these. While they may superficially resemble neoplasms, most cysts are pockets of foreign material or other types of cells rather than overgrowth; however, a cyst may also be neoplastic. Cysts are usually benign.

Benign and Malignant Neoplasms and Postmortem Considerations

Tumors are typically named based on the cells they morphed from. Tumor names typically end in *-oma*. Common tumor types include:

- **Chondroma**: benign connective tissue tumor
- **Osteoma**: benign bone tumor
- **Myoma**: benign muscle tumor
- **Adenoma**: benign epithelial cell tumor within gland(s) or duct(s); additional descriptive words specify tumor type (e.g., liver cell adenoma)
- **Sarcoma**: malignant connective tissue tumor (chondrosarcoma), bone (osteosarcoma), and muscles (myosarcoma)
- **Carcinoma**: malignant epithelial cell tumor (e.g., liver cell carcinoma)
- **Adenocarcinoma**: malignant epithelial cell tumor within gland(s) or duct(s)

- **Lymphoma**: malignant lymphoid cell tumor
- **Gliomas**: malignant glial cell tumor

Common postmortem considerations for decedents who had malignant tumors include:

- Effects of multi-drug or chemotherapies
- Emaciation, dehydration, and fragility
- Edema
- Jaundice

Blood Diseases or Conditions

Hematopoietic disorders are diseases of the blood. **Hyperemia** occurs when an overabundance of blood pools in a particular part of the body. **Anemia** is when there is a smaller than normal amount of erythrocytes (red blood cells), hemoglobin, or both. **Lymphoma** is a cancerous condition in which the immune system is attacked by malignant white blood cells. **Leukocytosis** is a condition characterized by a large number of white blood cells. **Leukopenia** is a condition characterized by a lower number of white blood cells. **Leukemia** is a cancerous blood disease affecting the bone marrow where blood cells are made. A **hemorrhage** is a condition characterized by blood escaping from the vascular system. A **hematoma** is a swelling or mass of clotted blood confined to an organ or space, caused by a ruptured blood vessel. **Hemophilia** is an inherited blood disease in which the person has a propensity for extreme and often unprompted bleeding. **Ischemia** is restricted blood flow. **Thrombosis** is when a blood clot (**thrombus**) forms in a blood vessel. An **embolism** is when a thrombus blocks a blood vessel. Circulatory **shock** is when there is not enough blood flow to supply the body with oxygen. There are four types of shock: hypovolemic, distributive, cardiogenic, and obstructive.

Diseases of the Heart and Blood Vessels

Atherosclerosis is when fatty deposits build up inside of arteries, resulting in decreased blood flow, which in turn leads to high blood pressure and increased risk of thrombi (blood clots) and emboli (moving clots). **Edema** is swelling from fluid retention. Edema may occur because of heart failure causing fluid to build up in the legs and feet and/or the lungs. Edema may also occur with kidney disease and severe allergic (anaphylactic) reactions. **Thrombophlebitis** is inflammation of a vein as the result of thrombi. The vein appears red, swollen, and tender and may spread emboli to other areas of the body, such as the brain (stroke) and heart (heart attack). **Heart failure** includes disorders of contractions (systolic dysfunction), filling (diastolic dysfunction), or both and may include pulmonary, peripheral, or systemic edema. The most common causes are coronary artery disease, systemic or pulmonary hypertension, cardiomyopathy, and valvular disorders. The incidence of chronic heart failure correlates with age. Uncontrolled heart failure leads to death. A **myocardial infarction (heart attack)** is when blood stops flowing to the heart, usually (95% of the time) because of a blockage in the arteries. Heart attacks can be fatal.

Review Video: Myocardial Infarction
Visit mometrix.com/academy and enter code: 148923

Diseases Impacting Postmortem Care

Gastrointestinal Diseases

Common diseases of the gastrointestinal tract and their impact on postmortem care include:

- **Dental cavities and gum disease**: Dental problems can lead to tooth extractions and the use of dentures or partial plates. The mouth is reconstructed to a normal appearance using the person's dentures, mouth formers, and/or cotton. Oral infections must be sanitized. Gum disease or eroding gums makes inserting dental ties with the needle injector difficult and may require sutures instead.
- **Gastroenteritis and inflammatory diseases** (e.g., Crohn's disease, IBS, and ulcerative colitis): Low body weight is common.
- **Neoplasms**: Tumors disrupt distribution of arterial fluid and can cause abnormal protrusions when large. Chemotherapy drugs impact the condition of the body.
- **Intestinal vascular diseases** (e.g., hemorrhoids, vascular lesions, and ischemia): These diseases impact arterial distribution.
- **Malabsorption diseases** (e.g., celiac disease, Whipple's disease, and intestinal ischemia): These diseases can cause low body weight.

Diseases of the Urinary Tract

Common diseases of the urinary tract and their impact on postmortem care include:

- **Metabolic disorders** such as diabetes mellitus affect the kidneys and can cause thickening of vessels, vascular stenosis, and an increase in uremia. These symptoms may complicate arterial injection.
- As the filtration system, the kidneys often are subjected to **bacterial infections** as they remove these bacteria from the blood. Bacteria can also infiltrate the urinary tract by entering the urethra. Medications and antibiotics used to treat urinary tract infections can impact the body, including causing circulatory issues and reducing preservation effects of arterial fluid.
- **Neoplasms** of the urinary tract tend to be malignant. These become more common with age.
- **Renal failure** occurs when the kidneys shut down and can no longer filter blood properly. As a result, toxins can build up within the body. Glomerular disease and polycystic kidney disease all decrease renal function. Medications, edema, and circulatory issues caused by kidney disease all impact postmortem care.

Diseases Affecting the Nervous System

Common diseases of the nervous system include:

- **Developmental diseases**: anencephaly, spina bifida, cerebral palsy
- **Cerebrovascular diseases**: stroke, ischemia, transient ischemic attack, intracerebral hemorrhage
- **Trauma**: traumatic brain injury from concussions, contusions, laceration, paralysis
- **Infection**: bacterial and viral infections that cause encephalitis, myelitis, meningitis, and cerebral abscesses
- **Neurodegenerative diseases**: Alzheimer's disease, Huntington's disease, Parkinson's disease, amyotrophic lateral sclerosis (ALS)
- **Neoplasms**: Gliomas, meningioma, neurofibromas

Postmortem considerations for nervous system diseases:

- Medicines and chemotherapies used to treat diseases impact the body's organs and circulatory system.
- Circulatory impacts include reduced blood flow to some areas, swelling in areas of hemorrhages, and facial asymmetry and drooping post-stroke.
- Degenerative diseases and neoplasms can lead to weight loss, low muscle mass, and emaciation.
- Prions are proteins that infect the brain, causing neurodegenerative disorders such as Creutzfeldt-Jakob Disease (CJD). Prion-based diseases are untreatable and fatal, difficult to kill (acids, autoclaving, sanitizing chemicals, or formaldehyde won't kill prions), can remain dormant on contaminated instruments/materials, and remain present and contagious in the eyes and brain tissue postmortem.

Diseases of the Reproductive Systems

Common diseases of the **male reproductive system** include:

- Infertility
- **Infections** caused by sexually transmitted diseases and pathogens entering the reproductive system through the urethra opening
- **Tumors** in cases of prostate and testicular cancer

Common diseases of the **female reproductive system** include:

- **Infections** caused by sexually transmitted diseases and infections from microbial pathogens ascending into the body
- **Hormone disorders** in which inadequate estrogen and progesterone levels impact menstrual cycles
- **Neoplasms** such as cancers of the cervix, vulva, uterus, and ovaries
- **Pregnancy complications**, for which pathological considerations include uncharacteristic fertilizations, atypical implantations, and maternofetal complications

Diseases of the reproductive system generally do not directly affect postmortem care. Postmortem considerations for these diseases involve the impacts of antibiotics, chemotherapies, and other medications that can alter a body's normal function prior to death. Tumors and extended illnesses can lead to weight loss and reduce musculature.

Diseases of the Skeletal System

Common diseases and issues of the skeletal system include:

- **Fractures** (broken bones)
- **Congenial deformities** such as achondroplasia, osteogenesis imperfecta, or osteopetrosis
- **Metabolic disorders** such as rickets, osteoporosis, osteomalacia, Paget's disease, or renal osteodystrophy
- Bacterial infections
- **Degenerative joint diseases** such as osteoarthritis or rheumatoid arthritis
- **Neoplasms** such as osteoma, osteosarcoma, chondroma, chondrosarcoma, or Ewing's sarcoma

Postmortem considerations include:

- Antibiotic and medicinal drugs impact the body's organs and circulatory system.
- Fragility from disorders causes a reduction in bone mass.
- Arthritis and osteoporosis cause joint deformation, reduced mobility, and muscle spasms, which can impact reposing the body in a standard manner. Fingers may be bent or contorted. The hand may not be able to open from a fist. Spinal curvatures prevent the person from lying straight and flat; blocks and additional supports are needed, along with modification to the casket, to achieve a natural pose.
- Fractures can alter the appearance and positioning of the decedent. They need to be reset prior to embalming so the surrounding muscles and features can fixate into a normal position to restore proper aesthetics.

Diseases of the Endocrine System

Common diseases and disorders of the endocrine system involve tumors, hyperfunction (increased hormone production), and hypofunction (decreased hormone production).

- **Pituitary gland**: Hyperfunction can lead to gigantism and acromegaly or metabolic issues resulting in hyperglycemia or hypercalcemia. Hypofunction is not as common and results from congenital defects, tumors, and ischemia.
- **Thyroid disease**: Hyperthyroidism is a result of autoimmune disorders (e.g., Graves' disease), hyperplasia, or tumors. Hypothyroidism causes congenital defects and inflammation (e.g., Hashimoto's thyroiditis). A goiter is when the thyroid becomes enlarged and swollen.
- **Adrenal gland**: Adrenal hyperfunction causes Conn's syndrome and Cushing's syndrome, while hypofunction causes Addison's disease.

Postmortem considerations for endocrine diseases include:

- Compacted bowels
- Edema
- Weight loss and reduced muscle mass
- Facial changes (e.g., drooping or puffy skin or periorbital edema) and hair changes (e.g., increased presence of facial hair or thinning, coarse, or brittle hair)
- Hyperpigmentation (in cases of Addison's disease)
- Round face, obesity, and other effects from use of steroids and other medications to treat these diseases

Diseases of the Integumentary System

Common pathologies of the integumentary system include:

- **Traumatic injuries** such as burns, wounds, and lacerations can be present. Burns are evaluated following the **rule of nines** to determine the percent of the body affected and course of treatment. In the rule of nines, the head, upper chest, anterior abdomen, upper and lower back, left and right arms, and anterior and posterior areas of the left and right legs are each estimated at 9% of the total body; the genital area is the remaining 1%.
- **Infections** can be caused when bacteria, fungi, viruses, and parasites breech the skin, entering hair follicles or sebaceous glands. Infections may present in numerous ways, including acne, athlete's foot, subcutaneous worms, or lice.

- **Autoimmune diseases** such as eczema, atopic dermatitis, psoriasis, or lesions caused by diabetes comprise another group of common pathologies.
- **Neoplasms** include melanoma, carcinoma, and Kaposi's sarcoma (dermal tumors that commonly occur in immunosuppressive diseases like AIDS).

Postmortem considerations include:

- Medicinal and chemotherapeutic effects may be present on the body's organs and circulatory system.
- Neoplasms and infections on visible areas, like the face and hands, require restoration measures and cosmetics after the tissue is chemically treated.

Diseases of the Lymphatic System

Common pathologies of the lymphatic system include:

- The lymphatic system plays a key role in the **metastasis of cancers**. Cancer cells enter the lymph vessels and are carried to other parts of the body. Lymph nodes are susceptible to developing tumors because they filter out cancer cells from the lymph.
- **Leukemia** causes anemia, bleeding, anoxia, and weakened immune systems.
- **Lymphoma**, both non-Hodgkin and Hodgkin types, consists of malignant cells that enter the lymph nodes, spleen, thymus, or bone marrow.
- Lymph nodes often swell during **infection** as the body fights back.

Postmortem considerations include:

- Medicine and chemotherapies used to treat infections and neoplasms affect the body's organs and circulatory system, which impacts arterial distribution and penetration into tissues.
- Weight loss, anemia, jaundice, and lymph node enlargement impact arterial and co-injection fluid selection along with treatment courses.

Microbiology

Microbiology studies life forms that require magnification to see. Microorganisms are microscopic, living, single- or multicellular organisms that include bacteria and viruses. There are five major divisions of microbiology. **Protozoology** is the study of single-celled animals. **Mycology** is the study of fungi, molds, and yeast. **Bacteriology** is the study of all bacteria (single-celled organisms without chlorophyll that reproduce asexually). **Virology** is the study of viruses, tiny non-cellular infectious agents that cannot be grown outside the living host. **Saprophytic bacteria** are microorganisms that ingest dead organic matter. A **microbial enzyme** is an enzyme produced by a microorganism; these enzymes contribute to decomposition by breaking down tissues.

Classification of Bacteria

Bacteria are single-celled organisms without a nucleus or organelles. They can live and function as individual cells or cluster together in a **colony.** Bacteria are classified according to their shapes. **Cocci** are sphere-shaped and responsible for food poisoning and pneumonia. **Bacilli** are rod-shaped and responsible for botulism, tetanus, and infections from *Escherichia coli* and salmonella. **Spiral** bacteria are further classified as **vibrios** (curved), **spirilla** (thick, unflexing spiral), or **spirochetes** (thin, pliable spirals). **Pleomorphic** bacteria are shaped based on their surrounding environment. Masses of bacteria are typed by arrangement**,** or how the group of cells looks. Bacterium can appear as **diplo-** (paired), **strepto-** (in a single strand), **tetrads** (four in a square, grouping with additional squares), **sarcinae** (eight form a cube), and **staphylo-** (sporadic groupings like grape clusters).

Bacterial Reproduction, Colonization, and Infection

Bacterial growth occurs in conducive environments. Bacterial cells require nutrients, carbon, water, nitrogen, and an energy source. Nucleic acids, lipids, and carbohydrates must be present to produce new cells. **Autotrophic bacteria** exist by self-sustenance, consuming inorganic materials for nutrients and using photosynthesis or chemosynthesis as a supply of energy. **Heterotrophic bacteria** exist by consuming organic (carbon-containing) materials as a supply of energy. Bacterial growth occurs by **binary fission**, which produces a new cell identical to the first. The cell divides by replicating its DNA while the cell grows larger. The chromosomes split in two, and a new cell wall forms between them as the cell pulls apart into two cells. Bacterial colonization is when bacteria are present in or on a host. Infection is when this colony causes disease.

Contamination and Disinfection

Contamination occurs when infectious materials such as soiled items are introduced to an area. An **opportunist** is a microorganism that does not typically cause disease in a healthy person but is potentially pathogenic in an unhealthy person. A **fomite** is an inanimate object, such as clothing or an instrument, that can transmit disease or organisms. **Sterilization** is the process of destroying any and all life forms on a surface area. **Disinfection** refers to the use of a **disinfectant**, a physical or chemical agent used to completely eliminate disease-causing microorganisms. This process is important for embalming instruments and is done with an **autoclave**, which sterilizes contaminated instruments with steam. Another method of sterilization is the immersion of an instrument in a suitable cold chemical sterilant. A **germicide** is a chemical that destroys microorganisms, a **viricide** destroys a virus, a **fungicide** destroys fungi, and a **bactericide** destroys bacteria. An **insecticide** is a solution or agent that destroys insects. A **bacteriostatic agent** is a biological or chemical agent that halts bacteria's ability to reproduce. **Quaternary ammonium compounds** are used as a topical disinfectant on the surface of the epidermis or on instruments. **Fumigation** is the use of a chemical gas to kill microbes.

Microbial Controls, Antiseptics, Disinfectants, and Chemical Controls

Microbial control can be accomplished using chemicals, physical means, or both in conjunction to **decontaminate** or eliminate microbes or microbial growth so they are no longer hazardous. Chemicals that kill microbes on living surfaces are called **antiseptics**, while those used on nonliving tissue are **disinfectants.** It is important to use the correct chemicals, following the manufacturer's instructions, for each situation to ensure that the decontamination process is effective. Factors that influence the effectiveness of antimicrobial chemicals are chemical concentration (high concentrations kill microbes quickly but superficially, while lower levels kill microbes slowly but soak deeper into the cells); temperature (high temperatures typically increase effectiveness, though the temperature must remain within the combustion limits); exposure time; microbial population (larger masses take longer to kill); and environmental influences (e.g., surface, suspension, and potential chemical interactions).

Chemicals are essential for disinfecting equipment, instruments, floors, and walls in the preparation room. They are also used to disinfect decedents topically and internally.

Chemical control methods include bactericides, fungicides, bacteriostatic chemicals, and fumigation.

Pathogens, Contamination, Virulence, and Toxins

Pathogens are bacteria, fungi, protozoans, algae, microbes, and parasites that cause disease in humans. **Infestation** is the unwanted presence of a large number of insects, rodents, or other animals. **Contamination** occurs when the human body or a surface is exposed to microbes. Exposure can be topical or internal through a wound, bite, food, or air. **Virulence** is a microbe's ability to infect an organism and cause disease within it. Pathogens cause and produce specific virulence factors that allow them to impact the host.

Toxins, products produced by microbes to harm the host cells and impact their ability to function normally, are a virulence factor. **Exotoxins** are proteins produced by bacteria that target a specific area of the body, causing damaging disease. **Endotoxins** are located within the cell walls of pathogenic microbes. They are typically lipopolysaccharides. When host cells or antibiotics attack bacteria, the cell wall breaks down and releases endotoxins. Upon release they can travel throughout the body but do not specifically target an area of the host like exotoxins. They are less toxic than exotoxins but harder to kill.

Infection and Transmission

An **infection** refers to the entrance, formation, and growth of a pathogen in the body or host organism, causing harm. A **nosocomial infection** is acquired in a hospital, nursing home, or rehabilitative facility. The earliest appearing infection in a host is called the **primary infection**. A **secondary infection** occurs after a primary one but is due to a different living organism. Elective localization, now called a **focal infection**, is when an infection is confined to a small area of the body such as a tooth or an eye. **Bacteremia** occurs when a decedent has bacteria in the blood. **Septicemia** is characterized by a bacterial infection that has spread through the vessels of the body. A **communicable** disease can be directly transmitted to another host. A **mechanical vector** is an organism (often an insect) or object that carries a disease on the exterior of its body and transfers it to a new host. A **biological vector** is a living carrier in which the disease-causing organism first grows or proliferates into increasing numbers before becoming infectious to a new host.

Disease and Pathogen Transmission

Pathogens enter the body at a **portal of entry**. **Exogenous** infections come from the exterior environment, while **endogenous** infections are caused by microbes normally in the body. Microbes can enter the skin via damaged areas (wounds, scrapes, or punctures) or natural openings (hair follicles or sweat glands). A protective mucous membrane layer covers the respiratory, gastrointestinal, and urogenital tracts. These membranes can be breached by microbes that are aerosolized, are present in food or liquid, or enter the body directly through an opening. They can be transmitted via parenteral routes such as sexual activity, placenta, or punctures.

Disease spreads when microbes pass through a **portal of exit** such as the gastrointestinal system (through vomiting or diarrhea) or the respiratory system (sneezing or coughing). The body expels the pathogens and infects another person through touching or direct contact with contaminated body fluids; through indirect contact via a reservoir such as contaminated tissues, bedding, towels, or needles; or through respiratory droplets expelled during exhaling, sneezing, or coughing.

There are many factors that influence an individual's susceptibility to infections. Genetics, age, gender, and race all play a role. Disease and medical treatments can also affect the immune system, not only increasing the risk of infection but also impacting how well the body fights off the infection.

Immune Response to Antigens

Antigens are anything that enters the body and evokes an immune response. Foreign materials, fungi, viruses, bacteria, protozoans, allergens, venom, and other toxins are examples of antigens. **Antibodies** are produced as part of an immune reaction to an antigen.

Immune Defense Mechanisms

The body has **innate** immune responses that are activated when an antigen is detected. These include the **first-line defense mechanisms** (physical and chemical barriers) and **second-line defense mechanisms** (phagocytosis, inflammatory response, or fever). When these responses cannot control the invasion, the **adaptive immune system** begins to work. This reaction is slower because it takes the body time to produce antigen-specific defenses. These **third-line defense mechanisms** include cell-mediated immunity and humoral immunity.

Cell-Mediated Immunity, Humoral Immunity, and Immune Sensitivity

Cell-mediated immunity involves **T cells**, which are lymphocytes specially created for defending the body against antigens. **Humoral immunity (antibody-mediated immunity)** involves **B cells**, which are white blood cells specializing in producing specific antibodies during immune responses. When a B cell discovers an antigen, it undergoes **clonal selection**, splitting into plasma cells and memory cells. Plasma cells produce antibodies, while memory cells aid in future immune response to the same antigen.

Hypersensitive immune responses cause an overreaction (allergic response), while hyposensitive immune responses (such as those caused by AIDS) underreact or completely fail to respond.

Common Bacterial Infections

Bacteria	Disease	Mode of Transmission
Staphylococcus aureus	Staph infection, including MRSA	Direct contact
Streptococcus pyogenes	Includes necrotizing fasciitis and toxic shock syndrome	Direct or indirect contact, ingestion, or inhalation
Streptococcus pneumoniae	Pneumococcal disease	Inhalation
Neisseria gonorrhoeae	Gonorrhea	Direct sexual contact
Neisseria meningitidis	Meningococcal disease	Extended direct contact
Clostridium tetani	Tetanus	Direct contact through a wound
Clostridium perfringens	Food poisoning	Ingestion
Clostridioides difficile (formerly *Clostridium difficile)*	C. difficile infection	Inhalation or direct contact with fecal material; usually only develops after taking antibiotics
Corynebacterium diphtheriae	Diphtheria	Direct contact with nasal, eye, or oral secretions
Salmonella enteritidis	Salmonella	Ingestion
Salmonella typhi	Typhoid fever	Ingestion
Francisella tularensis	Tularemia	Direct contact, ingestion, or inhalation
Mycobacterium tuberculosis	Tuberculosis (TB)	Inhalation
Mycobacterium avium complex	MAC infection	Inhalation
Treponema pallium	Syphilis	Direct contact with a syphilitic sore (chancre)

Bacteria	Disease	Mode of Transmission
Borrelia burgdorferi	Lyme disease	Bite from infected blacklegged tick (deer tick)
Mycoplasma pneumonia	Respiratory infection	Inhalation
Vibrio cholera	Cholera	Ingestion
Yersinia pestis	Plague	Bite from infected flea, direct contact, or inhalation
Klebsiella pneumoniae	Klebsiella infection	Direct contact
Clostridium botulinum	Botulism	Ingestion
Bacillus anthracis	Anthrax	Direct contact, ingestion, or inhalation
Leptospira interrogans	Leptospirosis	Direct contact with infected urine through a wound, or ingestion
Hemophilus influenzae	Includes Hib	Inhalation
Bacteroides spp.	Includes bacteremia and abscesses	Present in the gastrointestinal tract of all people; illness usually caused by escape into other systems
Proteus spp.	Includes urinary tract infections	Direct contact or ingestion
Pseudomonas spp.	*Pseudomonas* infection	Direct contact
Shigella	Shigellosis	Inhalation or direct contact with fecal material
Escherichia coli	E. coli	Present in all people; illness caused by ingestion
Campylobacter jejuni	Campylobacteriosis	Ingestion
Helicobacter pylori	Includes ulcers	Ingestion (present in most people)
Chlamydia trachomatis	Chlamydia	Direct sexual contact

Rickettsial Diseases

Bacteria from the order Rickettsiales cause a large number of diseases in humans. They are carried by **biological vectors**: ticks, mites, lice, and fleas. *Rickettsia* spp. are usually carried by ticks and can cause cat flea rickettsiosis and several forms of typhus and spotted fever. *Orientia* spp. are carried by mites and chiggers and cause forms of typhus. *Anaplasma* spp. are carried by ticks and cause anaplasmosis. *Ehrlichia* spp. are carried by ticks and cause ehrlichiosis. Symptoms of rickettsial infections vary but usually include headache, nausea, vomiting, fever, and often a rash. Many are caught while traveling and have an incubation period of 5–10 days. Due to the broad range of nonspecific symptoms and the lack of tests for many species, they can be difficult to diagnose. If caught early enough, they are generally treatable with the tetracycline class of antibiotics. Some **rickettsial diseases** can be fatal if untreated. There are no vaccines for rickettsial diseases.

Viruses

Viruses are microbes that are made up of DNA or DNA coated in protein. They reproduce by infecting cells of living organisms and using parts of those cells to make copies of themselves. This can make the organism sick. There are many viruses that infect humans. For many viruses, there are vaccines that can prevent or reduce the severity of illness. Viruses are frequently transmitted by respiratory droplets but can also be transmitted through direct contact or contact with body fluids.

Viral Diseases

Disease	Typical Symptoms	Mode of Transmission
Rubella (German measles)	Fever, sore throat, and a rash that starts on the face and spreads to the rest of the body	Respiratory droplets
Influenza	High fever, headache, muscle aches, dry cough, runny nose, and fatigue	Respiratory droplets
Coronaviruses	Cold-like symptoms, including a cough, runny nose, sore throat, and congestion	Respiratory droplets
COVID-19	A pandemic coronavirus that may cause severe symptoms	Respiratory droplets
Respiratory syncytial virus (RSV)	Nasal congestion, cough, sore throat, and headache; may be severe in infants	Respiratory droplets
Herpes simplex virus 1 (HSV-1)	Cold sores around the mouth	Close contact
Herpes simplex virus 2 (HSV-2)	Painful genital lesions	Sexual contact
Epstein-Barr	Infectious mononucleosis	Contact with body fluids
Measles	High fever, cough, congestion, conjunctivitis, Koplik spots (white spots in the mouth), and a rash consisting of flat red spots that start on the face and spread to the rest of the body	Respiratory secretions
Mumps	Painful swelling of the salivary glands	Saliva
HIV/AIDS	Flu-like symptoms, weight loss, and concurrent infections; death if untreated	Sexual contact or contact between mucous membranes and certain body fluids including blood

Review Video: Viruses and Antiviral Drugs
Visit mometrix.com/academy and enter code: 984455

Protozoa

Protozoa are microscopic, single-celled animals. Many protozoa are parasites and can cause diseases. **Malaria** is caused by a parasite from the genus *Plasmodium*. These protozoa are transmitted by the female *Anopheles* mosquito, which lives in tropical areas. **Giardia** is caused by the protozoan *Giardia lamblia*, which infects water supplies. It is the most common cause of non-bacterial diarrhea in the United States. **Toxoplasmosis** is a common infection caused by *Toxoplasma gondii* in undercooked meat or cat feces. Many people have no symptoms or flu-like symptoms, but people with weakened immune systems can have severe symptoms, including brain and eye damage.

Fungi

Fungi (singular: fungus) are organisms that feed on organic material and reproduce via spores. Mushrooms, yeasts, mildew, and mold are all fungi. Many fungal infections cause no symptoms in healthy people, but those with weakened immune systems may become ill. **Cryptococcosis** usually results from inhaling the fungus *Cryptococcus neoformans,* which is found in soil worldwide. It can also be caused by *Cryptococcus gattii,* which is associated with certain trees in the northwestern United States. People with cryptococcosis can have symptoms similar to pneumonia or meningitis.

Histoplasmosis is caused by inhalation of spores from the fungus *Histoplasma capsulatum*, which is found in soil and is associated with bird and bat droppings. It can cause flu-like symptoms. The fungus *Pneumocystis jirovecii* can cause pneumonia. Most people have been exposed to this by the age of 3 or 4. *Candida* is a type of yeast that may cause a variety of infections, including oral thrush, candidal esophagitis, candidal intertrigo (diaper rash), and candidemia. **Ringworm** is caused by the *Tinea* fungus. It appears on the skin as scaly, ring-shaped patches with normal centers. The patches may blister and ooze. It is transmitted by touching affected skin or through objects that have touched affected skin.

Funeral Practice Test #1

Want to take this practice test in an online interactive format?
Check out the online resources page, which includes interactive practice questions and much more: **mometrix.com/resources719/funeral**

Funeral Arts

1. The study of death and dying that places an emphasis on the psychological and social aspects is called:

a. Psychology
b. Psychiatry
c. Pathology
d. Thanatology

2. What is it called when someone makes funeral arrangements ahead of time for themselves or a loved one?

a. Aftercare
b. At-need
c. Near-need
d. Pre-need

3. What is a memorial service?

a. A service following cremation in which the cremated remains must be present
b. A service held without the decedent's body present
c. A liturgical and traditional service held prior to disposition
d. A non-religious service with or without the body present

4. When making funeral arrangements, when must the funeral director give the customer a copy of the General Price List (GPL)?

a. As soon as the customer sits down
b. After taking all the information for the death certificate
c. Before selecting the casket
d. When any mention of prices or costs is brought up

5. Funeral homes should conduct unannounced inspections and records reviews of a third-party crematory to:

a. Establish a contract between a between them.
b. Provide advice on operation standards.
c. Reduce liability, ensuring quality and legal operations standards.
d. See what other funeral homes use the crematory.

6. Which of the following is NOT a condition required for a negotiable instrument?

a. Must have an order to pay
b. Must be payable upon demand
c. Must be in writing
d. Must be conditional

7. Some cemeteries require cremated remains to be buried in:

a. An urn vault
b. A temporary container
c. A double urn
d. A niche

8. A will is an instrument for the ordered disposition of real and personal property that is to take effect upon death. Which of the following is a requirement for a will to take effect?

a. The will has a codicil.
b. The deceased was of legal age.
c. There was intestacy on the part of the legatee.
d. The will is notarized.

9. What company will ship human cremated remains?

a. UPS
b. FedEx
c. USPS
d. Any airline

10. The person with the authority and duty of final disposition who may or may not have actual custody (physical possession) of the deceased at a particular moment is considered to have what kind of custody?

a. Caveat emptor
b. Constructive
c. Consignment
d. Endowment

11. Having a grief counselor on staff at the funeral home for the families to speak with and to host bereavement groups is considered what type of aftercare?

a. Indirect aftercare services
b. Direct aftercare services
c. Information-oriented aftercare services
d. Therapeutic aftercare services

12. Funeral directors should encourage family ________________in funeral rites.

a. facilitation
b. participation
c. organization
d. bonding

13. Federal legislation that was designed to prohibit job discrimination on the basis of race, religion, color, national origin, and sex is called:

a. Age Discrimination Employment Act
b. Occupational Safety and Health Act
c. Immigration Reform and Control Act
d. Equal Employment Opportunity Act

14. What contributed to the popularity of cremation in ancient cultures?

a. Cremation symbolized releasing or freeing the spirit and allowed for easy transportation.
b. Cremation was easier to perform than burials.
c. Cremation was a quick way to dispose of the body.
d. Cremation was done because embalming was not around yet.

15. Who regulates crematories in the United States?

a. The federal government
b. The Cremation Association of North America
c. Crematories are unregulated
d. State and local government agencies

16. Which of the following is a liability?

a. The funeral home
b. Vehicles
c. Payroll
d. Office equipment

17. To begin the arrangement conference, the funeral director should:

a. Immediately gather information necessary for documents and records.
b. List the service options the funeral home offers.
c. Ask a question about the deceased to allow the family to begin opening up.
d. Present the General Price List to the family.

18. What does the Uniform Anatomical Gift Act regulate?

a. Paramount rights of disposition and disposition selection when someone dies intestate
b. Organ donation for donors and donees
c. Only how medical facilities can use anatomical gifts
d. The regulation of financial gifts to support organ donation programs

19. What is a cremulator?

a. A metal disc used for the identification of cremated remains
b. A pulverization machine
c. The combustion system within a crematory
d. The temperature regulation system on a cremation unit

20. During an arrangement conference, a family member says he would like to bring in a peanut butter jar for his father's cremated remains. What is the best way for the funeral director to respond?

a. Tell him that this is not allowed by law.
b. Explain that the crematory will not allow it.
c. Explain that if the jar is not large enough, the rest of the remains will have to be put into another container.
d. Suggest that the family purchase an urn on which a picture of a peanut butter jar can be engraved.

21. What type of pre-need contract has funds set aside and cannot be canceled?

a. Revocable pre-need contract
b. Non-guaranteed pre-need contract
c. Irrevocable pre-need contract
d. Guaranteed pre-need contract

22. Which of the following is a liability for funeral processions?

a. Inconsiderate and inattentive drivers outside of the procession
b. Funeral flags and amber lights
c. Police or traffic escorts
d. Four-way flashing lights

23. When does a funeral director's contractual liability begin?

a. With an oral agreement
b. With a written agreement
c. With either a written or oral agreement
d. When the decedent enters their care

24. Which of the following is true about pre-need law?

a. Pre-need funeral contracts can be established as non-guaranteed
b. Pre-need funeral contracts are not transferable
c. Pre-need funeral contracts must be established as irrevocable
d. The FTC regulates all pre-need funeral contacts

25. Due diligence is defined as:

a. The effort a business puts into recruiting another business to enter into a subcontract with them
b. A deadline given to a business to provide another with their procedure and policy manuals
c. A reasonable evaluation of a business, conducted prior to engaging in a business relationship, to ensure quality service and reduce liability
d. A liability one business has to another business to ensure they are operating within professional and ethical standards

26. What is the cornerstone of the Federal Trade Commission's Funeral Industry Practices Trade Regulation Rule?

a. The Funeral Rule
b. The General Price List
c. The Embalming Disclosure
d. The Statement of Funeral Goods and Services Selected

27. Which of the following should an adult do when a child is grieving?

a. Wait to tell them about the death until it is absolutely necessary.
b. Keep them from going to the cemetery.
c. Let them participate in the funeral if they want to.
d. Encourage them not to talk about it to other people.

28. Caskets use various lining materials. One material is a thin, crinkled cloth made of silk, cotton, rayon, or wool called:

a. Crepe
b. Satin
c. Velvet
d. Linen

29. What is a structure used to commemorate the life, work, and contributions of a decedent, named after the Latin word for *remind*?

a. Plaque
b. Memorial
c. Marker
d. Monument

30. Which of the following is NOT a trend associated with the increasing cremation rate?

a. Increasingly distinct regional differences
b. Shifted societal and spiritual principles
c. Increased life expectancy
d. Increasingly transient society

31. Providing the family with informational pamphlets, cards, books, and grief resources falls under which type of aftercare?

a. Information-oriented aftercare services
b. Direct aftercare services
c. Professional aftercare services
d. Basic aftercare services

32. Who has the paramount right to authorize disposition by cremation?

a. The oldest child
b. Spouse
c. Siblings
d. All children over 18

33. A funeral director can help a family with their grief by doing which of the following?

a. Tell them they do not need to write the obituary.
b. Offer to give the eulogy so a family member doesn't have to.
c. Explain that they do not need to go to the cemetery.
d. Allow them to bring in items from a collection their loved one had.

34. The reduction of the body in a controlled environment where accelerated decomposition is achieved using temperature, organic matter, and oxygen controls to facilitate microbial growth describes what form of disposition?

a. Alkaline hydrolysis
b. Cryonics
c. Natural organic reduction
d. Pyre

35. When recording personal belongings and effects, what should be detailed about jewelry?

a. Only the type of jewelry
b. Type of jewelry and observable details
c. Type of jewelry and materials (such as metal and stone type)
d. Record the details the family tells you about each item

36. Based on historical evidence, when did cremation first begin being used as a form of disposition?

a. 3000 BC
b. 400 AD
c. 2500 BC
d. 800 BC

37. What purpose does a car list serve?

a. Aids in parking cars at the cemetery
b. Guides the lineup of cars for the procession
c. Keeps track of funeral home fleet vehicles
d. Coordinates how the family will get to the funeral home

38. When someone pays a deposit or the entire amount for a preplanned funeral, all of the following can be done with the funds EXCEPT:

a. The entire amount can be deposited into the funeral home's bank account.
b. The funds can be deposited into an account at the local bank.
c. The funds can be deposited into the state funeral director association's trust fund.
d. In some states, the funds can be used for a life insurance policy for the deceased.

39. What is a *first call*?

a. The initial contact the family makes to other family members to notify them of their loved one's death
b. The initial contact made to the funeral home notifying them of a death to request assistance with disposition
c. The initial call police make to a family to notify them of a death
d. The initial call a sales representative makes to a funeral home to pitch new products

40. What is an alternative cremation container?

a. A combustible casket constructed with minimal metal elements and designed specifically for cremation
b. A cardboard container with interior fabrics that is used inside a casket shell
c. A simple receptacle, composed of easily combustible materials, used to hold a decedent prior to cremation and to ease placement into the cremation retort
d. A basic, industry-standard plastic container used to store cremated remains in lieu of an urn

41. Which of the following is NOT required to be on the Statement of Funeral Goods and Services Selected?

a. A disclosure identifying cash advances that are marked up
b. A list of all required items
c. The reason why embalming was selected
d. A signature of the person agreeing to pay for services

42. Who is eligible for burial in Veterans Affairs national cemeteries?

a. Eligible veterans and their immediate family
b. Only eligible veterans who are cremated
c. Eligible veterans, their spouses, and dependent children
d. Only honorably discharged veterans

43. Which of the following is NOT considered an asset when determining eligibility for Medicaid assistance and Supplemental Security Income?

a. Revocable pre-need funeral contracts over $1,500
b. Income from pre-need insurance policies
c. Irrevocable pre-need funeral contracts
d. Money intended for purchasing a burial space

44. Someone who exhibits atypical responses to grief or does not make progress on their grief journey to restructure their life without their loved one is experiencing what type of grief?

a. Maladaptive grief
b. Complicated grief
c. Normal grief
d. Advanced grief

45. Most crematories require the body of the deceased to be in a rigid container for the cremation process. Which of the following does NOT meet the definition of most crematories of a rigid container?

a. The deceased is in a mahogany casket.
b. The deceased is wrapped in a sheet.
c. The deceased is on a flat board.
d. The deceased is in a cardboard box.

46. Which of the following is not necessary information to gather during a first call?

a. Embalming permission
b. Decedent's name
c. Phone number for the place of death
d. Social security number

47. John dies and does not leave a surviving wife. He does, however, have nine children, and some of them express a desire to have his body cremated. In a state that requires the cremation process to be authorized by at least 60% of the children, how many of John's children must sign the authorization form?

a. Three
b. Five
c. Six
d. Seven

48. Similar to cremation, what major liability do alternative methods of disposition (natural organic reduction or alkaline hydrolysis) pose for funeral directors?

a. The processes are unknown, creating liability risks.
b. The processes increase liability with their rise in popularity because they are more environmentally friendly.
c. The processes are culturally and religiously controversial, creating the risk of community division.
d. The processes have liabilities surrounding decedent identification.

49. Under the Magnuson-Moss Warranty Act, what are funeral homes obligated to do?

a. Include indemnification of warranties on pricing documentation
b. Provide warranty information prior to the sale of a product
c. Display product reviews next to merchandise or compiled in a clearly labeled binder
d. Give adopted warranties on all products offered

50. What is *aftercare*?

a. Any additional treatment and care of the body after embalming preparation is completed to further prepare the decedent for the services
b. The process of preparing the cremated remains for burial or return to the family following the cremation process
c. Services, information, and support provided to grieving families following the funeral services
d. The work done at the cemetery to fill in and finish the grave after the committal service

51. When arranging for human remains to be shipped to a foreign country, what authenticates the government seals on the decedent's documentation?

a. A dry, raised, or impressed seal
b. The embassy's approval of the receiving country
c. The consulate's certification
d. An apostille

52. The federal government agency created to promote consumer protection, encourage free and fair competition, and prevent what regulators determine to be anti-competitive business practices is called:

a. FTC
b. ICCFA
c. OSHA
d. NFDA

53. Under the Bloodborne Pathogen Standard, employee training records must be retained for how many years?

a. 30 years
b. 25 years
c. 10 years
d. 5 years

54. What is a Reeves stretcher?

a. The backboard used on a stretcher to ease transferring the decedent on and off the stretcher
b. A flexible device used to secure and transfer a decedent out of tight quarters
c. An oversized stretcher used to accommodate obese decedents
d. A pulley device installed in the transfer vehicle to mechanically pull the stretcher into the vehicle

55. What is a section of a cemetery consisting of multiple interment spaces called?

a. Section
b. Lot
c. Block
d. Grave

56. Which of the following is NOT considered a liability associated with the cremation process?

a. Pulverizing cremated remains
b. Cremating personal possessions
c. Properly identifying the decedent and, later, their cremated remains
d. Securing authorizations

57. What is the legal definition of a dead body?

a. Any form of human remains
b. A human who is no longer breathing on their own
c. A human who is no longer alive but not completely degraded
d. Human remains reduced to skeletal remains

58. What liability do pacemakers implanted in the decedent pose for cremation?

a. The pacemaker could revive the person.
b. The pacemaker could shock the person handling the decedent.
c. The pacemaker battery can explode when subjected to heat, causing damage to the retort.
d. The pacemaker will beep continuously until it is disabled with a magnet.

59. Which of the following is NOT a manner of death on a death certificate?

a. Undeterminable
b. Accidental
c. Euthanasia
d. Natural

60. When funds have been prepaid for someone who is on Medicaid, they are deposited into an irrevocable account. If the funds in the account exceed the amount of the services provided when the death occurs, what happens to the leftover amount?

a. It is returned to the next of kin in a personal check made out to him or her
b. It must be sent to the Medicaid office
c. The funeral home can keep the entire amount
d. The institution where the money was deposited keeps it

61. There are three main factors that influence the grieving process. They are psychological, sociological, and:

a. External
b. Internal
c. Physiological
d. Illogical

62. What method can be used to calculate the relationship between the wholesale cost of merchandise and the combined cost of services and merchandise for the purchaser?

a. Gross profit margin
b. Merchandise value ratio
c. Consumer value index
d. Net profit margin

63. A person who is given a decedent's personal property based on a will is called a:

a. Consignee
b. Legatee
c. Devisee
d. Bailee

64. The science that studies various social groups and how individuals behave and relate to each other as a group to other social groups that can influence funeral service disposition arrangements is:

a. Funeralization
b. Ethnocentrism
c. Pathology
d. Sociology

65. Which of the following is NOT one of the five stages of grief presented by Dr. Elisabeth Kübler-Ross?

a. Acceptance
b. Bargaining
c. Anger
d. Shock

66. What is probate?

a. When someone dies without a will
b. Putting one's affairs in order prior to death
c. Settling and closing the estate of a decedent
d. Acknowledgement of a will and appointment of executor

67. What should be done following an identification viewing?

a. The next of kin should sign a statement or form acknowledging their identification of the decedent.
b. The next of kin should be given a photograph of the decedent to retain.
c. The next of kin should be given a memorial token.
d. The next of kin should sign a disclosure and indemnification form releasing the funeral home from liability related to their identification viewing experience.

68. When working with a family, you notice that one person seems to be struggling. When you approach this person, he says with strong hesitation, "I'm fine." This is an example of which type of nonverbal communication?

a. Facial expression
b. Paralanguage
c. Proxemics
d. Body position

69. A typical funeral cortege would be arranged in the following order:

a. Lead car, hearse, clergy, pallbearers, family cars/limo, and procession
b. Lead car, hearse, pallbearers, clergy, family cars/limo, and procession
c. Hearse, lead car, clergy, pallbearers, family cars/limo, and procession
d. Lead car, clergy, pallbearers, hearse, family cars/limo, and procession

70. Which of the following is a safety-labeling exemption in the preparation room?

a. Nonhazardous chemicals do not need to be labeled.
b. Chemicals mixes less than 10 gallons for immediate use do not need to be labeled.
c. Chemical mixes less than 10 gallons for use throughout the day do not need to be labeled.
d. There are no exemptions.

71. What do funeral homes use to create community cognizance, attract new customers, and maintain their client base?

a. Pre-need sales
b. Marketing
c. Community service
d. Aftercare

72. What is the removal of a dead body from its place of rest called?

a. Interment
b. Reinterment
c. Inhumation
d. Disinterment

73. The time-weighted average test monitors an employee's formaldehyde exposure levels, which must be less than __________ over an eight-hour period.

a. 0.75 ppm
b. 2.0 ppm
c. 0.5 ppm
d. 0.2 ppm

74. What is the definition of *vital statistics*?

a. The system for birth, marriage, and death record management
b. Information about the decedent used to complete legal documentation for government agencies to record, analyze, and track data
c. Data that funeral directors are required to retain on file at the funeral home for a state-regulated amount of time
d. Data collected to track disposition methods across the country

75. Depreciation can be claimed on which of the following?

a. Health insurance
b. Vehicles
c. Legal expenses
d. Payroll

76. What is the term used to describe a non-metal, non-ornamental receptacle used to enclose human remains?

a. Alternative container
b. Temporary container
c. Urn vault
d. Aron casket

77. Which of the following is NOT considered a form of aftercare?

a. Information regarding various grief journeys on the funeral home's website
b. Tribute ceremonies held for the bereaved during the holidays
c. Providing a list of local bereavement professionals to the family
d. Giving the family a laminated obituary of their loved one after the services

78. Grief that is excessive, does not come to a satisfactory conclusion, and is accompanied by the individual's awareness of their inability to resolve the bereavement process is called:

a. Masked grief
b. Delayed grief
c. Chronic grief
d. Exaggerated grief

79. During a procession into and recession out of a funeral chapel, church, or service location, which direction should the casket face?

a. The head end of the casket should enter the service room first while the foot end exits first.
b. The head end of the casket should lead in and out of the service room.
c. The foot end of the casket should lead in and out of the service room.
d. The casket can process into and recess out of the chapel facing any direction.

80. What type of property rights give the next of kin the right to treat a decedent as property, giving them the authority to make disposition decisions?

a. Real property
b. Quasi-property
c. Intellectual property
d. Personal property

81. Which of the following must be notified when you are planning a service that includes visiting hours, a funeral, and a burial?

a. The officiating person and the cemetery
b. The burial vault company and the cemetery
c. The officiating person only
d. The officiating person, the cemetery, and the burial vault company

82. Which of the following is NOT a sundry item?

a. Register book
b. Memorial folders
c. Honorarium
d. Clothing

83. "A civil violation of rights that results in damages" is the definition of:

a. Negligence
b. Liability
c. A tort
d. Mental anguish

84. The reduction of human remains to bone matter using a chemical mixture, high temperature, mechanical elements, and agitation refers to disposition by:

a. Aquamation
b. Terramation
c. Cryonics
d. Natural organic reduction

85. Which of the following statements is true about shipping human remains via common carrier within the United States?

a. They have to be embalmed.
b. They have to be sent prepaid.
c. They must be in a casket.
d. They must be accompanied by a burial/transit permit.

86. The legal principle by which precedents are established by prior decisions made by the court that also serves to provide insight into the potential outcome of similar cases is called:

a. Statute of limitations
b. Statutes
c. Equal Employment Opportunity Act
d. Stare decisis

87. What is a container consisting of a wooden base tray and cardboard top used to enclose casketed remains for shipping purposes called?

a. Temporary container
b. Combination tray
c. Air tray
d. Ziegler case

88. Which of the following is not an engineering control that reduces formaldehyde exposure?

a. Keeping the lid on the embalming machine
b. Securing lids on chemical products when not in use
c. Using a ventilation system to change air
d. Access to an emergency drench shower

89. In her book On Death and Dying (1969), Elisabeth Kübler-Ross identified and described the stages of dying. In order, these stages are:

a. Accept, express, adjust, and reinvest
b. Numbness, yearning, disorganization and despair, and re-organization
c. Shock, awareness of loss, conservation-withdrawal, and healing and renewal
d. Denial, anger, bargaining, depression, and acceptance

90. What is it called when a funeral home combines a set of services and merchandise together, offering them for a set price?

a. Itemized pricing
b. Package pricing
c. Economy pricing
d. Loss leader pricing

91. The relationship between the decedent and survivor, the nature of death, and prior experience with death are categorized by Beverly Rafael as what type of influences on grief?

a. Physiological
b. Sociological
c. Psychological
d. Biological

92. The common patterns and range of feelings and behaviors people exhibit after the loss of a loved one is called:

a. Grief syndrome
b. Guilt
c. Shame
d. Attachment theory

93. Which parties were influential in supporting the introduction and rise of cremation in the United States in the late 1800s?

a. Government officials and legislative bodies
b. Protestant clergy and medical professionals
c. Journalists and funeral practitioners
d. Catholic priests and sanitary health professionals

94. What personal effects should be removed from the decedent prior to the cremation beginning?

a. Clothing
b. Blankets, sheets, and pillows
c. Anything metal
d. Whatever the family requests

95. Which of the following are barriers that negatively influence a person's ability to effectively listen and process information?

a. Selective listening, bias, and exhaustion
b. Paralanguage, environment, and posture
c. Proxemics, body positioning, and eye contact
d. Awareness, rebuttals, and attentiveness

96. A wrongful act by a person for which damages can be sought by the injured party through a civil lawsuit is called a:

a. Tort
b. Mutilation
c. Obstruction
d. Replevin

97. Which of the following are the four fundamental principles of funeral management?

a. Planning, controlling, executing, and flexibility
b. Actuating, organizing, planning, and evaluating
c. Planning, coordinating, embalming, and cleaning
d. Inventory management, directing, organization, and rigidity

98. What is the rubber strip called that runs along the edge of the top body molding and between the lids of a half-couch casket and is used to seal the casket?

a. Gauge
b. Galvanized
c. Gasket
d. Gimp

99. Which of the following statements concerning the merchandise pricing strategy known as the declining price structure model is correct?

a. Creates a lower margin on the less-expensive caskets
b. Creates a lower margin on the most expensive caskets
c. Encourages the consumer to buy better merchandise since the consumer value index improves with higher-priced caskets
d. Both b and c

100. A casket constructed of various tree species such as willow, poplar, or cottonwood is called:

a. Single-hinged panel
b. Wood veneer
c. Selected hardwood
d. Pine box

101. What psychologist defined grief as the natural, necessary, and painful process of removing energy invested in a loved object that no longer exists to reinvest in something else?

a. Erik Erikson
b. Elisabeth Kübler-Ross
c. Sigmund Freud
d. Abraham Maslow

102. A trial balance helps a business owner do which of the following?

a. Keep track of inventory
b. Help with vehicle maintenance
c. Show profits and losses
d. Ensure accurate payroll

103. The entryway, foyer, or lobby to a funeral home or church is also called the:

a. Narthex
b. Nave
c. Niche
d. Sanctuary

104. Which of the following is a ferrous metal?

a. Copper
b. Stainless steel
c. Bronze
d. Zinc

105. Showrooms that have small sectional displays of caskets are called:

a. Fractional display rooms
b. Traditional display rooms
c. Quarter display rooms
d. Sectional display rooms

106. What percentage of pre-need funds do most states require to be placed into the financial trust or account?

a. 95%
b. 100%
c. 75%
d. 50%

107. Who established the first modern crematory, the basis of today's cremation units?

a. Dr. Hugo Erichsen
b. Sir Henry Thompson
c. Professor Ludovico Brunetti
d. Dr. Julius LeMoyne

108. Community outreach programs are an effective part of what aspect of a business?

a. Market research
b. Business management
c. Public relations
d. Advertising

109. A funeral director, acting in good faith, follows the directions of the next of kin based on the information they are provided. What disclosure protects the funeral director from liability in lawsuits resulting from inaccurate information or false next of kin representation?

a. Identification disclosure
b. Indemnification disclosure
c. Risk disclosure
d. Privacy disclosure

110. What is a non-traditional funeral service?

a. A non-religious service
b. A service without the body present
c. A service strictly following traditional religious rites
d. A contemporary religious service

111. A merchandise pricing method in which the funeral home uses a varied markup that increases for higher-cost items is called:

a. Fixed multiple factor
b. Declining price structure
c. Gradual recovery
d. Increasing price structure

112. The Jewish religion executes many rituals when someone dies. The preparation of the body for burial is called:

a. Shiva
b. Chevra kadisha
c. Yahrzeit
d. Tahara

113. What is a pall?

a. The stand used to hold the casket during services
b. A group of people who carry the casket
c. A cloth draped over the casket as a symbolic part of a religious funeral ceremony
d. The cloth skirt that is placed around the casket supports during a service

114. What is the most important part of displaying burial vaults?

a. Having a full-size vault in your selection room
b. Being able to explain the characteristics and advantages of each vault
c. Having a cross section of a vault
d. Showing pictures of vaults

115. What OSHA standard is the Needlestick Safety and Prevention Act regulated under?

a. Formaldehyde Exposure Standard
b. Bloodborne Pathogen Standard
c. Hazardous Communication Standard
d. General Industry Standard

116. Under common law, what is a nuisance?

a. Regulations that dictate what property within a particular area can be used for
b. A natural but atypical use of property which neighboring properties approve of
c. An uncommon and unusual use of property that disturbs neighboring properties
d. A classification of issues addressed and resolved by town or city counsels

117. Prior to closing the casket, what does the funeral director need to verify with the family?

a. In what order they want the cars for the procession
b. How they would like the decedent's hair and cosmetics done
c. What items remain in the casket and which items should be removed
d. How many rows of seating they want reserved in the service room

118. On the Statement of Funeral Goods and Services Selected, what category are cemetery fees placed under?

a. Additional services and facilities fees
b. Cash advances
c. Professional services selected
d. Alternative services

119. Which occurs first prior to a public visitation?

a. Family viewing
b. Prayer service
c. Committal service
d. Fraternal service

120. What act was issued by the Wage and Hour Division of the Department of Labor to regulate minimum wage, overtime, and equal pay?

a. Civil Rights Act
b. Equal Employment Opportunity Act
c. Fair Labor Standard Act
d. Age Discrimination in Employment Act

121. What are the average interior dimensions of an adult metal casket?

a. 86" × 30"
b. 75" × 23"
c. 84" × 29"
d. 78" × 23"

122. What authorizations must be secured prior to cremation?

a. A certified death certificate and a disposition permit
b. A certified death certificate, disposition permit, acknowledgement from an identification viewing, and next of kin authorization for cremation
c. Authorizations by next of kin and a certified death certificate
d. A certified death certificate, disposition permit, coroner or medical examiner authorization, and next of kin authorization

123. What is the top piece of an upright monument consisting of two pieces called?

a. Slant
b. Epitaph
c. Base
d. Die

124. Alkaline hydrolysis is also known as:

a. Cremation
b. Natural organic reduction
c. Cryonics
d. Aquamation

125. What type of closure creates a non-gasketed seal made by fusing the edges of the openings together?

a. Latched closure
b. Hermetically sealed closure
c. Chemical closure
d. Threaded closure

126. How should the funeral home employee or answering service speak during a first call?

a. Slightly slower speed than normal conversation
b. A sharp, short, and business tone
c. Soft, quiet speaking volume
d. Emphatic inflection and energetic tone

127. A community event hosted by the funeral home during the holidays to memorialize and pay tribute to the loved ones of the families they have served throughout the year is an example of what type of program?

a. Pre-need care
b. At-need care
c. Aftercare
d. Therapeutic care

128. The person who executes a promissory note is called the:

a. Maker
b. Payee
c. Drawee
d. Drawer

129. A ceremony provided by a social organization in conjunction with a funeral or memorial service is referred to as a:

a. Church service
b. Celebrant service
c. Fraternal service
d. Committal service

130. What function does the disposition permit serve?

a. Disposition permits are used to settle legal affairs.
b. Disposition permits are only used by cemeteries to record and document decedents who are traditionally buried.
c. Disposition permits are used to legally record and document the decedent's vital statistics and cause of death.
d. Disposition permits allow for and document transportation and disposition of decedents.

131. Failure to meet the legal duty a funeral director has to families and attendees to keep their premises safe and reasonably maintained falls under what legal category?

a. Tort liability
b. Zoning ordinances
c. Statutory duties
d. Contractual obligations

132. A deceased veteran must meet which of the following criteria in order to be eligible for military honors?

a. Have an honorable discharge
b. Obtained the rank of sergeant or higher
c. Died during wartime
d. Have a discharge other than dishonorable

133. Which of the following is true of Elisabeth Kübler-Ross's five stages of grief?

a. They do not always occur in order.
b. A grieving person usually completes them in about six months.
c. Each one takes about the same amount of time.
d. When people try to make a deal with God, it is called "denial."

134. When you record a payment made for a funeral, it will decrease the amount associated with which of the following?

a. Accounts payable
b. Accounts receivable
c. Expenses
d. Assets

135. An insolvent estate is an estate of a deceased person whose assets are not sufficient to pay the estate's debts, taxes, and administrative expenses. State statutes control the priority of these claims. In most states, the priority of claims—from top priority to lowest—is ordered as follows:

a. Taxes, funeral expenses, and medical bills
b. Medical bills, taxes, and funeral expenses
c. Funeral expenses, administration expenses, and taxes
d. Administration expenses, funeral expenses, and taxes

136. The amount by which a business's current assets exceed liabilities, defined as the operating liquidity of a business, is also known as:

a. Statement of operations
b. Working capital
c. Proving cash
d. Useful life

137. To communicate with those who are mourning the recent loss of a loved one to facilitate the bereavement process and help them move through the stages of grief is called:

a. At-need counseling
b. Grief therapy
c. Grief counseling
d. Both a and b

138. When entering a Catholic church for a Mass of Christian Burial, the casket is covered with which of the following?

a. A pall
b. A veil
c. A flag
d. A blanket

139. When a beneficiary brings in a life insurance policy to be used as payment for the funeral services, he or she signs a form. What is this form called?

a. An assignment
b. A consideration
c. A comfort letter
d. A mediation

140. The four items that affect an individual's views on death are religion, family, culture, and:

a. Gender
b. Race
c. Tradition
d. Financial status

141. Which of the following is the most important part of the arrangement conference?

a. Getting the death certificate information
b. Listening carefully
c. Writing the obituary
d. Explaining the costs

142. The summative experience of grieving and adapting to living after the loss of a loved one is called:

a. Mourning
b. Bereavement
c. Thanatology
d. Grief

143. When a funeral director begins talking to another director about purchasing his/her funeral home, the potential purchaser will probably be asked to sign which of the following types of agreements?

a. Collateral agreement
b. Confidentiality agreement
c. Consideration agreement
d. Collective agreement

144. How did funeral directors react to cremation as it began to increase in popularity?

a. They accepted and supported the cremation movement.
b. They began opening their own crematories.
c. They rejected and spoke out against cremation.
d. They looked for ways to meaningfully serve cremation families.

145. Which of the following religions prohibits cremation?

a. Catholicism
b. Islam
c. Buddhism
d. Judaism

146. What is natural organic reduction?

a. Reducing the body to bone matter in a pyre
b. Natural decomposition that occurs to the body as the casket deteriorates in the grave
c. Decomposition of a body in an accelerated, controlled, and contained environment
d. Reducing the dead with a natural alkaline chemical mixture

147. Which of the following individuals can sign the appropriate forms to authorize the cremation of a body?

a. An ex-spouse
b. A medical doctor
c. An agent assigned by the deceased in applicable states
d. The deceased's clergyman

148. Which of the following is an example of a material used for a biodegradable urn?

a. Marbelon
b. Metal
c. Plastic
d. Salt

149. Which of the following funeral rites is conducted without the presence of the casketed body?

a. Entombment service
b. Memorial service
c. Graveside service
d. Traditional or complete cremation service

150. How can a funeral director and funeral home reduce their liability in contracting with a third-party crematory?

a. Publish an indemnification disclosure annually.
b. Review records and perform visual inspections periodically.
c. Interview each employee at the crematory.
d. Oversee the cremation process.

151. What is the 1/8" thick (or thinner) velvety or woven material used to cover a casket called?

a. Doeskin
b. Broadcloth
c. Plush
d. Twill

152. If a woman deposits money in a preneed burial account at her local bank, the bank assumes which of the following roles?

a. Assignee
b. Devisee
c. Fiduciary
d. Distributee

153. What is a VA Form 21-2008?

a. Application for a United States flag
b. Application for a Presidential Memorial Certificate
c. Military discharge record request
d. Burial allowance application

154. Under the Hazardous Communication Standard, where must a collection of safety data sheets be retained, one for each chemical and product used in the preparation room?

a. In the preparation room
b. In the funeral director's office
c. In the main office and the preparation room
d. Everywhere chemicals are stored

155. When written laws and statues are not in place, what type of law is used to fill in legal gaps by referencing precedents, outcomes of previous cases, and universal principles?

a. Common law
b. Case law
c. Federal law
d. Constitutional law

156. In accordance with the orthodox Jewish funeral rite, the Chevra Kadisha performs what ceremony?

a. Tahara
b. Tachrichim
c. Tallitot
d. Torah

157. Throughout the funeral arrangements, the funeral director guides the family and acts as a:

a. Counselor
b. Therapist
c. Mediator
d. Legal advisor

158. Which of the following does NOT need to be addressed on the cremation authorization form?

a. Decedent identification information
b. Name of the funeral home
c. Final disposition directions
d. Communicable disease disclosure

159. There are various types of casket interior styles. In one style, the lining material is placed on a metal form. Weights are added, and the material is then steamed and attached to an upholstery or backing. This interior style is known as:

a. Masselin
b. Crushed
c. Extendover
d. Tufted

160. Crematories are required to have a standard operating procedure manual, a compilation of policies, documents, and procedures detailing facility operations, made available to which of the following?

a. Employees
b. Funeral directors contracting with the crematory
c. Any member of the general public
d. All of the above

161. A deceased veteran or reservist who was entitled to receive retired military pay qualifies to receive an American flag after the completion and submittal of the Application for United States Flag for Burial Purposes form, also known as:

a. VA Form 21-530
b. SSA-721
c. VA form 27-2008
d. VA form 40-1330

162. A funeral director can help family members by acknowledging their grief. Of the following family members, which person's grief is usually acknowledged the least by society?

a. A spouse
b. A sibling
c. A parent
d. A child

163. What type of survivor relationship is typically the least socially acknowledged loss?

a. Spouse
b. Parent
c. Child
d. Sibling

164. What type of wooden caskets come from deciduous trees?

a. Coniferous
b. Softwood
c. Hardwood
d. Particle board

165. What provides a grieving family with social and psychological support following a death?

a. Funeral rituals
b. The arrangement conference
c. Grief therapy
d. Hospice guidance

166. When is a casket protector used?

a. For mausoleum entombments
b. For in-ground interments
c. To protect against inclement weather
d. During casket deliveries

167. What is the best way to reduce identification liability prior to cremation?

a. Have a family member or family-appointed representative view the body to ensure it is properly identified.
b. Show photographs of the decedent to the family so they can identify the person.
c. Trust the hospital or facility identification tag.
d. Fingerprint all decedents prior to cremation.

168. Why is there more liability with disposition by cremation than by earth burial?

a. The cremation rate is higher than the burial rate.
b. Cremation is irreversible, while buried bodies can be exhumed.
c. Cremated remains are returned to the family, while buried bodies stay at a cemetery.
d. Cremation is not as environmentally friendly as burials.

169. A portable stretcher used by both ambulances and funeral homes to move the injured or deceased that is considered to be the most important item for transferring remains from a house or an institution is called a:

a. Cot
b. Flexible stretcher
c. Transfer vehicle
d. Church truck

170. Which of the following statements about outer burial containers is true?

a. All cemeteries require outer burial containers.
b. Vaults have sealing properties to protect caskets from outside elements.
c. Grave liners are not outer burial containers.
d. Fiberglass outer burial containers do not withstand heavy weight loads.

Funeral Science

1. The middle third of the face is designated by the measurement between what features?

a. The inner canthus of the eye to the upper lip
b. The superior margin of the eyebrow to the base of the nose
c. The bridge of the nose to the base of the nose
d. The zygomatic arch to the lip closure line

2. The femoral artery is ____________________ to the femoral vein.

a. medial and deep
b. posterior and deep
c. lateral and superficial
d. inferior and lateral

3. Additional and specific permission, outside of general embalming permission, must be secured from the family for any restorative alterations to the body EXCEPT:

a. Removal of malformations
b. Shaving facial hair
c. Treating body conditions such as edema and jaundice
d. Injecting feature builder to treat emaciation

4. How are the eyelids placed in a correct eye closure?

a. They meet in the middle.
b. The top lid meets the bottom lid two-thirds of the way down the eye.
c. The top lid closes all the way down over the eye to overlap the bottom lid.
d. The top lid closes all the way down over the eye to meet the bottom lid.

5. In preparing for a Catholic viewing at the funeral home, what should be set up on or near the casket?

a. Cross
b. Pall
c. Crucifix
d. Prayer shawl

6. The difference between the potential pressure reading and the actual pressure reading indicates the:

a. Vacuum pressure
b. Rate of flow
c. Differential pressure
d. Both rate of flow and differential pressure

7. A gelatinous tissue filler is not the only substance that can be used hypodermically to rebuild tissue. Which of the following can also be used?

a. Distilled water
b. Lip wax
c. Massage cream thinned with a little mineral oil
d. Tissue filler solvent

8. Post embalming, a tissue reducer can be used to:

a. Remove swelling and edema
b. Reduce neck swelling by securing it around the decedent's neck to apply weight and pressure to the area
c. Channel tissue to drain fluid to lower areas of the body
d. Procure tissue from organ donors

9. A type of bacterium that can cause tissue gas and can be transmitted from one deceased person to another as a result of improper disinfection of the trocar between uses is:

a. *Streptococcus pyogenes*
b. *Clostridium perfringens*
c. *Clostridium tetani*
d. *Staphylococcus aureus*

10. The widest part of the skull is measured between the:

a. Parietal eminences
b. Temporal bones
c. Zygomatic arches
d. Mental eminences

11. When shipping caskets in air trays on flights, how should the casket be closed?

a. Sealed
b. Taped closed
c. Left slightly ajar
d. Locked

12. Embalming is necessary in which of the following situations?

a. When the family chooses a direct burial
b. When the FTC Funeral Rule requires it
c. When the deceased will be shipped out of town
d. When the family requests it

13. What condition does existing tissue need to be in prior to beginning reconstruction with wax?

a. Malleable and dry
b. Soft and malleable
c. Firm and dry
d. Moist and firm

14. What is another name for the lips of the mouth where the exterior coloration is present?

a. Mucous membrane
b. Line of closure
c. Integumentary lip
d. Medial lobe

15. What is the name for rod-shaped bacteria?

a. Pleomorphic
b. Bacillus
c. Coccus
d. Vibrio

16. Using the theory of complimentary colors, what color of concealer will cover a bruise that is red?

a. Beige
b. White
c. Green
d. Brown

17. How should a funeral director return personal effects to the family?

a. Clean and organize items in an appropriate size bag
b. Remove and return items directly to the family
c. Remove and return all items to the family as soon as they come for arrangements
d. Store items in a sealed bag and return after the services

18. What facial feature changes the least throughout one's lifetime?

a. Mouth
b. Eyes
c. Nose
d. Ear

19. Cosmetics can be classified by their ability to allow light to pass through them. The type that does not allow light to pass through and is considered a concealing cosmetic is:

a. Translucent
b. Transparent
c. Opaque
d. Aerosol

20. There are seven basic shapes that describe the form of a head when observed from the front. The most common is where the cheekbones are wider than the cranium and the cranium is a little wider than the lower jaw. This shape is called:

a. Diamond
b. Oval
c. Round
d. Oblong

21. Antemortem chemotherapies and drug use impact embalming by:

a. Altering the properties of embalming chemicals
b. Increasing the permeability of cell membranes throughout the body
c. Decreasing the amount of arterial chemicals required for preservation
d. Decreasing the effectiveness of the arterial chemicals

22. The chemical secretions given off by the endocrine glands are called:

a. Hormones
b. Red blood cells
c. White blood cells
d. Bile

23. Aligning the trocar from the left anterior iliac spine with the point extending towards the right earlobe across the torso is the guide for reaching the:

a. Liver
b. Left side of the heart
c. Right lung
d. Right side of the heart

24. Which of the following does not necessarily suggest that the body should be reaspirated?

a. Received from another funeral home
b. Abdominal distention
c. Oral purge
d. Leaking cranial incision

25. The term for the condition in which excess blood is localized or pooled in an area that is not able to allow for the normal drainage movement of blood as a result of a disease is:

a. Thrombosis
b. Passive hyperemia
c. Active hyperemia
d. Embolism

26. The molecular movement of matter from an area of greater concentration to an area of lower concentration is:

a. Hydrolysis
b. Saturation
c. Diffusion
d. Compound

27. There are three types of blood vessels: arteries, veins, and:

a. Atria
b. Ventricles
c. Valves
d. Capillaries

28. Which of the following factors do not significantly influence arterial selection?

a. Trauma
b. Accessibility
c. Morbidity
d. Gender

29. What is responsible for the coloration of a person's skin?

a. Blood and carotene
b. Melanin, carotene, and adipose
c. Melanin, blood, and carotene
d. Carotene, blood, and adipose

30. What should be done with medical devices removed during embalming or after cremation?

a. Place in biohazard or medical waste disposal containers
b. Recycle metal components for profit
c. Return devices to the hospital
d. Autoclave metal devices

31. Gels used in the embalming process for an autopsied body have the same basic composition as which of the following types of chemicals?

a. Jaundice fluids
b. Cavity fluids
c. Humectants
d. Co-injection fluids

32. There are approximately six devices that can be used to inject arterial solution. Which of the following is NOT a device historically used during embalming?

a. Bulb syringe
b. Gravity bottle
c. Centrifugal pump
d. Hand pump

33. When a solution has all the solvent it can hold, this condition is known as:

a. Saturation
b. Sublimation
c. Inflammation
d. Binary fission

34. What is a postmortem examination conducted by a pathologist to determine the cause of death and manner of death for unattended, suspicious, accidental, or violent deaths called?

a. Hospital autopsy
b. Partial autopsy
c. Necropsy
d. Forensic autopsy

35. What type of arterial solutions should be used to treat anasarca?

a. Hypertonic arterial solutions
b. Arterial solutions with small colloidal molecules
c. Low strength arterial fluid
d. Hypotonic arterial solution

36. What is the structure that begins at the nasal wing and extends down to the same level as the line of closure called?

a. Angulus oris sulcus
b. Nasal sulcus
c. Nasolabial fold
d. Philtrum

37. Fluids that work well with arterial embalming fluids but have a higher concentration of preservatives and disinfectants are called:

a. Pre-injection fluids
b. Co-injection fluids
c. Cavity fluids
d. Venous fluids

38. How far down the orbital cavity is the line of closure of the eye?

a. Three-quarters
b. One-third
c. Two-thirds
d. Half

39. When a muscle of form and expression contracts, it pulls the skin creating what type of facial marking?

a. Smoothed skin
b. Furrow
c. Sulci
d. Eminence

40. Autopsies can be done on the complete torso and cranium, and on which of the following?

a. Thorax
b. Arms
c. Legs
d. Neck

41. In cases where it is necessary to use an electric spatula, it must always be used with which of the following?

a. Water
b. Massage cream
c. Soap
d. Nothing

42. When there is excessive swelling in the neck, a pattern of sutures can be made in the back of the neck. These points of entry and exit form which letter?

a. V
b. X
c. M
d. N

43. Using intermittent drainage during embalming will do which of the following?

a. Decrease saturation in the tissues.
b. Create clots.
c. Make aspirating the organs unnecessary.
d. Provide better distribution of the fluid.

44. Neurotropic diseases can be caused by infectious diseases that affect the nervous system and often create inflammation. The most specific term for the disease condition in which inflammation and swelling of the brain occurs is:

a. Encephalitis
b. Meningitis
c. Myelitis
d. Poliomyelitis

45. A common lesion such as a blister that forms an elevation on the skin and contains fluid is a:

a. Furuncle
b. Vesicle
c. Ulcer
d. Carbuncle

46. When do standard pacemakers need to be removed?

a. Prior to embalming
b. Prior to cremation
c. Prior to dressing and casketing
d. Prior to aspirating

47. There are several physical methods to control microorganisms. Which of the following physical methods is generally accepted as the least bactericidal?

a. Dry heat
b. Moist heat
c. Autoclave
d. Cold

48. Because of the chemical structure of embalming fluids, where is the best place to have an exhaust fan in the embalming room?

a. Close to the embalming table near the floor
b. In the ceiling
c. High on the opposite wall near the ceiling
d. Near the door

49. The branch of anatomy that studies how disease affects the structure and function of the body is:

a. Regional anatomy
b. Gross anatomy
c. Pathological anatomy
d. Systemic anatomy

50. When is the correct time to inject tissue builder with a hypodermic syringe?

a. After embalming
b. Before closing the mouth
c. After disinfecting
d. Before embalming

51. What treatments or procedures should be done at a minimum for an identification viewing without embalming?

a. Wash, set features, and dress the body
b. Set features and aspirate
c. Aspirate and inject cavity chemicals
d. Nothing, just unzip the stretcher cover and tuck it around the person's face

52. Where are the carotid artery and jugular vein located?

a. Posterior to the sternocleidomastoid muscle
b. Posterior to the trachea
c. Posterior to the sternum
d. Parallel to the ulnar artery

53. *Index*, as used in embalming, is defined as:

a. The ratio of formaldehyde, methyl alcohol, and water in a solution
b. The quantity of formaldehyde incorporated into 100 milliliters of a solution
c. The primary dilution strength of an arterial solution
d. The density of formaldehyde solution compared to the density of water

54. The hip contains a pair of coxal bones, and is made of three fused bones collectively known as:

a. The patella
b. The pelvic girdle
c. The phalanges
d. The circle of Willis

55. What chemicals or treatments should NOT be used in preparing a body for a delayed disposition?

a. Humectants
b. Preinjections
c. Vascular conditioners
d. Formaldehyde-based arterial fluids

56. What acquired facial markings occur between the eyebrows across the root of the nose or up from the root of the nose to the glabella?

a. Nasolabial sulci
b. Transverse frontal sulci
c. Superior palpebral sulci
d. Intercilliary sulci

57. What photographic angle provides a vantage that allows the eye to pick out a person's natural asymmetries and characteristics that may be unnoticed in other views?

a. Profile
b. Inverted
c. Three-quarter
d. Frontal

58. Carbon monoxide poisoning initially results in a:

a. Purple-red intravascular discoloration
b. Cherry red intravascular discoloration
c. Yellow intravascular and extravascular discoloration
d. Red extravascular discolorations in the form of dots

59. Which of the following is not a recommended point of entry for hypodermic tissue building along a sunken temple of the decedent?

a. Eyebrow
b. Hairline
c. Posterior to the anterior portion of the helix
d. Posterior to the superior part of the jawline

60. What is the convex area of the eye between the upper eyelid and the supercilium referred to as?

a. Superior palpebra sulcus
b. Supraorbital area
c. Naso-orbital sulcus
d. Orbital Pouch

61. Where should cranial hair restorations begin?

a. At the inferior margin
b. At the superior margin
c. At the center
d. At the medial margin

62. What is formaldehyde dissolved in water called?

a. Phenol
b. Index
c. Paraformaldehyde
d. Formalin

63. What instrument is used to remove thin layers of skin during tissue procurements performed by organ donation recovery teams?

a. Hemostat
b. Bistoury knife
c. Dermatome
d. Separator

64. Which of the following correctly describes the amount of movement associated with a synarthrosis articulation?

a. Not moveable
b. Somewhat moveable
c. Extremely moveable
d. None of the above; synarthrosis does not refer to articulation

65. Where is rigor mortis first observed on a decedent?

a. Large muscles
b. The muscles of organs
c. Muscles below the waist
d. Small muscles

66. Who is considered the father of embalming?

a. Joseph Henry Clarke
b. Dr. Thomas Holmes
c. Dr. Auguste Renouard
d. A. Johnson Dodge

67. What type of suture is used as armature or a reconstruction base?

a. Intradermal suture
b. Purse string suture
c. Baseball suture
d. Basket-weave suture

68. The center of the circulatory system is the:

a. Lungs
b. Heart
c. Arteries
d. Veins

69. In cases of delayed disposition of an embalmed body, what practice does not help maintain the body in ideal condition?

a. Appling massage cream to the hands and face
b. Spraying mold inhibitors on the body
c. Eliminating airflow
d. Keeping the decedent in a cool area

70. The bones that create the superior portion of the sides and the back of the cranium and account for the posterior two-thirds of the roof of the cranium are the:

a. Parietal bones
b. Occipital bones
c. Temporal bones
d. Zygomatic bones

71. What is the longest vein in the body?

a. Aorta
b. Inferior vena cava
c. Greater saphenous vein
d. Femoral vein

72. What are hexoses?

a. Fats
b. Emulsifiers
c. Carbohydrates
d. Organic acids

73. What legislative body regulates the use of refrigeration to delay disposition without embalming or prior to embalming?

a. Federal
b. State
c. Municipal
d. County

74. What type of modifying agent is used as an additive to arterial or supplemental fluids to specifically regulate pH within the vascular system and bodily tissues?

a. Humectants
b. Surfactants
c. Buffers
d. Borates

75. What type of wax is thick and slightly firm, used to fill surface blemishes or superficial areas requiring restoration?

a. Surface restorer wax
b. Lip wax
c. Wound filler
d. Restorative derma-surgery wax

76. What plastic garment should be used for protection when there is edema in the shoulders?

a. Sleeves
b. Unionalls
c. Capris
d. Coveralls

77. What effect do red or pink colored lights have on a cosmetized body?

a. They increase the red tones of cosmetics.
b. They decrease the red tones of cosmetics.
c. They decrease the reddish appearance of the body.
d. They highlight red tones in the cosmetics better.

78. What are embalming chemicals that are not used for arterial injection or cavity injection classified as?

a. Topical chemicals
b. Vascular chemicals
c. Supplemental chemicals
d. Accessory chemicals

79. What are the four steps of embalming case analysis?

a. Transport, embalm, dress, and casket
b. Observe body conditions, evaluate known information, select chemicals, and determine injection site
c. Disinfect, set features, inject, and aspirate
d. Observe, evaluate, implement, and assess results

80. Which of the following is considered an inexpert test of death?

a. Stethoscope
b. Electrocardiogram
c. Pulse
d. Evoked response

81. According to facial proportions, which of these equals the width of an eye?

a. The width of the base of the nose
b. One third the width of the mouth
c. One fourth the width of the face
d. One half the distance between the eyes

82. What is the term used for severe dehydration in which the body takes on a leathery appearance?

a. Desiccation
b. Imbibition
c. Ecchymosis
d. Crepitation

83. What is the center of drainage?

a. Left atrium
b. Right atrium
c. Left ventricle
d. Right ventricle

84. What is a source that causes an immunological response within the body?

a. Antiseptic
b. Antidote
c. Antibody
d. Antigen

85. What is the definition of *livor mortis*?

a. Temperature loss after death
b. Intravascular discoloration caused by settling of the blood to dependent areas
c. Areas of the body that have pressure restricting gravitational settling of blood
d. Extravascular postmortem staining

86. The four categories of embalming are cavity, arterial, hypodermic, and:

a. Co-injection
b. Autopsy
c. Surface
d. Pre-injection

87. What is the portion of the nose that extends from the forehead to the columna nasi called?

a. Glabella
b. Dorsum
c. Bridge
d. Root

88. Which of the following types of hepatitis is classified as highly contagious?

a. Hepatitis A
b. Hepatitis B
c. Hepatitis C
d. Hepatitis D

89. The most common of the basic linear forms of facial profiles is called:

a. Vertically balanced profile
b. Convex profile
c. Concave profile
d. Horizontally balanced profile

90. What is a metal cylinder with an interior rod used to expand the vein for drainage purposes called?

a. Angular spring forceps
b. Drain tube
c. Groove director
d. Trocar

91. The major source of formaldehyde in aqueous solution for human preservation purposes contains ____ percent HCHO gas by weight and ____ percent HCHO gas by volume in a compound commonly known as formalin.

a. 40; 37
b. 37; 40
c. 37; 30
d. 40; 27

92. What is the name of the muscle that is used as an anatomical guide for the common carotid artery?

a. Sternoclavicular articulation
b. Platysma
c. Omohyoid
d. Sternocleidomastoid

93. What is the thickest layer of an artery?

a. Intima
b. Media
c. Adventitia
d. Lumen

94. All of the following are types of arterial fluid preservatives EXCEPT:

a. Aldehydes
b. Phenolic compounds
c. Formaldehyde "donor" compounds
d. Humectants

95. Which of the following is the study of facial proportions?

a. Physiognomy
b. Physiology
c. Restorative art
d. Facial positioning

96. What is the post embalming discoloration of the body caused by formaldehyde reacting with hemoglobin called?

a. Biliverdin
b. Postmortem bruising
c. Formaldehyde gray
d. Formaldehyde burn

97. What is the second branch off the arch of the aorta?

a. Left common carotid
b. Brachiocephalic artery
c. Left subclavian artery
d. Right subclavian artery

98. A written record and sketch diagram of the condition of the body upon arrival to the funeral home, the method of embalming, treatments, the times at which the body arrived and preparations were completed, and the license numbers of the embalmers and assistants is called the:

a. Putrefaction case report
b. Sanitation case report
c. Decomposition case report
d. Embalming case report

99. Facial width is typically measured using which facial structure as a measuring standard?

a. The width of the base of the nose
b. The width of the eye
c. The width of the ear
d. The width of the mouth

100. There are four guides used in trocar aspiration. They serve to access the heart, cecum, urinary bladder, and:

a. Lungs
b. Liver
c. Stomach
d. Kidneys

101. A facial profile in which the forehead, upper lip, and chin all protrude to the same point is referred to as what type?

a. Concave
b. Vertical
c. Convex
d. Vertical convex

102. What is the norm used as a basis for the proportions of facial standards and a measurement for facial comparisons called?

a. Proportions of beauty
b. Beauty baseline
c. Classic proportions
d. Canon of beauty

103. In cases of jaundice, what causes bilirubin to turn into biliverdin?

a. Formaldehyde
b. Gluteraldehyde
c. Acidic pH
d. Basic pH

104. What is a connection between two blood vessels called?

a. Anastomosis
b. Vasa vasorum
c. Capillary
d. Aneurysm

105. Which of the following is one of the main arteries commonly used in embalming?

a. Iliac
b. Ulnar
c. Femoral
d. Aorta

106. A suture made around a circular opening or puncture that closes the margins when it is pulled is called a:

a. Basket-weave suture
b. Purse-string suture
c. Bridge stitch
d. Whip stitch

107. To calculate the number of ounces of fluid to use per gallon (128 ounces) of water for a 2 percent solution, which of the following formulas would you use?

a. 2 × the index of the fluid ÷ 128
b. 2 × 128 ÷ the index of the fluid
c. The index of the fluid ÷ 128
d. The index of the fluid × 128

108. What is a 10 inch long, 3/16" hollow bore instrument with a 90° curve used in aspiration called?

a. Autopsy aspirator
b. Hydro aspirator
c. Nasal tube aspirator
d. Trocar

109. What is the superficial suture used to reduce excess tissue by turning the margins of the incision under as they are brought together to create a flattened surface?

a. Intradermal suture
b. Worm suture
c. Purse string suture
d. Baseball suture

110. Before restoration can be done, what condition must be met?

a. Affected tissue must be firm and moist.
b. Tissue must be firm and dry.
c. Tissue must be soft and dry.
d. Tissue must be soft and moist.

111. What kind of brush would be used to simulate pores in the skin?

a. Tapered brush
b. Flat tip brush
c. Stipple brush
d. Pointed brush

112. Which of the following is a hollow organ?

a. Spleen
b. Brain
c. Kidney
d. Liver

113. What is the biggest issue that can result from short-term postmortem refrigeration prior to embalming?

a. Blood remains liquified
b. Superficial tissue dehydration
c. Rigor mortis slows
d. Livor mortis appears worse

114. Looking at the decedent straight on to observe direct facial characteristics provides what type of view?

a. Profile view
b. Frontal view
c. Inverted view
d. Three-quarters view

115. What is the chemical formula for formaldehyde?

a. HCOOH
b. HCHO
c. CHOCHO
d. CH_3OH

116. When embalming remains that have been autopsied, six arteries are usually used. Which of the following are two of them?

a. Right and left femoral
b. Right and left ulnar
c. Right and left iliac
d. Right and left jugular

117. When contracted, which direction does the zygomaticus major move the angle of the mouth?

a. Superior and posterior
b. Inferior and anterior
c. Inferior and posterior
d. Superior and anterior

118. When corneas have been donated, which of the following must be done?

a. Remove the materials left by the tissue bank in the eye socket and discard them.
b. Place an eye cap over the materials left in the eye socket by the tissue bank.
c. Carefully clean the outside of the eye and glue the eyelids to prevent any leakage only.
d. Excise any tissue remaining in the eye socket.

119. A blunt instrument used for tissue dissection and for determining the location and elevation of arteries and veins that is especially useful after the initial incision to locate the carotid artery and jugular vein is made is called.

a. Bistoury knife
b. Hemostat
c. Aneurism needle
d. Forceps

120. What type of mouth closure uses a suture that goes up into the left nostril from where the upper lip meets the maxilla, through the septum to the right side of the nose, and back down into the mouth, into the tissue where the lip and gum meet along the right side of the mandible, passing along to bone to the left side of the mouth before being securely tied?

a. Mandibular suture
b. Dental tie
c. Needle injector
d. Muscular suture

121. What are the contents of embalming drainage?

a. Blood and bodily fluids
b. Straight arterial solution
c. Blood, bodily fluids, and arterial solution
d. Blood and arterial solution

122. What is embalming fluid moving from the injection site throughout the vascular system to the capillaries called?

a. Diffusion
b. Distention
c. Distribution
d. Dilution

123. Funeral directors are ethically obligated to provide professional care that is:

a. Traditional and formal
b. Dignified and respectful
c. Quick and efficient
d. Legal and cheap

124. If a decedent develops blebs, what type of treatment should be done?

a. The decedent should be placed carefully in plastics to avoid rupturing the blebs.
b. The blebs should be drained.
c. The body should be reaspirated.
d. No additional treatment is necessary.

125. If there is not enough time or resources to do an adequate hair restoration, which of the following may be done?

a. Leave it as is and give an explanation to the family.
b. Use a scarf for a woman and a similar head bandage for a man.
c. Start the procedure and explain to the family that you didn't have time, but will complete it later.
d. Wrap a towel around the head.

126. The muscle that is the strongest chewing muscle of mastication and the one that assists in side-to-side movement of the mandible is the:

a. Temporal
b. Temporalis
c. Levator labii superioris
d. Corrugators

127. The decomposition of human remains is a chemical change in which matter is broken down into smaller types of matter. The most significant process related to this change is:

a. Vaporization
b. Diffusion
c. Adsorption
d. Hydrolysis

128. Casketed remains received from another funeral home should be:

a. Undressed to examine the condition of the body
b. Removed from the casket
c. Reaspirated
d. Refrigerated until the day of the services or disposition

129. What is secondary dilution?

a. Dilution of arterial embalming fluid as it enters the body
b. Dilution of embalming fluid when mixed in the embalming tank
c. Dilution of the embalming fluid as it drains from the body, mixing with table water
d. Dilution of the embalming fluid as it is bottled at the manufacturing plant

130. Which facial bilateral form is the main focal point for restoration work?

a. Forehead
b. Eyes
c. Nose
d. Cheeks

131. Which of the following bones are not procured as part of long bone donation?

a. Femur
b. Tibia
c. Humerus
d. Hemipelvis

132. The process by which blood settles or pools within the vessels to the dependent or lowest parts of the body as a result of gravitational movement is called:

a. Agonal hypostasis
b. Hemolysis
c. Intermittent drainage
d. Algor mortis

133. Which of the following are not arteries typically used for injection when embalming autopsied remains?

a. Left and right iliac
b. Left and right carotid
c. Left and right jugular
d. Left and right subclavian

134. What information can be used for the preembalming case analysis?

a. Distention
b. Drainage
c. Rigor mortis
d. Arteriosclerosis

135. What type of pressure measures the level of force within the tubing when the embalming machine is on "inject" and the stopcock is closed?

a. Rate of flow
b. Actual pressure
c. Injection pressure
d. Potential pressure

136. The natural facial marking that is a small convex distinction found lateral to the end of the line of closure of the mouth is called the:

a. Frontal eminences
b. Angulus oris sulcus
c. Frontal process of the maxilla
d. Angulus oris eminence

137. What is the final stage of embalming analysis?

a. Preembalming analysis
b. Postinjection evaluation
c. Cavity evaluation and treatment
d. Arterial injection

138. Calculate how much arterial fluid is needed per gallon to create a 2% solution using a 20-index fluid.

a. 12.8 oz/gallon
b. 10.5 oz/gallon
c. 16 oz/gallon
d. 8.2 oz/gallon

139. Using which of the following is NOT standard procedure in embalming a decedent who underwent an eye enucleation?

a. Preinjection
b. Restricted cervical
c. Slightly stronger arterial solution
d. Reduced rate of flow and injection pressure

140. In most states, all of the following people can observe the embalming process EXCEPT which of the following?

a. The attending physician
b. Nonparticipating embalmers
c. A family member of the deceased
d. The embalmer's non-licensed spouse

141. Hemorrhages can be classified based on where they actually occur. When there is bleeding inside the pleural cavity, it is known as a(n):

a. Epistaxis
b. Hemopericardium
c. Hemoperitoneum
d. Hemothorax

142. From where are coagulations and blood clots in embalming drainage removed?

a. Arteries and the heart
b. Veins and the heart
c. Arteries, veins, and the heart
d. Arteries and veins

143. What is the most common nasal profile form?

a. Convex
b. Concave
c. Roman
d. Straight

144. Under what circumstances can a funeral director refuse to let the next of kin view a decedent?

a. Immediate dispositions by cremation
b. Trauma or advanced decomposition
c. Drowning or burn victims
d. Never

145. Phalanges is the name used to classify bones in the distal portion of the:

a. Hand
b. Elbow
c. Toes
d. Ankle

146. What is intermittent drainage?

a. Drainage and injection are alternated
b. Drainage is stopped off and on throughout arterial injection
c. Drainage and injection occur simultaneously
d. Drainage is not taken

147. All living organisms are composed of one or more ____________, which regulate the structure and function of the organism.

a. cells
b. atoms
c. protons
d. molecules

148. What is the plastic garment that is pulled up over the legs, buttocks, back, and shoulders, also encasing the arms, before being zippered closed over the chest?

a. Coverall
b. Capris
c. Unionall
d. Shirt

149. Which of the following is the large opening at the base of the skull that is clearly exposed in a cranial autopsy?

a. Circle of Willis
b. Foramen magnum
c. Diaphragm
d. Interstitial space

150. Naturally occurring proteins that do not cease functioning when the body dies are called:

a. Catalytic enzymes
b. Autolytic enzymes
c. Digestive enzymes
d. Microbial enzymes

151. What type of dyes are used by manufacturers to distinguish arterial and supplemental chemical from one another?

a. Inactive dyes
b. Active dyes
c. Arterial dyes
d. Cosmetic dyes

152. What should be done with flower arrangements following a service?

a. Donate the flowers to a local hospital, hospice, or nursing home
b. Leave the flowers at the graveside
c. Follow family instructions for where the flowers should go
d. Deliver the flowers to the next of kin's house

153. What is the standard point of entry of the trocar for cavity aspiration?

a. Abdominal midline
b. 2 inches superior the umbilicus, midline
c. 2 inches superior and 2 inches to the left of the umbilicus
d. 2 inches superior and 2 inches to the right of the umbilicus

154. Multicolored blood clots with a dark layer of red blood cells beneath and clear layer of fibrin on top are referred to as:

a. Postmortem clots
b. Thrombosis
c. Postmortem coagula
d. Antemortem clots

155. For whom should an embalming case report be completed?

a. Decedents who are embalmed by the funeral home
b. Any decedent who enters the care of the funeral home, embalmed or not
c. Decedents who are embalmed and then shipped out to another funeral home
d. Decedents who are embalmed but later cremated

156. Which of the nine regions of the abdomen is located at the upper right section of the grid?

a. Right hypochondriac
b. Right epigastric
c. Right inguinal
d. Right hypogastric

157. Increased moisture, delicate skin, softer gums, small vasculature, and accessibility are all embalming challenges contended with in which of the following cases?

a. Infants
b. Children
c. Geriatrics
d. Trauma, all ages

158. What is one of the first things that needs to be done when a decedent enters the care of the funeral home?

a. Secure permission to transfer the decedent
b. Inventory personal effects
c. Embalm or box the decedent for cremation
d. Set features and prepare for identification

159. What is the term used to describe decomposition of body proteins?

a. Hydrolysis
b. Putrefaction
c. Proteases
d. Fermentation

160. Kaposi's sarcoma is sometimes seen in conjunction with which of the following?

a. Gangrene
b. Meningitis
c. COPD
d. AIDS

161. There are four major types of preservatives used in embalming fluids. One is formaldehyde. The other three are:

a. Aldehydes, alcohols, and phenols
b. Sterols, phenols, and alcohol
c. Sterols, lipids, and alcohol
d. Aldehydes, sterols, and phenols

162. When hemolysis of red blood cells occurs in a corpse and the result is post-mortem stain, the coloration made inside the body is referred to as:

a. Endogenous
b. Fomite
c. Atrophy
d. Exogenous

163. When reposed, the decedent's head should be straight or at what angle?

a. 15° angle to the left
b. 25° angle to the left
c. 15° angle to the right
d. 25° angle to the right

164. A condition in which there is a decrease in the number of white blood cells (leukocytes) that help fight disease circulating in the blood is:

a. Hemophilia
b. Leukemia
c. Polycythemia
d. Leucopenia

165. What is the opening of the ear called?

a. Tragus
b. External auditory meatus
c. Helix
d. Concha

166. What is the term used to describe death of the entire body?

a. Somatic death
b. Agonal death
c. Clinical death
d. Biological death

167. Bacteria are separated into three general groups according to their cellular shape. Which of the following is the term used to describe a bacterium that is rod-shaped or cylindrical?

a. Vibrio
b. Coccus
c. Spiral
d. Bacillus

168. What is the study of the properties, structures, and function of carbon and carbon-based compounds?

a. Organic chemistry
b. Inorganic chemistry
c. Biochemistry
d. Physical chemistry

169. Structures within the body that are used to locate another proximal structure are referred to as:

a. Linear guides
b. Anatomical guides
c. Anatomical limits
d. Anatomical margins

170. Syphilis is contracted in the four ways identified below. Which one accounts for approximately 95% of cases?

a. Sexual intercourse involving direct contact with fluids or lesions of an infected person
b. Placental transmission
c. Blood transfusion
d. Kissing

Answer Key and Explanations for Test #1

Funeral Arts

1. D: Thanatology is the analysis and study of death and dying and the states of affairs that are pressing on those involved. It evaluates how various factors integrate to influence a person's behavior. Psychology is the analysis and study of human and animal behavior and rationale, including how unique environmental circumstances influence behavior. Psychiatry is the scientific study of both mental and emotional abnormalities in people in order to provide treatment management options. Pathology is the scientific examination of diseases, including how the disease was contracted and how it affects physical well-being.

2. D: Pre-need arrangements are made prior to a death. They can be for the person making the arrangements or for a loved one. Pre-need arrangements help a person plan their final arrangements exactly how they want, allowing them to choose their method of disposition, service options, and merchandise and provide their own vital statistics. Some elect to write their own obituary. Pre-need can involve recording information and service selections, or it can include prefinancing. Near-need arrangements are done when a person is close to death; they are a subset of pre-need arrangements. Aftercare consists of services or information provided to family and friends following the services of a loved one. At-need arrangements are conducted following a death.

3. B: Memorial services are services conducted without the body present. They can be held prior to disposition, immediately after disposition, or months after disposition has occurred. Memorial services can be held for anyone regardless of their form of disposition (e.g., burial, cremation, body donation). They can be formatted however the family wants (e.g., traditional service, celebration of life, informal gathering, humanistic service) and can be held anywhere (e.g., church, funeral home, event locations, parks). When the body has been cremated, the cremated remains do not need to be present for the service to be classified as a memorial service.

4. D: The Federal Trade Commission's Funeral Rule requires that the funeral director provide the General Price List as soon as any mention of prices or costs is brought up. It doesn't matter if the customer asks about this as soon as they sit down or if it comes up within the order of topics that that the funeral director generally follows when meeting with a family. It must be provided as soon as the consumer asks questions about costs.

5. C: Conducting unannounced inspections of the crematory reduces the liability of a funeral home in contracting with a crematory. These inspections and reviews show due diligence in assuring that the crematory is operating professionally while meeting state and federal regulations. While many funeral homes do this prior to contracting with a crematory, it is not required for contract negotiations. Providing advice to the crematory for their operations policy is not necessary. Many third-party crematories serve other funeral homes in their area.

6. D: Negotiable instruments are in the form of either notes (promises to pay, like a loan) or drafts (orders to pay, like a check) and are considered an unrestricted (unconditional) guarantee that the writer will pay a specific amount of money to another party in exchange for goods or services. The Uniform Commercial Code is the model law that states have adopted into law regulating negotiable instruments. The requirements are that negotiable instruments must be in writing, must be signed, and must have an order to pay the holder in money upon demand. Missing information can either be implied or make the instrument invalid.

7. A: An urn vault is a receptacle used for retaining and protecting cremated remains that are buried in ground. The cremated remains are usually contained inside an urn or temporary container, which is then placed inside the urn vault for burial. Some cemeteries require urn vaults. Just like with outer burial containers, these protect the cremated remains and the urn from outside elements and weight loads. It also allows for the cremated remains to be disinterred more easily. Supply companies offer urn vault combinations to meet these requirements without having to purchase both an urn and urn vault as two units. The combination urn vaults are typically composed of marble, cultured marble, or a similarly durable synthetic material. Funeral directors should be aware of cemetery requirements so they can advise the family accordingly during the arrangement conference. If unaware of the cemetery requirements, disclose potential cemetery requirements to the family prior to them selecting an urn.

8. B: The deceased must be of legal age (generally over the age of 18, though there are exceptions) for the will to take effect. A will completed by a minor who dies while still a minor is not recognized as a legal will. A codicil is a formal addition to a will, but it is not a requirement for a will to take effect. The legatee is the person who is to inherit the personal property specified in the will. Intestacy is the condition that occurs when a person dies and has no will. Except in the state of Louisiana, wills do not have to be notarized.

9. C: The United States Postal Service is the only shipping organization that will ship human cremated remains. They must be shipped using either Priority Mail Express or Priority Mail Express International. The interior container must be sift-proof, not allowing any powder or particles to escape. The exterior container must provide protection and cushioning to withstand transportation. The box must then be clearly labeled as containing cremated remains.

10. B: *Constructive custody* in funeral service is the term applied to the custody rights that supersede actual custody rights, and they include the right of a party to control the disposition of the deceased. The person with actual custody may sometimes be a third party (such as a livery or common carrier), but someone else would maintain constructive custody at all times. *Caveat emptor* is Latin for "let the buyer beware." *Consignment* refers to merchandise shipped to an agent or to a customer. It does not take place as a result of an actual purchase, but under an agreement obliging the consignee to pay the consignor for the goods within a certain period of time once the merchandise is sold. *Endowment* refers to a permanent fund of property or money that is established to benefit an institution or person. An example is the sale of perpetual care cemetery property.

11. B: Therapy and counseling-based aftercare is considered a form of direct aftercare services. Direct aftercare can be individual, group, or event based. Information-oriented aftercare services consist of providing documentation (brochures, pamphlets, literature) to families and friends to help them navigate their grief journey.

12. B: Participation should be encouraged throughout the funeral process because it can be cathartic. Rituals of mourning refocus survivors, giving them specific tasks to complete and defined activities to channel their energy toward. Additionally, rituals bring comfort by reminding people of their beliefs and giving them a sense of community. Family participation can consist of picking songs, readings, and poems for the service; putting a picture collage or video together; lighting a candle as part of the ceremony; sharing stories and thoughts in a eulogy; dressing the decedent; participating in a cremation ceremony; bearing gifts; or acting as a pallbearer.

13. D: The Equal Employment Opportunity Act of 1972 was enacted to make any employment discrimination illegal. This included denying a candidate on the basis of race, religion, color, national origin, and sex. It was developed to ensure applications from all qualified candidates would be evaluated fairly by the potential employer. OSHA is the Occupational Safety Health Administration and the creator of the Occupational Safety and Health Act. Its role as a government body is to prevent work-related injuries, illnesses, and fatalities by developing written standards for workplace safety and health, making them available to employers, and enforcing penalties for non-compliance. The Immigration Reform and Control Act is national legislation that requires an employer to check and authenticate that job applicants are legally sanctioned to work in the United States, either because they are citizens or because they are approved aliens. The Age Discrimination Employment Act states that employer decisions regarding hiring, layoffs, merit increases, etc. can be classified as discriminatory and illegal if it is found that they were made on the basis that an employee was over the age of 40.

14. A: Across many cultures, cremation was selected because it symbolized releasing the spirit from the body. By doing so, the spirit would not haunt the family, and it could carry on its journey. For the ancient Greeks and other civilizations who frequently traveled far from home, cremations made transportation of the deceased back to their home easier. Cremations were not easy to do. The fires had to be maintained for a long time to properly reduce the body to ashes. Many cultures had elaborate cremation ceremonies and placed the cremated remains in ornate vases or urns. Burials were common among Christian and Jewish faiths. Although embalming as it is practiced today was not around, many cultures, such as those in Egypt and Peru, had their own means of preservation using elements from their natural environment.

15. D: State and local government agencies are tasked with regulating crematories within their jurisdiction. In 1996, the United States Environmental Protection Agency began investigating crematory emissions. Working with the Cremation Association of North America, they conducted a study to evaluate crematories. Upon conclusion of the study, it was decided that state and local authorities would be tasked with regulating crematories. Emissions are typically regulated by the state's environmental protection agency. Licensing, operating permits, zoning, documentation, and other business regulations are set by both state and local authorities.

16. C: Payroll is a liability; items owned by the funeral home are assets.

17. C: Beginning the arrangement conference with a few simple questions about the deceased helps the family feel more comfortable and shows empathy from the funeral director. Often this conference is the first time the family has the opportunity or time to discuss the death. Questioning whether the person had been ill long or if the family was present for the death opens the door for the family to begin telling the death story. Some people answer quickly and move on; others begin to provide insight into the death and life of their loved one. Listening and acknowledging their experience and feelings establishes a trusting relationship with the funeral director. Many directors begin by immediately asking questions to gather the necessary information; however, this is not as compassionate of an approach. The General Price List can wait to be presented until finances are discussed or the family inquires about financial information. Service options can be detailed when families ask what options are available or if the director senses the family might not be familiar with all the various options.

18. B: The Uniform Anatomical Gift Act was originally written as a model law but has been adopted as statute by all 50 states. The act covers and regulates all aspects of anatomical donation, including stipulating who can donate a body or body parts, how donations are made, what organizations can accept donations (donees), and what donor bodies and body parts can be used for. Anyone of legal age and sound mind can sign themselves up for donation or specify what organs they would like to donate upon death. Additionally, the person with paramount rights of disposition can also opt to donate a body or body parts for donation. Donees are stipulated in the act and include hospitals, medical and dental schools, storage banks, surgeons, physicians, and those in need of transplants. All donations must be used for research, education, and field advancement. The act also states that donations supersede the wishes of the survivors when the decedent prearranges their own donation. Those acting in good faith and in compliance with the act are exempt from civil or criminal action.

19. B: A pulverization machine used to break bones into small fragments after a cremation is called a cremulator. A cremation unit can be referred to as a cremation retort or cremator. Combustion chambers help remove odor and smoke from emissions prior to it entering the stack. Crematories have temperature regulation systems in place to control the main burner and afterburner. Metal discs with identification numbers are placed with the body to maintain an identification record throughout the cremation process.

20. C: A family member can provide a container for a person's cremated remains. A cemetery may have regulations for an urn vault if it will be buried, but there is no mention of a cemetery burial in the question.

21. C: Irrevocable pre-need contracts are established under terms stating that they cannot be broken. Money is specifically set aside for funeral expenses. The account can be established with a funeral home as guaranteed or non-guaranteed. Guaranteed accounts have money set aside for specific services that the funeral home is willing to guarantee at their current prices. Non-guaranteed accounts are established with a lump sum of money, usually based on current prices and anticipated inflation. At the time of death, the money and the accrued interest is applied toward the current funeral prices rather than the prices from when the account was opened.

22. A: Vehicles outside of the funeral procession are unpredictable and pose a safety risk for funeral processions. Liability during funeral processions can be reduced by giving the family and friends clear instructions at the conclusion of the service. While the cars are being lined up, staff members should speak to each car to ensure that they do not have any questions and are properly prepared for the procession (four-ways and lights on, flag secured in the proper location). Some cities have specific regulations for funeral processions to abide by. Amber or purple lights on the lead car and/or hearse help the procession stand out to other traffic. Police escorts are helpful in high-traffic areas and intersections.

23. C: Contractual liability can begin with either a written or oral commitment to providing an expressed or implied service or product. A breach of contract results in damages. In the case of funeral directors, breaches often cause mental anguish and emotional duress.

24. A: Pre-need funeral contracts can be established as either guaranteed or non-guaranteed. They can be either revocable (can be terminated by the client) or irrevocable (cannot be terminated). Trusts or accounts can be transferred from one funeral home to another; however, the funeral home receiving the contract can opt to honor price guarantees or use the money to go towards the cost of their services. State law regulates pre-need funeral contracts. The FTC only regulates funeral contracts that are established outside of a funeral home, classifying and regulating them under door-to-door sales laws.

25. C: Prior to engaging in a contract with another business, an effort must be made to ensure this business is operating within the industry's professional and ethical standards. Funeral homes and directors have a professional responsibility to ensure the third-party crematory they contract with meets these standards. Due diligence includes conducting inspections, interviews, and reviews of the crematories operating permits, policies and manuals, facility, equipment, and employees. This reduces the liability of the funeral home and their directors because it shows an assertive effort was put into ensuring the crematory operates within or above industry standards.

26. B: The Funeral Industry Practices Trade Regulation Rule, commonly referred to as the Funeral Rule, regulates many aspects of funeral service; however, the cornerstone of the Funeral Rule is the General Price List (GPL). This itemized list of services and prices of the funeral home must be given to the consumer before they make any financial decisions. The GPL must contain the name of the funeral home along with the address and phone number; effective date; the 16 specific goods and services laid out by the FTC; all other goods and services offered by the funeral home in addition to the designated 16; and 6 specific mandatory disclosures. The FTC further regulates the distribution protocols of the GPL. The embalming disclosure is mandated by the FTC to appear in specific wording on the GPL, acknowledging the consumer's right to select or decline embalming. The statement of funeral goods and services selected is given to the consumer to itemize all their selections, giving them an expense total of the services and merchandise.

27. C: Adults should let children participate in funerals if the child expresses a desire to do so. The child should be told of the death as soon after the death as possible, be encouraged to go to the cemetery, and be encouraged to talk to other people about it.

28. A: Crepe is a lightweight fabric lining cloth that has a slim, daintily crinkled or ridged facade made of silk, cotton, rayon, or wool. Satin is a fabric made of woven silk, nylon, or rayon that has a smooth, silky face. Velvet is a fabric made of woven silk, cotton, or rayon that has an evenly distributed, short, substantial, and dense pile. It is typically found in costlier caskets. Linen is a fabric made from the flax plant or non-flax fibers that are woven into a cross-section contour that contributes to the coarse consistency of the fabric.

29. D: A monument is erected to memorialize a life lived, telling the living of the departed's accomplishments and contributions. They are typically composed of metal and/or stone. A marker is a small headstone used to mark an individual's grave. A memorial is an object erected and displayed to remind the living of a person, group of people, event, or accomplishment (good or bad).

30. A: Cremation rates have increased over the years because regional differences across the United States have been decreasing; traditions have changed or aren't adhered to as strongly; people are more educated and environmentally conscious; life expectancy has increased; society is more mobile, which decreases traditions and community roots; and, over all, cremation has become more socially accepted.

31. A: Aftercare presented as publications is considered information-oriented aftercare. These documents can be displayed in an accessible part of the funeral home, allowing family and friends to look them over or take them home. They can also be given to the next of kin as part of an "after the funeral" packet of information and resources. Professional aftercare services fall under direct care services and would be facilitated by someone who has grief therapy or grief counseling training.

32. B: The surviving spouse has the paramount right of disposition by cremation. The order of authorization goes as follows: surviving spouse, children over the age of 18, parents, then siblings. If there are multiple people at the highest level of kinship, they should all agree and authorize the cremation; however, some states do allow cremation to proceed with only a majority of the next of kin agreeing. Authorizing agents must be of sound mind. Exemptions can be made for special relationships such as an unrelated friend or caretaker who has provided care and support for years. In these cases, blood relatives may be estranged without contact or the decedent may have appointed this person to take control of disposition. People can waive their authorization rights.

33. D: Allowing the family to bring in personal items will help them in their grief. It will be helpful not only to have the items at the services, but also to gather them at home. All of the other choices are offers of assistance intended to make things easier, but they don't help the family deal with their grief.

34. C: Natural organic reduction is a form of disposition only legal in a few states. Certified facilities place the body in a specially designed receptacle along with organic matter such as wood chips, alfalfa, straw, and flowers (the exact contents vary based on the facility). The temperature and airflow through the receptacle are then regulated to facilitate an accelerated decomposition process. Upon completion, the family can opt to receive the organic matter (soil) of their loved one or donate it. The process results in around a cubic yard of organic matter (700–1,600 lb based on the moisture content). Alkaline hydrolysis is the reduction of body to bone matter using chemicals, water, agitation, and pressure. Cryonics uses cryogenic temperatures to freeze the dead, or parts of the dead, in specialized vessels in hopes of restoring life decades or centuries later. A funeral pyre is a fire cremation that takes place in the open air, not retained or controlled within a retort.

35. B: Property and personal belonging inventory records should consist of observable details. For jewelry, the type of item (e.g., ring, earrings, necklace, pin) should be documented along with observable details. Do not make assumptions about the materials the jewelry is composed of (e.g., type of metal and stones). Write down what color the metal is and what color the stones are (e.g., write *yellow* instead of gold, and *clear* instead of documenting a stone as a diamond). Other observable details can include the brand (e.g., a watch might have a visible brand name on it), inscriptions, and shapes. Additional information that should be recorded includes the date the items were received, from whom the items were received, and the anticipated disposition of the items. When the items are returned to the next of kin, they should sign the document to acknowledge the receipt of items while authorizing the remaining items, if any, to stay with the decedent.

36. A: Cremation has been around for centuries; across the United States and Canada, it started increasing in popularity over the last few decades. Historians believe that cremation began in Europe around 3000 BC. During the Stone Age, cremation spread to Eastern Europe and Russia. Cremation was seen across Western and Northern Europe (today's Spain, Portugal, and Ireland) around 2500 BC, Greece around 1000 BC (by 800 BC it was the most common disposition for Grecians), and the Roman Empire around 27 BC. Burial remained the method of disposition within Christian and Jewish faiths. Cremation remained popular until around 400 AD, when Christianity began to spread and burial again became the primary method of disposition. Asian cultures commonly used cremation throughout history. In the late 1800s (AD), a new cremation movement began in Europe, England, and America as part of a call for health and sanitation reform. Today, over 30 countries practice cremation, some with increasing prevalence while within others it remains a rarity.

37. B: The procession, or cortege, is the line of cars traveling from the service location to the cemetery. Some services have a procession from the funeral home to the service location and then to the cemetery. The funeral director should ask the family in what order they would like the cars to be arranged. This list can be just a person's name or can have additional details like vehicle make, model, and how many people are in the car. A cortege usually assumes the following order:

1. Lead car with the officiant
2. Officiant car if driving separately
3. Pallbearers if driving together
4. Hearse
5. Closest family members
6. Additional guests

38. A: The funds can be deposited into a state funeral directors' association's trust fund, an account at a local bank, or, in some states, in an insurance policy or annuity. Under no circumstances is it legal for the entire amount to be deposited into a funeral home's bank account.

39. B: A first call is the beginning of a funeral director's services. This initial notification of a death can come from the next of kin, a friend, the coroner/medical examiner, facility employee, or hospice staff. Specific information about the decedent, their location, release, and next of kin should be secured during this call. Upon receiving a death notification from a facility or hospice group, the funeral director should contact the next of kin prior to transferring the body.

40. C: A person must be placed in something for the cremation process. An alternative container is typically composed of cardboard but can also contain composite materials or wood for support. A cremation casket is composed of combustible materials and minimal metal components. Ceremonial caskets are used for viewings and services prior to a cremation. The outer shell of the casket is reused, while the cardboard insert is removed and used to facilitate the cremation. A temporary container refers to an industry-standard receptacle for cremated remains when an urn is not selected. This plastic container, which holds the cremated remains inside a plastic bag, is typically in a cardboard carrying case.

41. D: The Statement of Funeral Goods and Services Selected is not required to be signed by the next of kin or person in charge of paying for funeral expenses. Funeral homes often have the next of kin or financially responsible person sign the statement, making it a contract. The statement must itemize all services and merchandise selected from the General Price List, giving the family a breakdown of their expenses. Packages can be listed as a single charge on this document; however, everything included in the package must be individually identified on the document. Cash advance items need to be listed on the statement also. Any cash advances that are marked up by the funeral home or any discounts the funeral home receives for items must be disclosed in this section. The statement must contain the mandatory embalming disclosure in addition to the reason why embalming was selected. It is also required that the funeral home disclose what items are legally required, required by the funeral home, or required by other parties based on the services they select. A copy of the statement must be given to the family at the end of the arrangements.

42. C: Eligibility requirements and stipulations are regulated by each individual Veterans Affairs national cemetery. National cemeteries accept eligible veterans (based on service records, type of discharge, and rank), their spouses, and dependent children either under the age of 21 or under the age of 23 if they are a full-time student or have a mental or physical disability that began before the age of 21. Some national cemeteries can only accommodate cremated remains due to limited space. Depending on the cemetery, the eligible person may have the option of an inground casket burial, burial of cremated remains, entombment of cremated remains in a columbarium, or scattering cremated remains in a scattering garden.

43. C: When filing applications for eligibility for Medicaid and Supplemental Security Income, all assets must be disclosed for governmental evaluation. Funded pre-need funeral contracts can be excluded from a person's assets and resources if the accounts are established correctly. Irrevocable pre-need funeral contracts established by a funeral director (or specifically designated in an account with a banking/financial institution for funeral expenses, depending on state law) are not considered part of a person's assets. In most states, these accounts do not have a maximum dollar amount, allowing them to be opened with any reasonable amount of money. Reasonable is determined by considering any funeral-associated costs (services, merchandise, transportation, cemetery costs, cash advances, monument expenses, obituary publication costs, even luncheons) that would be culturally, geographically, and financially appropriate for that individual person. There is a *burial space exclusion* which prevents burial spaces, merchandise, and other related products from being considered part of a person's assets if proof can be shown that they have already been purchased. This exclusion clause is often used in states that limit the use of irrevocable pre-need funeral accounts. In addition to the burial space exemption, the *burial funds exclusion* will exempt $1,500 set aside in burial trusts, revocable accounts, and assets when they are designated for covering funeral expenses. The insured does not receive income from insurance policies.

44. B: Complicated grief occurs when grief causes a person to feel overwhelmed, start unhealthy behaviors, or remain stagnant, not moving towards reconciling their bereavement. Exaggerated, delayed, masked, and chronic grief are all expressions of complicated grief. They can include new fears, extreme lifestyle changes, extended raw emotions, obsessions, avoidant behavior, and physical changes. Complicated grief can be seen when someone suffers a loss that is sudden, unexpected, traumatic, or young. If the relationship between the person and the decedent had a high level of intertwined attachment, it can result in a complicated grief journey. Early professional intervention is the best way to help someone struggling with complicated grief.

45. B: The body must be placed in a rigid container for cremation. Just imagine the awkwardness involved in getting a body into the retort wrapped in a sheet, with nothing sturdy underneath it to get it in safely.

46. D: Information to be gathered during a first call includes the decedent's full name and age; location of the decedent, including the facility/location phone number; release and permission to transfer; name of caller and their phone number; the next of kin name, address, and phone number; certifying physician; and whether the person died of a communicable disease. When speaking with the family, the funeral director inquires as to what kind of services they will be assisting the family with. The funeral director can verbally verify permission to embalm or not based on the service that is being requested. Additionally, knowing if the family is present, size of the deceased, and potential obstacles or challenges for the transfer team is helpful. Vital statistics do not need to be secured during the first call. Some callers provide extensive information during this conversation, while others do not.

47. C: To determine the number of John's 9 children who must agree to the cremation, find 60% of 9 and then round up. Sixty percent of 9 is 5.4, which means that at least 6 of the children must agree to the cremation.

48. D: Just like with cremation, the processes of natural organic reduction and alkaline hydrolysis reduce the body to unidentifiable organic matter or fine bone matter. Funeral homes should follow the same identification viewing process in order to reduce their liability. Due diligence inspections and evaluations of alternative disposition facilities should be performed to ensure they are meeting legal, ethical, and professional operating standards. It should be ensured that the facility has an identification process established to properly identify the decedent throughout the disposition process. These alternative methods of disposition are not legal in every state and are not always supported by communities or religions. They are relatively new methods of disposition, so ensure that the family understands the entire process, associated costs, and transportation involved. The next of kin should sign an authorization form and indemnification statement, similar to the cremation authorization process.

49. B: The Magnuson-Moss Act is a federal statute regulating both implied and expressed warranties. By providing merchandise and goods to clients, funeral homes must abide by these regulations. Simply by offering merchandise, the funeral home is implying that the product will successfully function as it was presented and intended (e.g., urns should competently hold cremated remains just like caskets should a decedent). Under this act, funeral homes must either display warranty information next to the product or have a clearly labeled and visible binder compilation of warranties for all offered products. Warranties must be available to consumers prior to purchase. Express warranties are guarantees that are clearly stated and advertised (typically by the manufacturer). Adopted warranties are when the seller is presumed to be providing the warranty to the consumer. Warranty disclaimers are typically printed on pricing documents and indemnify the funeral home from claims made by the manufacturers. Some states do not allow sellers to make warranty disclaimers.

50. C: Aftercare services can vary from giving the family information (brochures, cards, books, contact information for bereavement professionals) to sponsoring and hosting grief-support events. Providing the bereaved with support is a way to continue to help the families after the funeral services are complete. It is important because not everyone has a support system of family and friends that they can rely on throughout their grief journey.

51. D: An apostille is a document that is included with the required travel documents that verifies the authenticity of the signatures and seals on said documents. This signed document is issued by the state that issued the government seal on the travel documentation. The embassy or consulate of the country where the remains are being shipped should be contacted to verify their current shipping requirements. An impressed, raised, or dry seal is placed on the original legal documents by the issuing agency of notary.

52. A: The Federal Trade Commission (FTC) is the government agency created to promote consumer protection and fair competition, and also to prevent anti-competitive commerce practices. The ICCFA is a national trade association for funeral homes and cemeteries, and serves as a resource for cemetery/funeral service professionals and the public. OSHA is the Occupational Safety and Health Administration, and is a government agency created to prevent work-related injuries, illnesses, and fatalities by issuing and enforcing standards for workplace safety and health. The NFDA is the National Funeral Directors Association. It is not a government agency but instead a trade association for funeral directors. It serves as a resource for funeral service professionals and the public.

53. D: Employee bloodborne pathogen training records must be retained by the funeral home for 5 years. Medical records must be retained for 30 years. Under the Bloodborne Pathogens Standard, the funeral home must provide training to employees upon hire, when changes are made, and annually thereafter. The Bloodborne Pathogen Standard also mandates that funeral homes have a written exposure control plan; make the hepatitis B vaccine available for employees who are exposed to bloodborne pathogens and other potentially infectious materials at no charge; have personal protective equipment available for exposed employees; training programs; exposure follow-up protocol; and recordkeeping that documents employee training and medical records (containing name, Social Security number, hepatitis B vaccination record, exposure incidents, and exposure follow-ups).

54. B: A Reeves stretcher, or Reeves flexible stretcher, is essential for facilitating transfers through tight or narrow spaces. It is made out of a synthetic material with wooden slat inserts to provide support while maintaining flexibility. The device has straps to secure the decedent tightly and carrying handles to ease handling. Once the decedent is removed from the challenging area, the Reeves stretcher, with the decedent still secured to it, can be placed and secured on the stretcher. The flexible stretcher can be used to remove decedents from small spaces, up or down stairs, through narrow hallways, or around furniture. These stretchers are much lighter in weight than transfer cots/stretchers.

55. B: A cemetery *lot* is defined as a division within a cemetery consisting of a group of multiple grave spaces. A *block* is a division of a cemetery consisting of multiple lots. A *section* is a group of several blocks together within a cemetery. A *grave space* is the area allotted for containing a single interment (some cemeteries will allow for multiple interments within one grave space with double-depth graves, allowing cremated remains to be buried above casketed remains, or two sets of cremated remains in a traditional size grave space). An excavated area for the purpose of burying human remains is called a *grave*.

56. A: Pulverizing cremated remains is not a liability associated with cremation. The details of the pulverization process are required to be on the cremation authorization form. Therefore, families are already aware of how the bones are reduced into finer matter. Cremating personal possessions, proper identification of the decedent, labeling the cremated remains, cremating without proper authorization, co-mingling cremated remains, cremating medical devices, and neglecting to return the cremated remains in full are all liabilities surrounding cremation.

57. C: A dead body is defined by three qualifications: human, no longer alive, and not completely degraded. Legally, a completely decomposed body, reduced to skeletal remains or bone fragments, is not considered a dead body. Medically, the definition of *dead* was changed from the cessation of life (respiration and the heart both stop), to the irreversible cessation of brain function, including the brain stem. The definition was altered with the development of artificial life support in which the heart and lungs can continue to function with mechanical intervention. The term *corpse* is legally synonymous with *dead body*.

58. C: Pacemakers are surgically implanted superficially in the upper chest on the left side. They have one, two, or three wire leads that are inserted into the heart to help stabilize irregular heart activity. These pacemakers are large and battery operated. They must be removed prior to cremation to prevent a damaging explosion when the battery is subjected to intense heat. Leadless pacemakers are inserted via a catheterization procedure through the femoral vein and placed into the right ventricle of the heart. These pacemakers do not need to be retrieved; they can be cremated with minimal battery reactions because they are very small.

59. C: There are five options for manner of death that are listed on death certificates. Natural deaths occur by natural causes. Accidental deaths are the result of misfortunate events. Suicide is when a person ends their own life purposefully. Homicide is when a person kills another person. Undeterminable deaths are cases in which the investigative parties are unable to clearly state how the person died. Pending investigation deaths are awaiting further analysis and examination. State law regulates that death certificates are signed and filed within a specific time frame following death; when investigations and analysis take longer, a pending certificate is issued while waiting for additional information and results. Euthanasia is a medically assisted suicide to alleviate long-term pain and suffering from an irreversible or untreatable disease. It is not a legal manner of death on a death certificate, nor is it legal in most states.

60. B: If a person on Medicaid dies and has a burial account, the funds must be paid to the Medicaid office. Before all of a person's assets and funds are exhausted through paying the costs of their own nursing home or other care, they are permitted to set aside funds to pay for their own funeral expenses. Medicaid then takes over the financial responsibility of paying the high cost of their care. It is only fair, then, that the amount not used for its intended purpose be returned to the agency that has paid thousands of dollars for care. The other choices are prohibited by law.

61. C: Internal factors are psychological and external factors are sociological. Although illogical behavior may be displayed during grief, it is not one of the three main factors.

62. B: The merchandise value ratio (MVR) can be calculated by dividing the wholesale cost by the total amount the consumer is charged for services and merchandise. This percentage shows the funeral home's merchandise expense compared to what the consumer is paying for both services and merchandise. Gross profit margin is calculated by subtracting the wholesale price from the retail price. This shows the profit margin for the item. Net profit margin factors in all costs associated with a product and deducts them from the consumer's price. For example, calculating the net profit of an urn, the wholesale cost of the urn, taxes, and shipping fees would be subtracted from the retail cost. The consumer value index (CVI) is calculated by dividing the wholesale cost by the retail cost of a product. This measures the value the purchaser gets from the amount of money they've spent, enforcing the philosophy "spend more, get more."

63. B: A legatee is a person who inherits personal property based on the terms of a will. A consignee is the individual to whom goods are shipped, usually via a common carrier. A devisee is a person who inherits real property (land or objects attached to the land, such as a house). A bailee is a person who receives personal property on a temporary basis, such as for safekeeping.

64. D: Sociology is the science that studies various social groups and how individuals behave and relate to each other as a group in relation to other social groups. This can influence funeral service disposition arrangements. Funeralization is the practice of the funeral itself, including a variety of activities linked to the final disposition. This includes the type of service and the merchandise needed to accommodate the funeral service. Ethnocentrism is the belief that one's ethnic or cultural group, nation, race, or culture is better than all other groups. Pathology is the science that studies the origin, nature, and track of diseases.

65. D: Dr. Elisabeth Kübler-Ross developed the five stages of grief after observing people who were terminally ill. Denial, anger, bargaining, depression, and acceptance are the stages people go through when faced with their own mortality. People do not need to progress through these stages in a specific order. These stages can be brief or last days or weeks. Shock, alarm, disbelief, yearning, searching, disorganization, and resolution are the stages of grief associated with children.

66. D: Probate is when the will of a decedent is recognized as valid and an executor or administrator is appointed to execute the will. This representative is sworn in and can then proceed with dividing and dispersing assets to beneficiaries under the direction of the will. Probate law and the process of probate vary from state to state. Eighteen states follow the Uniform Probate Code, a standardized probate process. The term *intestate* is used to describe someone who has died without having a will established. Estate planning involves putting affairs in order prior to one's death.

67. A: Following the identification viewing, the next of kin (or appointed representative) should sign a form that acknowledges the decedent was positively identified. The form should contain the name of the decedent, date of death, name and relationship of the next of kin, and viewing date and time. If an appointed person is used, the next of kin should sign a statement giving permission in writing for this person to act on their behalf. If identification is done by photograph, the next of kin should sign and date the back of the photograph. The photograph should be retained in the decedent's file, not given to the family. Some funeral homes give a memorial token to the family, but it is not a standard practice. An indemnification disclosure is only suggested if the funeral director strongly advises against an identification viewing because it may cause trauma and mental distress, but the next of kin insists. Often in these causes of traumatic or violent death, the coroner or medical examiner will sign as the identifying agent on behalf of the family.

68. B: Although facial expressions, proxemics, and body position are all types of nonverbal communication, paralanguage is when a person's words do not match the tone of their speech.

69. D: Although some states may have requirements for processions to have a police car in the lead, the order of the cortege is typically: lead car, clergy, pallbearers, hearse, family cars/limo, and procession.

70. B: Chemicals that are mixed for immediate use do not need to be labeled as long as they do not exceed 10 gallons of total volume. Any chemical mixture removed from the original packaging needs to be labeled if stored, no matter the volume, for any duration of time (not immediately used in full). Even if the product is not hazardous, the chemical needs to be labeled if it is stored in a container other than the original manufacturer's container. For example, soap bought in bulk and stored in smaller squeeze bottles for ease of use needs to be relabeled. Labeling needs to consist of the product name, manufacturing company, address of the manufacturer, and hazardous warnings.

71. B: Marketing is used by businesses to encourage people to purchase their products and utilize their services. There are many forms of marketing that can be used by funeral homes to promote their business and increase their client base. Successful marketing plans need to be well thought out and organized with a clear objective for a specific audience. Advertising can be in the form of commercials (radio or television), printed brochures (mailed or strategically placed in a publicly accessible location), newspaper and publication advertisements, business cards, websites, and online forums.

72. D: Disinterment is when a body or cremated remains are exhumed from a place of rest. Disinterments, although typically avoided by the courts, are deemed necessary in cases of public interest or allowed for private reasons. Public interest cases can be confidential, or reasoning for the exhumation may be publicly announced. These types of disinterments are granted by the courts to assist with procuring evidence in criminal and civil cases. Following examination and processing, the body is reinterred in the same place. Private disinterments are conducted in accordance with the wishes of the next of kin. Typically, private disinterments are to move the decedent from one location to another, either within the same cemetery or to a different one.

73. A: The time-weighted average (TWA) monitor must be worn during testing for the duration of the time in the preparation room, up to eight hours. This device monitors the air quality and level of formaldehyde exposure through the embalming or work shift. The time-weighted average permissible exposure limit is 0.75 ppm. The short-term exposure level monitors the presence of formaldehyde for a 15-minute period and has an exposure limit of 2.0 ppm. The action level is 0.5 ppm. If the TWA exceeds 0.5 ppm, the action level is exceeded; even if the TWA limit is not, steps must be taken to reduce the formaldehyde level, and testing should be repeated until it is below the action level.

74. B: Vital statistics consist of specific information collected for legal documentation. It is used by various government agencies to collect and analyze data surrounding life events. Vital records include death certificates, fetal death records, birth certificates, marriage records, and divorce records. Some examples of vital statistics compiled on death certificates are legal name, maiden name, parents' names, legal address, marital status, date and place of birth, and race. Death certificates are state specific but require similar information throughout the United States.

75. B: Depreciation can be claimed on tangible assets that will decrease in value, such as vehicles. Health insurance, legal expenses, and payroll are all intangible liabilities.

76. A: Alternative containers are composed of combustible or biodegradable materials such as cardboard, composite woods, fabric, or canvas. They are made without metal and usually do not have ornamental details or interior linings. Alternative containers can be used for burials or to facilitate the cremation process. Temporary containers house cremated remains following the cremation and pulverization process. Urn vaults house cremated remains and have protective qualities. Aron caskets are wooden caskets created without the use of metal; they are commonly used within Jewish funeral rites.

77. D: Providing the family with memorial or keepsake items, such as a laminated obituary, is not a form of aftercare or grief support. Memorial and tribute ceremonies throughout holidays, informational brochures, lists of local resources and events, and information about grief or links to bereavement resources on the funeral home website are all forms of aftercare support.

78. C: Chronic grief is excessive and continues for an extended period of time. The individual is aware that their grief does not seem to be resolving, and they cannot move on emotionally. Masked grief is when a person is oblivious to the fact that their symptoms (physical and behavioral) are related to a loss. The person does not permit oneself to express grief. Delayed grief is when a person deliberately postpones or suppresses the natural grief reaction. Exaggerated grief is an escalation of a normal grief reaction. It can result in various medical conditions, including clinical depression or anxiety disorder.

79. C: The casket should be rolled into the service area feet first. Following the service, the casket should recess out of the church feet first. The positioning of the casket for the service is dependent on the religious denomination, facility space, and requests of the presiding officiant. Typically, at funeral homes, nonreligious venues, and many Protestant churches, the casket is positioned parallel to the altar or front of the service space. In Catholic and Lutheran churches, the casket is positioned perpendicular to the altar. Catholic priests are the exception for entering and exiting church; they enter and exit head first. For church services, always speak with the officiant first to confirm procession and recession procedures (some churches don't do this; rather, the casket is set up ahead of time) and casket positioning.

80. B: Quasi-property is used to mimic property rights, allowing another person to take possession and control of a dead body to proceed with disposition. Quasi-property is also considered to apply to cases in which affording someone rights similar to property rights benefits the public, like making the dead property to ensure prompt disposition. Personal property is considered transportable physical and tangible things a person can own such as clothing, furniture, and vehicles. Real property is defined as land, structures, and houses. Intellectual property assigns control of intangible ideas and creative thoughts to a person.

81. D: The officiating person, the cemetery, and the burial vault company must all be notified when planning a service that includes visiting hours, a funeral, and a burial.

82. C: Sundry items are miscellaneous products provided by the funeral home, for free or for purchase, that are used in conjunction with the services being provided. The following are examples: register books; prayer cards; memorial folders; bulletins (service folders); religious, fraternal, or military items; thank you cards; clothing purchased from the funeral home; and flowers. The honorarium is the money the funeral home provides to the service participants for their time. This includes officiants, musicians, singers (cantors), professional pallbearers, etc. Honorariums are charged to the family as a cash advance (money the funeral home pays to third parties on behalf of the family). There are times when the family opts to pay these people directly.

83. C: A tort is a civil violation of rights that results in financial or other personal damages and may be remedied by monetary compensation to the wronged party. Negligence is when a reasonable standard of care is not met. Liability is when a person is legally responsible for something. Mental anguish is emotional duress caused by another person's actions.

84. A: Alkaline hydrolysis, also known as aquamation, uses an alkaline chemical mixture in conjunction with water and other controls to reduce the body to liquid and bones. The liquid is drained out of the receptacle after the process. Once the bones are dried, they are pulverized into fine bone matter like cremated remains. This process is considered by many to be ecofriendly even though the process uses chemicals which, along with the liquified body, are released into the septic or sewer system. Using around 300 gallons of water per person, the process is not considered to be water-conservation conscious.

85. D: Remains must be shipped with a burial/transmit permit. They do not have to be embalmed or casketed, and prepayment is not required by law, though it may be required by the common carrier.

86. D: Stare decisis is the theory of law that purports that an established past court decision can be a model to provide insight for a future case since the court is likely to uphold the basis of law used to make the previous conclusion. A statute of limitations is a law that creates a set time limit to pursue legal action and certain forms of litigation after the action in question occurred. Statutes are legal policies formed by legislation that direct the administration of acceptable behaviors in a state, city, or country. The Equal Employment Opportunity Act of 1972 was enacted to make any employment discrimination illegal. This included denying a candidate on the basis of race, religion, color, national origin, and sex. It was developed to ensure applications from all qualified candidates would be evaluated fairly by the potential employer.

87. C: An air tray has a wooden base for the casket to sit on while the cardboard top sets down over the casket, secured with straps, to provide protection while traveling. A combination case is used to transport human remains without a casket. This unit is composed of a wooden base tray, wooden slats used to create side walls, and a cardboard top that sets down over the wooden sides to protect and cover the remains. A Ziegler case is a hermetically sealed, metal receptacle used to transport human remains. A temporary container is typically a plastic container containing bagged cremated remains and held by a cardboard carrying case.

88. D: Workplace controls, engineering controls, and good hygiene practices all help ensure that formaldehyde exposure is limited. Examples are keeping the lid on the embalming machine, chemicals, and garbage cans; using a ventilation system to exchange air with fresh, clean air; keeping a clean workstation on the embalming table with running water; closed drainage systems; and respirators. OSHA requires preparation rooms to be equipped with emergency drench showers, eye wash stations, and first aid kits; however, these measures do not reduce formaldehyde exposure.

89. D: Denial, anger, bargaining, depression, and acceptance are the five stages of dying identified by Dr. Elisabeth Kübler-Ross in her book *On Death and Dying*. Accept, express, adjust, and reinvest refer to the Tasks of Mourning outlined by J. William Worden. In this theory, he described the route whereby the person accepts the reality of the loss and experiences the expressive pain, then adjusts to the condition where the deceased is not there, and finally re-invests into another relationship. Numbness, yearning, disorganization and despair, and reorganization refer to the four phases of mourning described by John Bowlby. Shock, awareness of loss, conservation-withdrawal, healing, and renewal refer to the phases of the mourning process as described by Catherine Sanders.

90. B: Rather than itemize services and products individually (itemized pricing), package pricing is when the funeral home groups items and services involved in a specific type of service together. This is allowed by the FTC as long as the package price is also listed on the General Price List and details exactly what products and services it entails. The most common package funeral homes have is a direct cremation package. Economy pricing is when the funeral home uses the method of offering the lowest price in the area to attract clients. They are often referred to as discount funeral homes. Loss leader pricing is when a low price is advertised with the hope that the client will actually make a more expensive purchase. This is only legal if the low-priced options are available to the client and the funeral director does not pressure them to select higher-end options.

91. C: Psychological influences of grief are internal struggles and influences. Beverly Rafael separated psychological factors that affect grief into three groups. The relationship between the decedent and the survivor influences the grief journey depending on the level of love, attachment, and dependency. The nature of the death influences a person psychologically as they make sense of and come to terms with their loss. Extended illnesses and other anticipated deaths give the survivor time to reflect and begin processing their emotions prior to the death while unexpected deaths and stigmatized deaths (suicide and drug overdoses) cause complicated psychological grief work. The third influence is how a person's prior experience with loss plays a role in them coping with a new loss. Unresolved losses can compound upon new ones further complicating grief. Sociological influences of grief are external influences like community support, family structure, and religion. Physiological influence are biological factors such as sleep, nutrition, and health.

92. A: *Grief syndrome* is the term used to describe the most common and ordinary patterns and assortment of feelings and behaviors people exhibit following the loss of a loved one. Guilt is blaming oneself for something that has occurred. Shame is the assumption of blame aimed at oneself in the presence of others. Attachment theory is John Bowlby's concept that for safety and security reasons, people develop long-lasting attachments to specific persons when they are very young.

93. B: In the 1870s, a burial reform movement started across the United States. The movement was led by medical professionals, Protestant clergy, and Germanic communities throughout the US. These groups began forming cremation societies and began publishing articles to educate the public. The first crematory was opened in Pennsylvania in 1876 by Dr. F. Julius LeMoyne. By the 1900s, there were around 24 crematories in 15 states. The Catholic church remained opposed to cremation until 1963. Clergy, medical professionals, and sanitation advocates lobbied for the government to establish a system and agency (state and/or federal) to oversee sanitary controls and issues regarding public health in the wake of epidemic outbreaks (cholera, yellow fever). States began to establish their own health agencies beginning in 1869. This health and sanitary reform then lead to burial reforms. The government did not specifically lobby for cremation, and funeral directors did not support the cremation movement this early.

94. D: The family should be asked what they would like back from the decedent prior to cremation. Removal of requested items should be followed as long as the request is reasonable, legal, ethical, and without excessive burden. They may want the clothing, bedding, or the decedent's special blanket, or they may want those items to be cremated with their loved one. Jewelry should all be removed prior to cremation. Some families may request it to be cremated with the person; however, this is an immense liability. In these cases, suggest putting the jewelry in the urn with the cremated remains after the cremation process if they want it to remain with the decedent's remains. This way they can retrieve the jewelry if they change their minds later without it having been damaged in the cremation process. Other metal items can be removed if the family requests it (e.g., they want the belt or shoes back). Metal items (medical implants, casket pieces, buttons, etc.) are removed post cremation and prior to pulverization.

95. A: Effective listening can be negatively impacted by the following barriers: selective listening (the listener hears what they want to hear or takes things out of context), bias, exhaustion, environmental stimulants and interruptions, informational overload, feeling rushed for time, emotional stress, and defensiveness (caused by prejudices and judgements before the understanding is reached). Funeral directors need to be effective listeners by actively listening, showing empathy, being open and nonjudgmental, staying focused and attentive, and being aware of nonverbal communication. Nonverbal communication consists of proxemics (the spatial separation between people), facial expressions, paralanguage (tones), eye contact, attire, gestures, and posture.

96. A: A tort occurs when a person takes a wrongful action against another person or property, and is a civil law matter. Mutilation as it relates to mortuary science is inflicting bodily damage or injury on a deceased person or animal by removing or destroying body parts. Obstruction occurs when a person or a situation creates an impasse or hinders someone from doing something. Replevin is an action to pick up goods or property by somebody who claims to own them and who promises to have the claim later tested in court. It does not apply to human remains.

97. B: Funeral management is defined as motivating people and resources within the funeral home to accomplish goals and objectives. The four cornerstones to successful funeral management are planning, organizing, actuating, and evaluating staff and resources. Planning entails developing a mission, goals, and objectives. Organization involves dividing the goals and objectives of the business between staff members and allocating resources to accomplish these tasks. Actuating or directing is the management and coordination of the systems, plans, staff, and resources. Evaluation is reflecting on the success of the process, employees, resources, and overall results of obtaining the goals of the business, positive or negative. From there, the manager must restructure as needed.

98. C: A gasket is a rubber strip along the top lid and top of the casket base that is used to seal the casket. Half-couch caskets also have a strip along the seam between the head and foot ends of the lids. Gauge is the measurement used to define the thickness of metal. Galvanized steel contains a layer of zinc to resist rusting. A gimp, or fold, is a cloth, plastic, or metal attachment to the interior panel of the casket to conceal the roll anchors.

99. D: The declining price structure model incorporates a lower margin on higher-priced caskets so the consumer value index improves as they spend more. Choices B and C are both components of the declining price structure model. The modified declining model places a lower margin on less-expensive caskets.

100. C: *Selected hardwood* is a phrase used to describe a casket made of various trees, such as willow, poplar, or cottonwood. A single-hinged panel is a casket lid that is in two sections. Wood veneer refers to the method of using glue during assembly to join a thin layer of superior wood to a layer of less costly wood so the superior wood is on top. A pine box is a casket made of wood from a pine tree.

101. C: Sigmund Freud wrote *Mourning and Melancholia* in 1917. He theorized that the grief process involves the internal struggle of letting go of invested energy (which he defined as libido) from objects that no longer exist. He describes it as a painful, natural, and necessary process. Freud's work set the foundation for psychologists to begin defining normal and abnormal grief work. Erikson organized developmental theories into eight stages of conflict and resolution, ranging from infancy to death in late adulthood. Kübler-Ross developed the five stages of grief. Abraham Maslow is known for his hierarchy of needs.

102. C: A trial balance shows the profits and losses of a business. It does not track inventory, help with vehicle maintenance, or ensure accurate payroll.

103. A: The narthex is the entryway to the funeral home or church, and is also known as the lobby or foyer. The nave is the seating or audience section of the church. A niche is a permanent resting place for cremated remains, typically found in a church or cemetery. A sanctuary is the area in the church where the public are seated during the service, and can also describe the area around the altar.

104. B: Ferrous metals are composed of iron (Fe) and other elements. Steel is made from iron and carbon. Gauge is the term used to refer to the thickness of the metal, defined as the number of sheets needed to create one inch. The lower the gauge, the thicker the metal. 20-gauge caskets (need 20 sheets to form an inch of thickness) are usually the least expensive metals. 16 gauge (16 sheets to form an inch of thickness) is the most expensive version. Ferrous metals will rust and are often magnetic. Stainless steel is composed of steel and chromium and can also include nickel. To be considered a stainless steel, there must be a minimum of 11% chromium in it. Stainless steel is more durable against corrosion but doesn't withstand the elements as well as copper or bronze. Most caskets are made of either 400 series stainless steel (steel, 11–12% chromium, and no nickel) or 300 series stainless steel (steel, 18% chromium, and 8% nickel). Bronze is composed of 90% copper with tin and sometimes zinc. Copper caskets are composed of a seamless mass of copper.

105. A: Fractional display rooms show segmented sections of a casket. They can be 1/4 or 1/8 models (featuring the corner and a panel section) or just the end section of the caskets. Both sectional options will showcase enough of the casket for the customer to see the coloring, shading, shape of the corners, and the handle, arm, and lug features. Traditional display rooms have full-size caskets displayed. Display rooms can showcase caskets from one company or multiple. They can also use a combination of fractional and traditional displays.

106. B: Over half of the states in the United States have laws requiring 100% of pre-need money be secured in a trust or financial account. Third-party funeral merchandise providers have been challenging these laws as it is not uncommon for 20 or more years to pass between establishing a funeral trust and using it. Many states have upheld their 100% trust laws, even while acknowledging that they prevent the seller from covering operating costs, to help prevent fraud and misuse of pre-need funds.

107. C: After years of experimentation, professor Ludovico Brunetti showcased the model of the first modern-day cremation retort at the 1873 Vienna Exposition. Dr. Hugo Erichsen was the founder and first president of the Cremation Association of America in 1913. Sir Henry Thompson, a surgeon advocating for sanitary health reformation, supported disposition by cremation; he organized the formation of the Cremation Society of England. Dr. Julius LeMoyne opened the first crematory in America in 1876.

108. C: Public relations programs introduce the public to information and resources on funeral options, grief, and preplanning. They can involve participating in and supporting community events unrelated to the industry. The goal is to gain public awareness of the funeral home, establish the funeral home as an industry leader, and build a positive business image, all of which maintain current clientele and help gain new clients while supporting the community.

109. B: An indemnification disclosure is a statement releasing the funeral home, crematory, and staff members from any legal issues resulting from their actions based on the information they have been provided. One of the sections on the cremation authorization form that the next of kin signs certifies that the information they have provided is correct and they indemnify the funeral home, crematory, and staff from liability if any of the information is incorrect.

110. D: Non-traditional services are modern religion-based services personalized to the deceased to include favorite music and readings. Traditional services closely follow religious rites with minimal adaptation. Humanistic services are not religion based. Memorial services can follow any of these styles but are conducted without the decedent's body present. They typically are held after disposition has occurred.

111. C: Gradual recovery is a pricing structure in which the markup changes based on the wholesale cost of the product. There is a direct relationship between the wholesale cost and the markup: as the merchandise increases in cost, so does the markup. This method of merchandising makes lower-priced items the best value. Fixed multiple or times factor uses the same markup across all merchandise. The declining price structure method reduces the markup as the wholesale cost increases (an inverse relationship). This method decreases the price gap between high-end and low-end merchandise, encouraging spending on higher-end items.

112. D: Preparation of the body in the Jewish rite is called tahara, and is done by the chevra kadisha, or holy society. Shiva is the period of mourning after the death and the yahrzeit is the first anniversary of the death.

113. C: The pall is used during the funeral ceremony as a symbolic covering for the casket in some religious denominations. Depending on the religion, a pall can represent religious concepts like baptism or equality in the eyes of God. Casket bearers, or pallbearers, carry the casket throughout various parts of the ceremonies. A bier is used to hold the casket in lieu of a church truck at the funeral home; it is typically composed of wood. Some people also use the word *catafalque* synonymously with *bier*; however, some use the word *catafalque* for the skirt of material or drape used to conceal the church truck under the casket.

114. B: Although many funeral homes display full-size vaults, cross sections of vaults, or vault photos, the most important part of displaying burial vaults is being able to provide a knowledgeable, accurate description to the consumer of each, including their advantages.

115. B: The Bloodborne Pathogen Standard addresses the Needlestick Safety and Prevention Act. Under this regulation, funeral homes are required to have a needlestick exposure control plan enacted to reduce employee sharps risks. Sharps are defined as any object that is pointed, has a risk of being contaminated, and has the potential to cause injury. Trocar points, needles, scalpels, glass, and debris are some examples. The Formaldehyde Exposure Standard regulates employee exposures to formaldehyde by monitoring air quality, access to personal protective equipment, sanitation controls, emergency response plans, employee training, and record management. The

Hazardous Communication Standard identifies the employer's obligation to keep their employees safe through hazard awareness, training, written control plans, safety labeling, and access to safety data sheets. The General Industry Standard regulates general safety measures for businesses such as fire extinguishers, signage and posted locations, and electrical safety regulations.

116. C: A nuisance is any property use that causes distress to neighboring properties as a direct result of anomalous, unreasonable, or peculiar activities. Activities, business, or conditions must be hampering neighbors' comfort and general happiness to be considered a nuisance. Often, public nuisances are declared when the health and welfare of the surrounding population and property owners are determined to be jeopardized, resulting in emotional distress and contention. Legal precedents have been established protecting funeral homes from being considered a nuisance in general because the court deems them necessary to public health and safety. Zoning regulations restrict residential housing, businesses, and establishments and dictate what properties within designated areas can be used for. Although funeral homes traditionally are not deemed a nuisance, they can be considered one if their operations conflict with the established zoning ordinances (e.g., a funeral home operating in a residential area). Some funeral homes are grandfathered into residential areas but face opposition when they try to install a crematory or make other significant changes that will impact neighboring properties.

117. C: Prior to closing the casket, the funeral director needs to verify with the next of kin in charge what items are staying in the casket and what items need to be returned. This information is typically discussed during the arrangement conference or when the family brings in clothing, jewelry, and personal possessions. Because people can change their minds, it needs to be readdressed to ensure that the proper items are being removed or added to the casket. Some families want items worn or displayed for the viewing but then returned to be retained as a keepsake. Others want the decedent to keep these possessions as grave goods.

118. B: Cash advances are services and fees the funeral home pays to third parties on behalf of a family. Cemetery fees are considered a cash advance and are listed as such on the Statement of Funeral Goods and Services Selected. Cemetery fees can consist of the grave opening and closing, a layout fee for marking out the grave, weekend/holiday/afterhours fees, or even the purchase of a grave space. Some funeral homes will advance these fees, while others prefer the family pay the cemetery directly for their services. Grave openings are not always paid to the cemetery when another party does the excavation on behalf of the cemetery.

119. A: The family viewing is the first time the decedent is viewed by close family members. Typically, the family arrives at the service location at least an hour prior to the start of the public visitation. The funeral director should greet the family and let them gather in a room until they are ready to go into the viewing area. When ready, the funeral director should walk them into the room. Some directors will walk the family in and be a presence in the back of the room, while others will escort the family into the room and up to the casket. During this time people may react in many ways: being calm, being quiet, crying, sobbing, shaking, collapsing, or with anger or frustration. Prayer services and fraternal services can be held privately (with just the family) or publicly prior to the public visitation, or they can be held at the conclusion of a visitation. Prayer services are typically reserved for before the visitation, after the visitation, or before the funeral service. Fraternal services can be held at these times or before, after, or during the service. Committal services are usually held at the graveside; however, some are held at the conclusion of the service if there is not going to be a place of interment.

120. C: The Fair Labor Standard Act was created to regulate minimum wage, the lowest amount an employer can pay an employee, overtime requirements after 40 hours in a designated work week (funeral directors as professionals are typically exempt from the overtime payment requirements), and equal pay (regulates discrimination in wages). Both federal and state-specific regulations are enacted on funeral homes. The Civil Rights Act regulates discrimination based on race, religion, gender, pregnancy, and nationality. The Equal Employment Opportunity Act regulates fair treatment of employees. The Age Discrimination in Employment Act regulated discrimination based on age, specifically 40 years old and up.

121. D: The average interior dimensions of an adult metal casket are 78" × 23", while wooden caskets are slightly smaller, with an interior of 75" × 22". The interior height of a metal casket is 16–24", while wooden caskets are 16–22" high. When determining if a person will fit in a standard size casket, the interior dimensions need to be considered. The exterior dimensions of an adult casket are 84" × 29". As caskets increase in size to accommodate larger people, the funeral director needs to anticipate additional complications, including interior vault dimensions (86" × 30"), grave space dimensions, doorway and hallway widths, elevator dimensions, and strength and number of pallbearers.

122. D: A death certificate and a disposition permit must be complete prior to cremation. Authorization should be secured from all next of kin within the highest level of kinship, although some states have a "majority rule" that permits cremation without unanimous consent. An authorization from the coroner or medical examiner from the place of death must be given in writing or verbally, followed by a written document (depending on local regulations). Identification viewings and a signed acknowledgement of identification are strongly recommended but not required.

123. D: The tablet, or die, of a monument is the vertical or upright portion of the monument. This is where the engraving is usually located. The front (face) or back of the monument can be straight or slanted at a 45° angle. Slanted monuments are typically 16–18" high while upright monuments have more of a height variance; both styles can be used to mark single graves, double graves, or family plots. The base is the stone foundation that the upright or slanted monument sits upon for support. An epitaph is the engraved inscription on the monument.

124. D: *Aquamation* is a term used interchangeably with *alkaline hydrolysis*. It reduces the body to bones similar to the remains after a fire cremation. With both fire cremation and aquamation, the remaining bones are then pulverized. Because of this similarity, aquamation/alkaline hydrolysis has also been referred to as *water cremation*. Cryonics uses extremely low temperatures (−196 °C or −320.8 °F) to freeze the dead. Natural organic reduction uses a controlled environment to reduce the body at an accelerated speed, mimicking decomposition. It is also referred to as human composting or terramation.

125. B: Hermetically sealed closures on caskets or containers are considered airtight and impenetrable by external and internal fluids, odors, and gases. The type of sealing method used depends on the composition of the materials being sealed. Latched closures secure the lid of caskets with a basic latch that snaps together when the lid is pressed down onto the casket base. Chemical closures are when products such as epoxies and glues are used to secure the lid to the base. This closure method is used for some brands of infant caskets and urn vaults. Threaded fasteners are used on caskets with hinge caps to twist or screw the lid closed.

126. A: It is important that the funeral director or employee answering the telephone speaks clearly and slightly slower than in normal conversation. This allows the caller to more easily understand and process the information they are being provided. Speaking quickly can overwhelm and confuse the caller. Speaking clearly, at a normal volume, and with some inflection helps ease communication by telephone. A monotonous, gloomy, or energetic tone should not be assumed by the director. Using a sharp, business-like tone of voice is not appropriate either. During the first call the director must use their tone of voice, volume, and dictation to convey assurance, compassion, and professionalism to the caller.

127. C: Memorial gatherings held for the community and families a funeral home has served is an example of aftercare. Aftercare is the contact and support that a funeral home offers to families after services are completed. It can be in the form of newsletters, emails, informational pamphlets, community events, support groups, counseling sessions (with a trained mental health professional on staff), or a telephone call to check in. Pre-need care covers education for funeral planning; it can be in person, over the phone, or at hosted community events. At-need care is when services are provided at the time of a death.

128. A: The maker of a promissory note is the entity or individual who makes the guarantee to pay, and is the signer of the promissory note. The payee is the entity or individual to whom the pledge of monies is made. The drawee is the entity or individual selected and required to make the payment of finances. It is from their monies that the draft is drawn. The drawer is an entity or person that draws or executes an order for the disbursement of money.

129. C: A fraternal service is organized and conducted by a social organization to honor the decedent's dedication and commitment as a member of the group. The service can be held at the beginning or end of calling hours; before, during, or after the service; or at the graveside. Fraternal services are typically not allowed to be conducted as part of a service at church. A celebrant service is officiated by a certified celebrant, a person who is trained to organize and conduct unique and personalized funeral services for people from all backgrounds, beliefs, and religions. A church service is conducted in church. A committal service is held at the graveside. Occasionally, officiants will do the committal service ceremony at the service location when the family is not able to travel to the cemetery, there is inclement weather, or there is not an interment location.

130. D: Disposition permits are issued by a government agency and completed by the funeral director. Once completed with decedent information and disposition information, they are approved by a government agency or locally appointed registrar. The exact information collected for the permit and the completion/processing procedures vary from state to state. Most states have electronic filing systems in place. Disposition permits also allow and authorize the decedent to be transferred from one location to another. Every decedent needs a disposition permit regardless of the type of disposition.

131. A: Tort liabilities address damages that occur resulting from the failure to meet contractual obligations or breach of legal duties and obligations. The duties of a funeral director include not impeding the right of burial and putting reasonable effort into maintaining and ensuring their property is reasonably safe for the public. Funeral homes have a high degree of duty to the families and service attendees on their property because they have been invited onto the property. In cases when someone enters the property uninvited, a low degree of responsibility is held. Additionally, tort law also covers wrongful withholding of a body, loss of a body, mutilation of a body, and liability related to the safety of pallbearers and clergy.

132. D: Any veteran with a discharge other than dishonorable is entitled to military honors. This means that any veteran with an honorable or general discharge is eligible. Rank is inconsequential, as is whether death occurred during wartime.

133. A: The five stages of grief do not always occur in the order in which they are usually listed. Because everyone is different, so is their grief. Individuals take different amounts of time to get through each stage and the total process of grief. Making a deal with God is called "bargaining."

134. B: Amounts owed for funeral services are included in accounts receivable. Therefore, the amount in accounts receivable will decrease when an amount that is owed is paid.

135. C: In most states, the funeral expenses of the deceased take top priority. This claim is immediately followed by the administration fees associated with settling the estate. Taxes come last. Taxes are not a preferred claim expense over the funeral expenses of the deceased in most states. Medical bills owed do not supersede taxes or funeral expenses in most states. Administration expenses are given less priority than funeral expenses and taxes in most states.

136. B: Working capital is the tangible working liquidity that is accessible for use by a company. The statement of operations, also called the income statement, is a written statement that identifies the financial profitability of a company over a precise period of time. Proving cash is when a business authenticates that the cash it has on hand and in the bank is equal to the amount listed in the accounting documentation. Useful life is the number of years that a business asset or piece of property can be depreciated, and is established by the IRS.

137. C: Grief counseling involves communicating with those who have lost a loved one recently and are mourning to facilitate the bereavement process and help them move through the stages of grief. At-need counseling is providing informational services to families subsequent to the death of a person. An example is when a funeral director provides a GPL to quote prices on various service selections. Grief therapy is typically one-on-one counseling for those who are unable to move through and complete the stages of mourning. Typically, the person in need of this type of therapy is having a delayed grief reaction or an exaggerated grief response, or is demonstrating physical or behavioral symptoms that remain unresolved.

138. A: The cloth covering that is placed on the casket in a Catholic church is called a pall. If a flag is on the casket going into the church, it must be removed before the pall can be placed on the casket. A flag cannot be placed under or over the pall.

139. A: When a person gives someone else the right to claim something that belongs to her, it is known as an assignment. She is assigning it, or signing it over, to someone else.

140. C: Tradition is also a big influence on a person's perspective. Gender, race, and financial status may be factors in other facets of life, but ideas about death are more influenced by religion, family, culture, and observed and experienced traditions.

141. B: Although getting the death certificate information, writing the obituary, and explaining the costs are all components of the arrangement conference, the most important one is listening carefully. A funeral director cannot make arrangements for services that will meet or exceed the customer's expectations unless he or she practices careful listening.

142. B: Bereavement is the experience a person goes through subsequent to a loss when they are grieving and mourning the loss of a loved one. Mourning is the process one goes through after the loss of someone as they reorganize their life without the person. Thanatology is the study of dying, death, and grief. Grief is the emotional reaction that results from the loss of a loved one.

143. B: A confidentiality agreement makes the prospective purchaser promise to keep all information discussed, financial and otherwise, confidential.

144. C: Funeral directors were very resistant to the cremation movement that began in the late 1800s and continued into the 1900s. They often shared the belief, along with most of the American population, that cremation was not a respectable or honorable form of disposition. In the 1960s, with the shift of spiritual and social trends, cremation began to increase in popularity. Instead of embracing the change and looking for ways to meaningfully serve cremation families, funeral directors dug in their heels. Some went as far as to decline to serve cremation families. The 1980s brought a rise in cremation companies that catered specifically to cremation families. After losing clients to these companies, funeral homes began to more readily offer and advertise cremation services in addition to traditional services.

145. B: The Islamic faith prohibits cremation because Muslims believe in the resurrection of the body. Both Catholic and Jewish faiths have traditionally been apprehensive of cremation; however, today both religions accept cremation as a method of disposition within their faith. The Buddhist and Hindu religions use cremation as the primary means of disposition.

146. C: Natural organic reduction (NOR) is a form of disposition in which the body is placed into a specialized receptacle with organic matter to facilitate accelerated decomposition of the body using temperature controls and air flow to encourage rapid microbial growth. Funeral pyres are open-air cremations that use fire and combustible materials to reduce the body to bones. Alkaline hydrolysis (also called aquamation or water cremation) uses alkaline chemicals and water to reduce a body to bones. Natural organic reduction, funeral pyres, and alkaline hydrolysis are only legal in some states.

147. C: A legal divorce severs the relationship that once made the former spouse the next of kin. Medical doctors and members of the clergy do not have the legal ability to sign a cremation authorization (unless they are next of kin to the decedent). Many states now recognize an agent assignment made by the deceased during his life that gives the agent specific powers. The assignment must specify the right to authorize cremation in writing.

148. D: There are many options for retaining cremated remains when families want something eco-friendly and biodegradable. Examples are urns composed of sand, salt, heavy paper, cardboard, cornstarch, salt, unfired clay, plant-based materials, and untreated wood. Some of these options degrade quickly when subjected to the elements of the ground or water; others degrade over time. Marbelon is a synthetic marble-like material often used in urn vaults or urn vault combination units. These protect the cremated remains from the elements and do not degrade. Metals and plastics are not biodegradable either.

149. B: A memorial service is always held without the casketed body. *Funeral rite* is a term that can describe both funerals and/or memorial services. *Funeral*, on the other hand, describes a service conducted when the body is present. During an entombment service, the casketed body is placed in a crypt. A graveside service is one in which the deceased is in a casket. It is held at the cemetery interment site (grave) instead of a church or chapel. The casketed body is present at a traditional or complete cremation service, but at the end of the service the deceased is brought to the crematory to be cremated instead of to the cemetery for burial.

150. B: Funeral directors/funeral homes should review a third-party crematory's licensure, permit and renewals, maintenance logs, and records. Additionally, an unannounced visual (onsite) inspection should be done periodically to ensure quality care is being provided and the facility is in good working order. While interviewing the operations manager is helpful, interviewing every employee is not necessary, nor is staying for the duration of each cremation.

151. A: Doeskin, also called moleskin, is used as a type of material for cloth-covered caskets. It is 1/8" thick or less and composed of a rugged cotton that is velvety or suede-like in texture. Broadcloth is a twilled, napped, or wool material, typically cotton, silk, or rayon, that creates a dense and smooth cloth covering for a casket. Plush cloth coverings consist of those that have a pile or nap greater than 1/8". Twill is a material that is woven to create diagonal lines.

152. C: A fiduciary is a person or institution who keeps money for someone else. An assignee is someone who assigns goods to another person. A devisee is a person designated in a will to receive real property. A distributee is one who receives property from the deceased's personal representative.

153. A: VA Form 21-2008 is the form requesting a United States flag to be used for burial purposes relating to a qualified veteran. The application can be filed at a local Veterans Affairs office or US post office. The flags are used to drape the casket or displayed with the casket/urn during services. At the cemetery (or designated service location) the flag can be folded and presented to the family as part of military honors. The family members typically retain the flag as a memorialization of their loved one's dedication and service to their country. VA Form 21-530 is an application for burial benefits such as burial and plot-interment allowances. VA Form 40-0247 is a request for a Presidential Memorial Certificate. A DD 214 is a discharge record of military service.

154. C: According to the Hazardous Communication Standard, a binder with safety data sheets (SDS) for every chemical and product used in the preparation room (hazardous or not) must be located in two places: the preparation room and the main office of the funeral home. This allows for easy access to the chemical and product information in both the preparation room and the main office in case of an emergency. The Hazardous Communication Standard, in addition to SDS, regulates employee training, container labeling, and the funeral home's written hazardous communications program.

155. A: Common law is unwritten law that has often been used for hundreds of years and is based on universally accepted principles and precedents. Common law is used to support the gap in coded or written laws and statutes. Case law is used to set precedents; it is the court's interpretation and application of written laws and statues to specific cases. Federal law consists of regulations set by the federal government that all states must abide by. Constitutional law is written laws and statutes written and enforced by either the federal government or state government.

156. A: The tahara is a ceremony where the decedent is washed, dressed, and casketed while prayers are recited. The Chevra Kadisha is a group of people, the same gender as the decedent, who perform the tahara. The tachrichim is a burial shroud the decedent is dressed in. These are simple garments made of white material to show equality in the eyes of God. A tallitot is a prayer shawl. The Torah is the religious book of the Jewish faith. It is composed of the first five books of the Christian Bible and includes teachings, traditions, and laws of the Jewish faith.

157. A: A funeral director wears many hats throughout the arrangement conference and services they offer. They can guide families in making appropriate selections and choices that will help them navigate their grief; in this sense, they are acting as funeral or grief counselors. They provide emotional support and professional guidance as the family says goodbye to their loved one. Funeral directors will actively listen and validate emotions throughout the process. It is important not to cross any professional lines. Funeral directors are not grief therapists and should not act as such. They may mediate by providing suggestions and alternative options, but decisions need to be left to the family to resolve. Funeral directors should understand mortuary laws regulating their state and be familiar with the legal processes involved in disposition; however, legal advice should always be sought from legal professionals and not given out by a funeral director.

158. D: A cause of death or communicable disease disclosure is not a mandated requirement on a cremation authorization. The following are required: decedent identification information, name of the receiving funeral home, next of kin proclamation (certifying that they are the nearest and dearest with right of disposition) and signature, medical device disclosure, disposition (post cremation) instructions and unclaimed property policy, directions for personal possessions, description of pulverization, and indemnification statement for the funeral home and staff.

159. B: Casket interiors featuring a crushed style have a lining fabric placed on a metal form. Weights are added, and the material is then steamed and attached to an upholstery or backing. Masselin is the paper used in layers of sheets that is pressed and made up to provide an upholstery or backing. The extendover is the segment of the casket interior that extends over the top body molding. A tufted casket interior is made by inserting a padded material between a lining material and a backing material. Stitches are then added to create raised puffs.

160. D: The policies, forms, procedure, and standard of care must be in writing and made available to any inquiring person. Funeral directors and funeral homes contracting with a crematory should review this manual as part of their due diligence inspection. This should be done prior to engaging in business and reviewed annually to monitor changes.

161. C: The Application for United States Flag for Burial Purposes, also known as VA form 27-2008, is the accepted document to apply for an American flag. The Application for Burial Benefits is the form to apply for burial benefits at the Veterans Administration. The Statement of Death by Funeral Director is a form completed by the funeral director to notify the Social Security Administration of the death. It is unrelated to the Veterans Administration. The Application for Standard Government Headstone or Marker is for a memorial issued by the Veterans Administration.

162. B: Grief experienced by all survivors is significant, but the grief of family members who survive the death of a sibling is often diminished or overlooked. It is a specific and unique grief, and needs to be acknowledged.

163. D: Society at times struggles to support and relate to specific types of death. The effect of a death on a sibling, especially during childhood, is often overlooked by society. In these cases, much of society focuses on the parent who lost a child. Even that (death of a child) focus is limited because to most people it is unrelatable, and they don't understand how complex the grief is; it is not something that is quickly "gotten over" or moved on from. Societal expectations set grief work to be completed within one year; grief is much more complicated and can take significantly longer depending on the age (of the decedent and/or survivor), nature, type, and expectancy of death. Often society bases their knowledge of death on media depictions, which frequently portray death unrealistically.

164. C: Hardwood caskets are made from angiosperm (reproduce through flowering with an encased seed) and deciduous trees (lose their leaves annually). Hardwood trees are slow-growing and therefore denser and typically more expensive than softwood. Examples of hardwood are birch, poplar, oak, cherry, maple, mahogany, cherry, and walnut. Softwood caskets are made from gymnosperm (reproduce with open, unprotected seeds) and coniferous trees (have needles and produce cones). They grow faster and are lighter in weight than hardwoods. Examples are pine, cedar, and spruce. Particle board and fiberboards are manufactured woods composed of woodchips from primarily softwoods but can at times have some hardwood mixed in.

165. A: For centuries, funeral rituals have provided the grieving with social and psychological support that helps them along their grief journey. Rituals give the family something to focus on, give them tasks to do, and allow them to acknowledge the death publicly. They give the public a place to come and show support to the surviving family. The shift away from traditional rituals has impacted people's grief journeys and can leave them feeling isolated and their loss unacknowledged.

166. A: Casket protectors are used by mausoleums to help prevent odor, infestations, and fluid leakage from mausoleum entombments. They are composed of a chemically treated fiberboard base tray with an absorbent liner, which the casket is placed on and then covered with a specialized plastic covering that is sealed around the casket. Outer burial containers are used to maintain weight loads and meet cemetery requirements for in-ground interments. Vaults are outer burial containers that meet cemetery requirements and also seal, providing protection from the outside elements. Some funeral homes use a plastic cover when transporting the casket during rain or snowstorms to protect the exterior of the casket. Most caskets are delivered with cloth coverings to protect the exteriors during transportation; once the casket is off the truck, the delivery person takes the covering off to reuse.

167. A: Conducting an identification viewing allows the family or their appointed representative to positively identify the decedent. This can be done at the place of death when the funeral home arrives to transfer the person if the family is present, or it can be done later at the funeral home. Photographs can be taken if legal permission is granted by the family; however, this is complicated because sharing photographs of the dead can be traumatic or can negatively impact the grief journey if families have constant access to the pictures (if they are emailed to or retained by the family). Identification tags from the place of death can help with identification, but they can also be incorrect, or people can have the same name. Fingerprints are only useful in identification if you run the fingerprint and the person had fingerprints in a database to match.

168. B: Once the cremation has begun, it is irreversible. This creates an immense amount of liability for funeral homes and crematories. It is essential to limit liability by securing proper authorizations, establishing identification, and verifying what is to be cremated with the decedent. Burials have less liability because they are reversible; a person can be exhumed.

169. A: The mortuary or ambulance cot is the most important item for transferring remains. It is a portable stretcher that has wheels, a mattress, and belts. It is used by both ambulances and funeral homes to move the injured and deceased. A flexible stretcher is a collapsible stretcher that folds so it can be carried up and down stairs. It can then be opened on site. The deceased can be placed on it and strapped in until they can be transferred to the cot. It is not the most important item for transfer since it is only used in special circumstances when access is difficult, such as in stairwells or elevators. The transfer vehicle refers to the actual motorized vehicle that transports the deceased from the place of death to the funeral home. The church truck is the portable device on wheels that can be extended to serve as a resting apparatus to display or move a casket in church or a funeral home.

170. B: Vaults have sealing properties to protect the casket from outside elements and withstand cemetery weight loads. Outer burial containers are required by most cemeteries (not all) to help with ground maintenance, helping to prevents the ground from caving in as the casket deteriorates and to withstand passing weight loads as cemetery equipment drives over and around graves. Grave liners are a non-sealing type of outer burial container. All outer burial containers are designed and manufactured to withstand the weight of the earth around the casket and passing weight loads. Common materials for outer burial containers are concrete (lined or unlined, reinforced with steel or not), steel, stainless steel, copper, polypropylene, and fiberglass.

Funeral Science

1. B: The middle third of the face is designated by the distance between the superior margin of the eyebrow and the base of the nose. This measurement is equivalent to the length of the ear, and the distance from the lateral eye to the tragus. The first third extends from the natural hair line, down the forehead, to the superior margin of the eyebrows. The lowest third extends from the base of the nose to the inferior margin of the chin. The lower third can be broken into three equal subsections: the base of the nose to the lip line, lip line to the superior margin of the chin, and the superior margin of the chin to the inferior margin of the chin.

2. C: Within the femoral triangle, the order from lateral and superficial to medial and deep is femoral nerve, femoral artery, and femoral vein. Most arteries are medial to, and deeper than, their corresponding vein. However, the layout within the femoral triangle is different. The lateral border of the triangle is the medial aspect of the sartorius muscle. The medial border is the adductor longus muscle. The superior border is the inguinal ligament. The femoral artery and vein are located under the fascia lata. If a vein is found superior to the fascia lata, it is presumably the greater saphenous vein, which connects to the femoral vein.

3. C: Oral and/or written permission must be given prior to embalming a decedent. Technically, any alteration made to the decedent should have specific permission granted by the family, not just restoration procedures that significantly alter the appearance of the decedent. Most funeral homes use the embalming authorization to cover basic embalming and restoration measures such as setting features and repositioning the body in a reposed position. Bodily conditions treated during arterial injection, such as edema, jaundice, and emaciation treatments using humectants, fall under the basic restoration procedures of embalming. For advanced or extreme restoration procedures, formal permission should be secured in writing. Malformations may be normal for that decedent and removal would alter the appearance beyond recognition. A family may not want any alterations or corrective measures performed for this reason. For recent malformations, disfigurements, and traumas, the family may specifically request that corrective measures be taken. If the family does not suggest restorations, always ask and secure specific permission.

4. B: If the eyes are closed correctly, the eyelids meet two-thirds of the way down the eye but do not overlap. The top lids are not pulled all the way down as is commonly believed.

5. C: The crucifix should be set up by the casket for the viewing of a catholic decedent. The location the crucifix is placed varies based on the traditions of the area and type of caskets used. Typically, it is placed by the head of the casket or centered behind the closed foot end cap of a half couch casket. If the casket is closed, the crucifix is usually centered behind the casket. A crucifix is a religious cross that depicts Jesus on it. There are different variations of the crucifix depending on the religious sect (Orthodox, Roman, Russian, Ukrainian, etc.). A cross is a religious Christian symbol of two perpendicular pieces, vertical and horizontal, intersecting, without Jesus depicted on it. A pall is a Catholic drape for the casket used during a funeral mass at church to represent the decedent's baptism. Other Catholic equipment that may be set up or used for the visitation in addition to the crucifix are the kneeler, candles at the head and foot of the casket, mass tray, rosary beads, and prayer cards.

6. D: Differential pressure is the difference between the potential pressure reading and the actual pressure reading. It is a gauge of the rate of flow, which is the amount of embalming solution that enters the body in a given period. A vacuum breaker is an accessory device that prevents water from flowing backwards into an unintended water source, which would result in contamination or pollution.

7. C: Massage cream thinned with a little mineral oil works well to fill in tissue subcutaneously. Water will not fill in tissue, and will probably make the condition of the tissue worse. Wax is too thick to inject hypodermically, and tissue filler solvent will not fill in tissue.

8. A: A tissue reducer, or tissue dryer, is used to remove fluid from areas of the body subjected to trauma and edema. The tissue reducer needs to be heated up with the selected tip (sizes vary based on working area, methods, and treatment goals). Apply massage cream liberally to the area that will be exposed to the heat. The tissue reducer is applied to the skin and pulled/pushed to move fluid out of an area. The tissue reducer can also be used to smooth out skin or recreate facial wrinkles and characteristics. A water collar can be filled with water or sand and secured around a swollen neck to reduce the size with pressure and weight. A trocar or baby trocar are used to channel tissue to help drain fluid out of an area. Procurement teams use a dermatome to remove thin shavings of skin off organ donors.

9. B: *Clostridium perfringens* is a bacterium can cause tissue gas when it is present in a deceased body (postmortem). This bacterium is easily transmitted from one body to another if the trocar is not disinfected between uses. The bacterium *Streptococcus pyogenes* can be transmitted from large respiratory droplets, and infected persons can develop streptococcal sore throat or rheumatic fever. *Clostridium tetani* is a bacterium transmitted by spores that can enter the body through needle sticks and puncture wounds. It is also called tetanus (lockjaw). *Staphylococcus aureus* is a bacterium often present in skin abscesses, furuncles, and carbuncles, and can be transmitted by infiltrating lesions in the skin and mucous membranes.

10. A: The parietal eminences, located on each of the parietal bones, are the widest part on each side of the skull. When determining a skull's width, the measure is taken between the left and right parietal eminences. These eminences are located superior to the posterior ear. The parietal bones are located on the superior sides and top of the cranium. The temporal bones make up the inferior sides and base of the cranium. The zygomatic arch is the cheekbone. It attaches to the temporal bone at a portion of it called the squama. The lateral aspect of the zygomatic arch is the widest part of the face. The mental eminence is the triangular prominence on the medial aspect of the mandible (the chin).

11. D: Caskets should be locked or securely latched. If the casket is metal with a gasketed seal, it should be locked but the cap for the locking mechanism should not fastened. The end of the gasket where the crank opens and closes it should be left open to accommodate air pressure changes. If the cap is secured in place on a locked casket, it creates a seal which can damage the casket with changing air pressures during the flight. Wooden caskets, like the metal ones, should be latched or locked to secure the lid. Wooden caskets do not have a risk of compression damage during flights because they are not airtight.

12. D: If a family asks for the body to be embalmed, it must be performed. If they choose services such as direct burial or direct cremation, embalming is not necessary. The FTC Funeral Rule does not require embalming. Remains do not have to be embalmed to be shipped out of town because religious or other customs may allow the deceased to be shipped using dry ice or other means of preventing decomposition en route.

13. C: Ideally, the base tissues for reconstruction are firm and dry. It is essential that they are dry. Moist tissue is not suitable for reconstruction because tissue and cosmetics will not adhere to it. Soft and malleable tissues are difficult to use as a base for reconstruction because they move when trying to apply wax. Firm tissue allows wax to be applied and manipulated into shape easier.

14. A: The often reddish, exterior protrusion of the upper and lower lips which round convexly from the line of closure to the integumentary lip is called *vermillion*. In embalming and restorative art texts, it is referred to instead as the *mucous membrane*. Technically, the anatomy of the upper and lower lips has mucous membrane, vermillion, and cutaneous parts. In mortuary studies, the vermillion is referred to simply as *mucous membrane* because it is composed of a modified mucous membrane. The cutaneous surface of the lips in this context is referred to as the integumentary lip. Outside of this context, mucous membranes are found throughout the body and function as the lining of many cavities and organs throughout the digestive and respiratory systems. The oral mucosa, the interior of the mouth, is composed of mucous membrane. The line of closure is where the upper and lower mucous membranes (vermillion) meet when the mouth is closed. The upper integumentary lip extends superiorly from the upper mucous membrane while the lower extends inferiorly from the margin of the lower mucous membrane towards the chin.

15. B: Bacteria are prokaryotic, single-celled organisms that can live and function independently or in colonies. Bacilli are rod-shaped bacteria that cause diseases such as anthrax, botulism, and tetanus or infections such as *E. coli* and *Salmonella*. Pleomorphic bacteria vary in shape and size based on environmental factors. Cocci are sphere-shaped and responsible for causing some types of urinary tract infections, toxic shock syndrome, and pneumonia. Vibrio are a type of spiral bacteria that have a curved, comma-like shape. They can cause cholera, septicemia, and gastroenteritis. Other types of spirals are spirilla (thick, rigid spirals) and spirochetes (thin, bendable spirals).

16. C: On the color wheel, the complimentary color to red is green. Although the most common color for concealer is beige, complimentary colors work best on discolored areas. Once these areas have been neutralized in this manner, they can then be covered with a natural color of makeup.

17. A: Personal possessions must be removed from the decedent, washed, labeled, inventoried, and prepared for being returned to the family. The family may want specific items to remain with the decedent for the services. These items may be returned to the family after the service, prior to disposition, or the family may want them to stay with the body. The requests of the family and disposition of the possessions should be documented on the inventory list. The list should then be reviewed with the family. Often, funeral homes will have the next of kin sign off, authorizing disposition or acknowledging the receipt of the possessions. Any items the family wants back can be returned once they are clean and organized for the family. This may be at the arrangement conference after the list is reviewed with the family, or at a later time. Do not store items without reviewing them with the family. Problems could arise if the family wanted to bury or cremate something with the decedent, but it was removed and stored past disposition without their knowledge.

18. D: The ear is subject to the least amount of change throughout a person's life because it is composed of cartilage and covered with smooth, taut skin. The lobe consists of adipose and areolar tissue. This composition subjects the lobe to the most change over time compared to the rest of the cartilaginous ear. Other facial features are comprised of combinations of bone, muscle, cartilage, and adipose tissues covered by integument. These compositions allow for natural folds and sulci while the repetitive movement of facial muscles causes acquired furrows, grooves, and sulci to develop over time.

19. C: Opaque cosmetics are used to cover something like a blemish or discoloration from view since they do not permit light to pass through them. Translucent cosmetics are used to diminish the appearance of something but not hide it from view since they allow diffused light to pass through. A transparent cosmetic is one that is used when there is no need to hide any blemish or discoloration. An aerosol is a medium for spraying a product that uses a gas propellant. In the case of cosmetics, an aerosol can spray products that are opaque, translucent, or transparent.

20. B: The oval head shape is the most common head shape. When viewed from the front, the cheekbones are wider than the cranium and the cranium is a little bit wider than the lower jaw. The diamond head shape is the widest when viewed from the front. It is also characterized by wide cheekbones and a narrow forehead and jaw line. The round head shape is short and features full cheeks, a full jaw line, and a rounded cranium. The oblong head shape is long and narrow. The forehead and the chin may be rounded or square.

21. D: Chemotherapies and drugs (medicinal or recreational) impact the body by causing physiological changes which in turn decreases the effectiveness of embalming chemicals. For example, drugs can reduce the permeability of cell membranes, making it more difficult for embalming fluid to enter the cell to achieve preservation. Drugs and chemotherapies can also cause liver failure, resulting in jaundice, or kidney failure, causing an increased amount of nitrogenous waste to be present in the body. The chemotherapies and drugs do not alter the embalming chemicals and their properties. More arterial fluid is needed to ensure preservation.

22. A: The endocrine system manufactures hormones from various glands. The hormones are transported all over the body and direct chemical communication in the body. Red blood cells are formed in the bone marrow. White blood cells are created in the bone marrow. Bile is a solution formed by the liver that accumulates in the gall bladder and is discharged into the small intestine through the bile ducts.

23. D: When aspirating, the right side of the heart can be tapped by aligning the base of the trocar along the left anterior iliac spine with the point extending across the torso and directed towards the right earlobe. The liver is located in the right upper quadrant of the abdomen. The left side of the heart would be tapped by aligning the base of the trocar below the standard point of entry and directing the point of the trocar towards the left earlobe. The lungs are aspirated by directing the trocar in a fanning motion throughout the chest cavity within the ribcage.

24. D: Cranial incisions from an autopsy may leak if the sutures are not secured tightly, the incisions and tissues are not fully chemically cauterized, or with excessive movement or pressure. Plastic should be kept under the head (between the head and pillow) in the casket to provide a protective barrier. Absorptive pads can also be utilized. The physical movement from moving the body from the table to the casket can cause the sutured area to weep. The positional change (the angle and incline of the body) between the table and casket can also spur leaking. If a there is abdominal distension, the body needs to be reasipriated to remove gas and prevent additional buildup of gases that can lead to nasal and oral purge. Leaking sutures along the carotid incision (or even the femoral) can be a sign of increased pressure from gas or fluid in the torso. All bodies coming from another funeral home should be reaspirated to ensure the body was not only treated properly initially but to alleviate any fluid or gas buildup that occurred during transportation.

25. B: Passive hyperemia is a condition that occurs when a malady causes excess blood to stay in a body part, preventing normal drainage. Thrombosis is the condition of reduced blood passage due to a blood clot (thrombus) inside a blood vessel. Active hyperemia is the condition when surplus blood is purposefully taken by blood vessels to an area such as a muscle during exercise. It is not the result of a disease. An embolism is a condition that occurs when a thrombus causes a stoppage in the flow in a blood vessel by blocking the passageway.

26. C: *Diffusion* refers to the movement of molecules from a region of high measurable concentration to a different locale with low measurable concentration. Hydrolysis is a chemical change that occurs as a result of the introduction of water. Cell walls burst and their water is released. It is a very significant component of tissue decomposition. Saturation is an explanatory term used to describe a solution that has absorbed all the solvent it can. A compound is matter that contains two or more components that are chemically integrated.

27. D: Capillaries are the third type of blood vessels. The atria and ventricles are part of the heart but are not blood vessels. Valves are found in the heart and the veins, but are not vessels themselves.

28. D: Arterial selection is influenced by many considerations and observations made during the initial preembalming case analysis and the reevaluations throughout the embalming. Initial arterial selection is influenced by pathologies, trauma, cause of death, malformations and disfigurements, age of the decedent, and morbidity. Vessel accessibility and practicality are influenced by these factors. Throughout the embalming, if distribution to specific areas of the body is not successful, less practical or convenient vessels will need to be considered to obtain sufficient distribution. Gender has little influence compared to the other factors of vessel selection. Some embalmers select the femoral as the primary injection site for females so the neckline of clothing does not need to be limited or restricted. Alternatively, some embalmers opt to use more discreet sutures such as the worm or intradermal suture in visible (or potentially visible) areas.

29. C: Skin coloration is affected by the amount of melanin deposited in the cells of the epidermis and the coloration of blood within the superficial vasculature. Another pigmentation that impacts a person's skin tone comes from the superficial fascia (fat or adipose) within the hypodermis; this coloration is called carotene. The level of a person's carotene fluctuates throughout life. In the elderly, carotene can cause a yellow or gray appearance. The deeper a person's pigmentation, the more melanin is present within the cells comprising their epidermis. Exposure to sun deepens the pigmentation as a natural defense mechanism of the body. Moles and freckles are areas of deeper pigmentation.

30. A: Medical devices should be removed prior to embalming when they are attached or secured to the face or if they will interfere with embalming. Devices such as intravenous lines may act as counter pressures to prevent leaking during arterial injection when left in place. Once removed, these medical devices are disposed of as biohazardous medical waste. All removed medical devices are documented on the embalming report. Internal hardware and medical devices are left intact. If a person is cremated, the metal is removed following the cremation, prior to pulverization. Some states allow crematories to sell metal removed from the body to recycling companies. State law regulates the profit from this, donation of profit, and disclosures that need to be made to families prior to cremation. Hospitals do not want used medical devices back. Occasionally, the family or the medical team will ask for a medical device back for evaluation, research, or to conduct testing on it. This is not the norm though. Autoclaves are used to clean medical instruments.

31. B: Autopsy gels have the same chemical composition as cavity fluid but are in a gel form to make applying the gels to the autopsied surfaces of the body and viscera easier.

32. C: The centrifugal pump is a relatively contemporary device because it uses an electric pump to produce pressure that can be delivered with or without a pulsating effect. The bulb syringe was a device that was used in the past in embalming. It was manually squeezed to deliver and release pressure and the ensuing flow. The gravity bottle was a frequently used historic technique of embalming that used the force of gravity to move embalming fluids. The hand pump was another device historically used for embalming that relied on the manual action of one's hand to create pressure and move fluid.

33. A: Saturation is an explanatory term used to describe a solution that has absorbed all of the solvent it can. Sublimation is the direct conversion of a solid to a gas. The matter does not go through the liquid phase. Inflammation describes the condition of a living body that has stimulated itself into a state of resistance in which engorgement and calor (heat) become noticeable physical characteristics. Binary fission is the means by which most bacteria reproduce.

34. D: Forensic autopsies are ordered by the coroner or medical examiner to determine the cause and manner of death for deaths that are unattended, suspicious, violent, traumatic, or accidental. They can be conducted with or without permission from the family. A pathologist, forensic pathologist, or medical examiner conducts the examination and testing. Hospital autopsies are conducted with the permission of the family, when a medical diagnosis has not been determined prior to death, experimental treatments were used, following a death during a diagnostic surgery or childbirth, in the case of a contagious disease, or under other undeterminable or suspicious circumstances. Partial autopsies are performed on a specific area or areas of the body, rather than on the entire body. They are typically categorized as thoracic, abdominal (abdominopelvic), vertebral (ventral or dorsal), and cranial autopsies. *Necropsy* is another word for autopsy but commonly used to describe postmortem examinations of animals rather than humans.

35. A: Anasarca, generalized edema present throughout the body, should be treated with a hypertonic solution or solution containing large colloidal molecules to displace the excess fluid present within the tissues of the body. Using strong arterial fluid concentrations to account for secondary dilution, high index fluids to cause dehydration, and specialized edema coinjections containing salts all help draw excess fluid out of the tissues and into the vascular system to be drained. Hypotonic solutions are used in cases of dehydration to retain moisture within the tissues of the body.

36. C: The nasolabial fold extends from the superior, lateral nasal wing and extends down laterally to the line of closure. The fold forms a crucial aspect of the anterior cheek. The lateral aspect of the nasolabial fold is seen from the profile view, while the medial aspect is hidden from view. When the fold has significant projection, the angulus oris eminence and angulus oris sulcus are also blocked from view. The angulus oris eminence is a small protrusion lateral to the line of closure where the muscles converge. The angulus oris sulcus is a crease in the eminence where it meets the line of closure. The nasal sulcus is the groove that extends from the superior portion of the nasolabial fold and curves down around the exterior margin of the nasal wing. The philtrum is a natural facial crease that extends from the lateral aspects both sides of the columna nasi down the upper integumentary lip to the upper mucous membrane.

37. C: Pre-injection and co-injection fluids also work well with arterial preservative fluids, but cavity fluids have higher concentrations of preservatives and disinfectants.

38. C: The line of closure for the eye is where the upper and lower eye lids meet when the eye is closed. The upper eyelid extends two-thirds of the way down the orbital cavity before meeting with the lower eyelid. The lower eyelid therefore extends upwards from the bottom one-third of the space. The line of closure begins at the inner canthus and extends in an arced line to the outer canthus.

39. B: Furrows, grooves, folds, hollows, prominences, and depressions (dimples) are all created when facial muscles and muscles of expression contract, pulling at the skin. The insertion point of a muscle is this movable attachment while the opposite end of the muscle is the origin, the immovable attachment point to bone or cartilage. Furrows, grooves, or wrinkles are creases that appear on an otherwise smooth surface in reaction to a muscle contraction. Furrows appear perpendicular to how the muscle runs; if the muscle runs vertically, the furrow appears horizontally. This repeated movement of muscles of form and expression create acquired facial markings. Natural facial markings are characteristics that a person is born with such as sulci, eminences, folds, and dimples.

40. A: A partial autopsy may be done on the thorax and/or the abdomen. There are no autopsies done on appendages, and the neck is usually part of an autopsy of the torso.

41. B: Because of the heat it emits, an electric spatula can cause burns unless it is used carefully and massage cream is liberally applied to the skin before use.

42. B: The points of entry and exit form the letter "X," and this pattern of stitches can help reduce swelling in the neck.

43. D: Intermittent drainage will provide better distribution of the fluid, increase saturation in the tissues, and help with the removal of clots. It will not affect the organs enough to make aspiration unnecessary.

44. A: Encephalitis is a neurotropic viral disease that affects the cranial cavity by causing an engorgement and swelling of the brain tissue. Meningitis is a bacterial or viral ailment that results in an irritation of the protective membranes encasing the brain and spine (meninges). Myelitis is a disease characterized by irritation of the spine, which negatively impacts the functionality of the central nervous system. Poliomyelitis (polio) is a viral malady that impacts the function of nerve tissue and can lead to limited or complete paralysis.

45. B: A vesicle is a diminutive lesion of raised skin with fluid inside of it, such as a blister. A furuncle is an infection deep in the skin, such as an abscess or boil. An ulcer is a necrosis confined to a small area on the skin or on a mucous membrane. A carbuncle is two or more adjacent furuncles located in the deeper layers of the skin.

46. B: Most pacemakers and other medical devices with batteries need to be removed prior to cremation. The intense heat during cremation can cause the batteries to explode. These explosions will damage the brick and interior of the retort. The pacemaker can stay in place during embalming (injection and cavity treatment). If the person is going to be cremated after services that require embalming, the pacemaker can be removed prior to dressing and casketing (before the services), or it can be removed immediately prior to the cremation. Leadless (wireless or Micra) pacemakers are inserted via the femoral vein and implanted directly into the heart. They contain a battery, but it is too small to create a damaging explosion during cremation, so they do not need to be removed.

47. D: The use of reduced temperatures, including the use of freezers, will not destroy bacteria. Cold is not bactericidal; it has only been demonstrated to be bacteriostatic because it merely slows the growth of bacteria. Dry heat involves the use of a hot-air oven. It is more effective at destroying bacteria than cold. Moist heat is more bactericidal than dry heat or cold, and it is faster than both of them. An autoclave uses steam under pressure, and is the most bactericidal of the physical methods listed.

60. B: The natural convex area between the supercilium (eyebrow) and upper eyelid is called the supraorbital area. Its inferior margin is along the superior palpebra sulcus, the acquired crease along the superior margin of the upper eyelid. The naso-orbital fossa is the natural concave space between the root of the nose, medial edge of the upper eyelid, medial side of the supraorbital area, and medial inferior margin of the supercilium. The orbital pouch is the acquired area inferior to the lower eye lid, extending from the oblique palpebral sulcus (natural curving crease off the inner canthus) in an arc back up to the supraorbital area. This pouch can be puffy in some decedents or may appear as a concave, dark area in those who struggled with extended illness or emaciation.

61. A: Cranial hair restoration begins at the inferior margin where the hair loss begins. The space can be filled working in either direction (medial to lateral or lateral to medial), working across the area first and then working upwards following the direction the hair lays. Typically, hair is applied in small sections or increments. The hair should be applied at longer lengths and trimmed once in place. The direction of the hair (how it lays, combs, or styles) does impact how the restoration should begin. At the top of the head, the restoration begins at the posterior margin and works forward towards the face.

62. D: Formalin is a solution in which formaldehyde is dissolved into water or water and methyl alcohol. Formaldehyde is a colorless gas at room temperature. A measured 37.0-37.3% mass (or 40% volume) of formaldehyde gas and 7% methyl alcohol are used to create formalin. The remainder of the solution is water. Paraformaldehyde is the solid form of formaldehyde. Index is the number of grams of formaldehyde gas dissolved into 100 mL of a solution of water or water and methyl alcohol. Phenol is a preservative, germicide, and bleaching agent primarily used in cavity fluids and as a cauterant, bleaching, reducing, and drying agent applied topically or injected hypodermically. Embalming machines are typically labeled with warnings to not use them to inject fluids containing phenol.

63. C: A dermatome is an instrument used to procure a thin layer or shaving of skin from a donor. Typical areas of procurement for skin are the back, buttocks, thighs (front and/or back), and calves. Sometimes a thick layer of skin is procured from the shoulders, down the back to the top of the buttocks, rather than just a thin shaving. A hemostat is a locking forceps used to clamp tissue and vessels with either a straight or curved end with a smooth or serrated edge. A bistoury knife is a type of scalpel used to incise tissue and vessels. A separator is used to raise vessels above the level of the skin. It is fished under the vessel and is long enough to rest on both sides of the incision, keeping the vessel accessible above the surface of the skin.

64. A: Synarthroses are skeletal links that are not moveable, are unbending, and are held together by unyielding connective tissue. Amphiarthroses are skeletal links that are somewhat moveable. They are held together by connective tissue that allows some articulation. Diarthroses are skeletal links that are very moveable, allowing for a full range of articulation in a joint.

65. D: Rigor mortis is the stiffening of the muscles throughout the body as lactic acid increases and the body no longer processes adenosine triphosphate (ATP). Although rigor occurs in all muscles, affecting them at the same time and rate, it can be observed first in the smaller muscles such as facial muscles (e.g., eyes, jaw, face), then becomes apparent over time in larger muscles of the torso, upper extremities, and lower extremities. Primary flaccidity occurs prior to onset of rigor when the body muscles are relaxed immediately postmortem. Secondary flaccidity occurs post rigor when the muscles begin to relax again as proteins are broken down.

66. B: Dr. Thomas Holmes (1817-1900) is credited with being the father of embalming. Prior to the Civil War, Holmes was a medical physician and coroner who experimented with embalming techniques and chemical mixtures. Techniques sometimes involved arterial injection without drainage or cavity treatment. Other times, hypodermic injection was used along with opening the cavity to treat the viscera. During the Civil War, Holmes opened an embalming practice in Washington, DC and embalmed over 4,000 bodies, including many prominent and highly ranked soldiers. Following the war, he operated a drug store and only performed embalmings sporadically. Dr. Auguste Renouard (1839-1912) started using a new technique for arterial embalming and was widely praised for the appearance of his bodies. In 1878, he published the first embalming textbook written in the United States and was instrumental in opening and heading multiple embalming schools throughout his career. Renouard advocated for the use of both arterial embalming and cavity treatment. Joseph Henry Clarke (1840-1916) was a casket and embalming fluid salesperson who performed demonstrations and embalming classes, eventually founding the Clarke School of Embalming in Cincinnati, OH. A. Johnson Dodge (1848-1926) wrote three embalming textbooks, owned a traveling embalming school, and later started another school of his own. He eventually opened Dodge Chemical Company in Boston, MA.

67. D: Basket-weave sutures are used to secure tissue together and span gaps, giving filling materials support in areas that have been subjected to trauma or excision. These sutures are made intradermally when the tissue needs to be filled in rather than built up. If the tissue has been undercut and will need to be built up further with wax, the basketweave suture can be stitched back and forth, weaving in and out of the skin. The suture pattern begins from the anchoring stitch, across the expanse of the wound, and back. The spacing of the stitch depends on how firm and supportive the underlying tissues are. Once the expanse is filled, sutures are then made in the perpendicular direction. For example, if the first set of sutures went from the lateral to medial borders of the margin, the second set would go anterior to inferior. Sutures will be applied to the deepest tissues and worked superficially toward the surface of the expanse. Armature is the framework or support used in reconstruction (wire, metal, plastic, plaster of paris, cotton, sutures, or a combination of materials).

68. B: The heart is the center of the circulatory system. The lungs are central to the respiratory system. Although arteries and veins are part of the circulatory system, they cannot operate without the heart.

69. C: Airflow should not be eliminated when storing a body for delayed viewing or disposition. Sufficient airflow is needed to help keep the body dry and prevent mold growth. Putting the body on bridges or body blocks allows air to flow under the body. If the body is flat on the table, air will not be able to pass underneath. Without the blocking, the body would also lay in any fluid that leaks out, leading to faster deterioration of the body. If the body is exposed to too much airflow, it will dehydrate. It is important to keep the hands, face, and neck coated with a massage cream to help prevent dehydration. The body should be sprayed with a chemical wetting agent and draped with a gown dampened with the wetting agent to prevent dehydration and mold growth.

70. A: The parietal bones are the two area bones of the cranium as well as the apex piece of the cranium. The occipital bones are situated in the lower back region of the cranium. The temporal bones includes the lowermost sides and base of the cranium. The zygomatic bones are the diamond-shaped bones that outline the cheekbones.

71. C: The greater saphenous vein is the longest vein in the human body. It extends from the medial marginal vein located on the dorsum of the foot, around the medial aspect of the knee, and connects to the femoral vein within the femoral triangle. The largest-diameter vein in the body is the inferior vena cava, which connects to the lower right atrium of the heart. Veins from the lower body move deoxygenated blood from the tissues of the body, connecting to other veins, increasing in size as blood is pumped back towards the heart, then conjoining with the inferior vena cava. The aorta is the largest artery in the body, connected to the left ventricle of the heart by the aortic root. The sections of the aorta as it leaves the heart are the aortic root, ascending aorta, aortic arch, descending aorta, thoracic aorta, and abdominal aorta which bifurcates into the left and right common iliac arteries.

72. C: Hexoses are simple sugar carbohydrates composed of six carbons. They are found throughout the body as glucose in the blood and galactose in brain and nerve tissue. Lipids are fats created when an aldehyde reacts with fatty acid. Lipids contain hydrogen, carbon, and oxygen but can additionally contain other components such as nitrogen or phosphorous. Emulsifiers are compounds used to mix two or more compounds together that normally do not mix. Organic acids are organic compounds with acidic properties and have a general formula containing a carbon double bonded to oxygen, ending in a hydrogen (−**COOH**).

73. B: State law regulates when refrigeration should be used for retaining the dead. There are legal requirements for how long a decedent can be held without being embalmed, cremated, or sealed in a casket for burial without embalming. In many states, this time is 24-48 hours. Delays past these times often involve requiring refrigeration (or a means of refrigeration such as dry ice or ice packs) until disposition can proceed. State law will also regulate how long the decedent can be removed from refrigeration prior to proceeding with disposition.

74. C: Buffers are used in supplemental chemicals such as preinjections or coinjection chemicals and even added to arterial fluids by manufacturers. Buffers help prepare the vascular system and tissue to effectively receive preservation by balancing the pH within the blood and tissues. Buffers do not contribute preservation qualities. When buffers are used within arterial chemicals, they aid in correcting pH and maintaining a close to neutral balance. Some buffers can also act as water conditioners and anticoagulants. Anticoagulants can be preinjected or used as coinjections to treat postmortem coagulations and blood clots that form as the body dehydrates and fluid gravitates postmortem. Water conditioners are used to treat hard water (water is added to the embalming fluid during primary dilution), address medications and drugs within the body, create a slightly alkaline condition during injection, and work as anticoagulants. Water conditioners can also act as buffers. Humectants are used to prevent dehydration of the tissue during and after the embalming process. These emollients retain moisture and give the tissue a soft, life-like appearance.

75. D: Restorative derma-surgery wax has a medium thickness and firmness. It is made to fill in surface blemishes or shallow restorations. Wound filler is a firm and dense wax for larger, deep restorative work. Surface restorer is used for minor blemishes on the skin such as razor burn or abrasions. Lip wax is ideal for restoring features of the lips. Wax can be bought or tinted in different colors. Environmental factors such as temperature and humidity will impact the firmness and density of the wax.

76. B: When a body has problematic shoulders or has edema in the shoulders, the most protection against leakage will be provided by unionalls. Any leakage from the shoulders will be wicked down the back. Absorptive powders should be placed inside the unionalls to absorb any of this liquid that may escape the body. Plastic shirts could be used to cover the shoulders. However, they may not provide protection from wicking and gravitating fluid. Shirts used in conjunction with other plastics (tucked into pants, capris, or coveralls) may prevent leaking. Sleeves only cover the arms from above the wrist to the armpit. Sleeve coverage does not adequately extend over the shoulder to provide efficient and secure protection.

77. B: Using red or pink lights in the viewing room will make the body appear redder in color overall, effectively washing out the red tones of cosmetics used to highlight warm areas of the face. When using these lights, it is necessary to apply a significant amount of red coloring to warm areas to make them stand out more under the red or pink lights. This creates an exaggerated or theatrical look under normal white lighting. Red lights are helpful in jaundice cases because they cast an overall red hue on the decedent. Incandescent bulbs with eggshell or ivory shades can complement cosmetics by adding a natural yellow, common in some skin tones. Lighting color and strength is important because it affects coloration (e.g., darken, lighten, redden, yellow), washes coloring out, or creates natural or unnatural shadows.

78. D: Accessory chemicals are used to support preservation, disinfect, control leaking, cauterize, and bleach. They can be used internally (autopsies, surgical wounds, organ donation), topically (wounds, abrasions, skin slip), or injected hypodermically (discolorations, areas lacking preservation). Accessory chemicals come in the form of sealing agents, powders, gels, liquids, and creams. Topical chemicals are a type of accessory chemical. Supplemental chemicals are preinjection chemicals and co-injection chemicals which are used as vascular conditioners, modifying agents, anticoagulants, dyes, and treatments for body conditions. They support arterial fluid but do not offer any preservative qualities.

79. D: Case analysis is when the embalmer observes the body, factors in known information (e.g., medical history, service period, family requests), and determines what methods and techniques will achieve the best results. During the initial case analysis and throughout the embalming, there are four steps to implement: observation of the body condition, evaluation of known information, and implementation of a treatment course (chemical selection, injection and drainage selections, restoration approach), which ideally results in a sanitized, temporarily preserved, and viewable body. Continuous observation and evaluation throughout the entire embalming may lead to changes to the original strategy and implementation of different methods to ensure satisfactory results.

80. C: Checking for a pulse is considered an inexpert test of death. Inexpert tests are conducted by those without medical expertise or when medical equipment is not available. Other inexpert methods include a ligature test, ammonia injection test, and listening to or observing respirations or heartbeat by ear. Expert death tests are conducted by trained medical professionals legally allowed to declare a person dead (this is determined by specific state law). Expert tests include using a stethoscope, ophthalmoscope, electroencephalogram, electrocardiogram, or evoked response testing. Embalmers and funeral directors are not legally responsible to conduct death tests. However, there are times when knowing how experts conduct death tests and how to conduct inexpert death tests is beneficial.

81. A: In standard facial proportions, the width of the base of the nose equals the width of the eye. The eye is one-half the width of the mouth, one-fifth the width of the face, and equal to the distance between the eyes.

82. A: Desiccation is severe dehydration of the body, resulting in a leathery appearance to the skin. Areas where the skin is thin are apt to show signs of desiccation first. These areas include the lips, fingertips, toes, eyelids, ears, and nose. Arterial injection and hypodermic injection will do little to correct this extensive dehydration, especially in severe cases. The lips will turn black and recede. Other areas will turn yellowish-brown and then black as they shrivel with dehydration. The skin loses its elasticity, becoming very hard in addition to changing color; this makes rehydrating the tissue difficult even with hypodermic treatment. Imbibition occurs postmortem when the body absorbs the liquid portion of blood out of the vascular system, causing postmortem edema.

Ecchymosis is the flat bruising or discoloration of the tissue from a ruptured vessel. Crepitation is the crackling and popping sensation when touching areas where gas is trapped within the tissues of a decedent. Examples of this are subcutaneous emphysema or tissue gas caused by clostridium perfringens.

83. B: The center of drainage is the right atrium of the heart. When using the right internal jugular as the primary drainage site, the drain tube or angular spring forceps are inserted towards the heart. They are often long enough to reach into the upper portion of the right atrium. Blood enters the right atrium from the superior vena cava and inferior vena cava, travels through the tricuspid valve to the right ventricle, and through the pulmonary valve into the pulmonary artery to the lungs. Once oxygenated, blood travels back through the pulmonary vein, into the left atrium, through the mitral valve, and into the left ventricle, then is pumped out through the aorta. When drainage is from a different location, such as the femoral vein, the instruments are directed towards the heart.

84. D: An antigen is something that enters the body and causes an immune response. An antibody is a protein produced by the body when exposed to an antigen. It is part of the immune response to fight off the invasion of the antigen. An antidote is a treatment that neutralizes a poison. An antiseptic is used for disinfecting surfaces such as the skin.

85. B: Livor mortis (also called postmortem lividity or cadaveric lividity) is the intravascular discoloration of dependent areas of the body caused by hypostasis, which is gravitational settling of the blood. Discoloration begins postmortem as a red color, which deepens and darkens over time to a reddish, purple, or blue color. Lividity is impacted by the blood volume and blood viscosity. Embalming will remove or reduce lividity because it is intravascular. Extravascular postmortem staining occurs when blood (technically heme, which results from hemolysis, the breakdown of hemoglobin within the blood) is pulled out of the vascular system by gravity, into the dependent tissues. Extravascular stains are not removed with arterial embalming so other methods to reduce the staining must be implemented. Tardieu spots are extravascular heme discolorations caused by small vascular ruptures or petechial hemorrhages that are also not removed during arterial injection. Contact pallor is when a dependent area is not subjected to lividity because of pressure on the area. Examples are the bend of an elbow or the back where the body weight is pressing on the table. Temperature loss postmortem is called algor mortis. The cooling rate of the body is impacted by intrinsic (e.g., body mass, surface area, and body temperature at time of death) and extrinsic (e.g., ambient temperature, environment, and clothing) factors.

86. C: Pre-injection and co-injection are not categories of embalming, but are part of the arterial embalming process. Autopsy embalming is not an embalming category.

87. B: The dorsum of the nose extends from the glabella down the entire length of the nose and continues as it curves around the tip, ending at the columna nasi. The dorsum consists of the root, bridge, protruding lobe, and tip of the nose. The nasal profile extends down the dorsum from the root to the tip of the nose. The glabella is the eminence on the forehead directly superior to the root of the nose. The root is located at the superior portion of the dorsum at the natural dip where the frontal bone and nasal bone meet. The bridge is the area of the nose covering the nasal bone, inferior to the root.

88. A: Hepatitis A is classified as highly contagious, hepatitis B and C are mildly contagious, and there is no such thing as hepatitis D.

89. B: The convex profile is the most common profile form among human beings. In this form, a person's forehead posteriorly recedes from the eyebrows and the chin recedes from the upper lip. A vertically balanced profile is when the chin, forehead, and upper lip are all aligned, so none of them protrude or recede more than the other two features. A concave profile is when the forehead protrudes further than the eyebrows and the chin protrudes beyond the plane of the upper lip. There is no such thing as a horizontally balanced profile.

90. B: A drain tube is a hollow cylinder with an interior rod, inserted into the vein to control drainage. The interior rod is used to break up clots. The tube can be opened or closed to allow drainage to exit the vein or closed to build pressure within the vascular system. A rubber hose can be attached to the drain tube to aid in keeping a clean workspace. Drain tubes are available in assorted sizes, with or without angles, so they can be used in various veins. Angular spring forceps are an instrument used to hold or grasp tissue by manually pinching the handle to close the two-piece end. They function as a drainage instrument and come in various sizes and lengths. They hold the vein open and can be pinched to grab and pull clots out. Groove directors are instruments inserted into a vein or artery to hold it open while the drainage or arterial instrument is inserted. Trocars are large cylindrical, hollow instruments with a point on the end, used to remove fluid from the cavity during aspiration. The trocar can also be inserted directly into the right atrium of the heart, from the standard insertion point, for an alternative method of drainage. It should be used as a secondary drainage method, to work in conjunction with a primary drainage method, rather than as the primary drainage method.

91. B: The 100 percent formalin mixture used in embalming is 37 percent HCHO gas by weight and 40 percent HCHO gas by volume.

92. D: The medial boarder of the sternocleidomastoid muscle is used as the anatomical guide to locating the carotid sheath, which contains the internal jugular vein, vagus nerve, and common carotid artery (ordered lateral and superficial to medial and deep). The platysma is the thin, superficial cutaneous muscle, functioning to move the skin of the neck to contribute to facial expressions, which is incised through to expose the anterior triangle. The omohyoid muscle runs superficially across the carotid sheath. This is a helpful guide for the embalmer as they dissect deep towards the vessels. The sternoclavicular articulation is the joint where the medial aspect of the clavicle conjoins with the sternum.

93. B: Arteries and veins both have three layers. The thickest layer of an artery is the tunica media, the middle layer. which is composed of muscle and elastic tissue cells. This composition allows for the artery to expand and contract to regulate blood flow. The outermost layer, the tunica adventitia or tunica externa, is made of connective tissue. The inner layer is the tunica intima and is composed of endothelial cells. This inner layer is what capillary walls consist of. The hollow space within arteries is called the lumen. Arteries are thicker than veins because they accommodate blood at higher pressures than veins. Veins have venous valves to prevent backflow of blood while arteries do not.

94. D: Humectants are not arterial fluid preservatives but modifying agents, which work with arterial fluids to help offset dehydration.

95. A: Physiognomy is the study of facial proportions. Physiology is the study of the functions of living systems. Restorative art is the practice of restoring something to its original state. Facial positioning is a meaningless term.

96. C: Formaldehyde gray is the discoloration to the skin caused by a reaction of the formaldehyde used during arterial injection with the hemoglobin in the blood, which creates methylhemoglobin. This occurs in cases with poor drainage or when sufficient drainage (blood) is not removed from the body. Aspiration also aids in removing large amounts of blood left within the heart and cavity of the body. Keeping the head elevated above the chest prevents blood from setting out of other parts of the body into the face, which would cause this gray discoloration to appear there. A formaldehyde burn is a raised area that occurs during arterial injection where the capillaries have broken, causing an excessive amount of fluid to enter the tissue. This swelling typically reduces after a few hours; the discoloration can remain depending on the dyes that were used in the arterial injection. Biliverdin is caused by a chemical reaction between the bilirubin within the vascular system and tissue of a decedent and the acidic environment that injection chemicals cause as they bond to the tissues of the body. Postmortem bruising is caused when capillaries are damaged when subjected to pressure (similar to the cause of an antemortem bruise).

97. A: The arch of the aorta has three branches. The first branch is the brachiocephalic artery, which bifurcates into the right subclavian artery and the right common carotid artery. The second branch is the left common carotid artery. The third branch is the left subclavian artery. The aorta then curves down behind the heart, transitioning into the descending aorta, thoracic aorta, and then the abdominal aorta, which bifurcates into the left and right common iliac arteries. The ascending aorta is connected to the left ventricle at the aortic root and transitions into the aortic arch.

98. D: The embalming case report is the all-encompassing written record that includes a drawn sketch diagramming the condition of the body. It identifies the deceased and the embalming practitioner, as well as the chemicals used, the time elapsed, and the funeral home procedures performed. Putrefaction is a term used to describe the decomposition of proteins by diverse enzymes as well as the actions of anaerobic bacteria. It is not the title of a case report. Decomposition is the breakdown of compounds into simpler substances by microbes and autolytic enzymes. The level of decomposition is one finding listed in the embalming case report. Sanitation refers to the documentable efforts to provide for personal and environmental hygiene while working around a deceased body. The body and its immediate environment are unsanitary, and create a hazardous condition that could result in an infection to the embalming practitioner. Sanitation is not addressed in a separate report, but the use of chemicals should be listed in the embalming case report so that there is a record of sanitization efforts.

99. B: Facial width is measured using the width of the eye as a standard. Facial width constitutes the measurement from one ear to the other. This width is equivalent to the width of five eyes. The space between the left and right inner canthi, across the root of the nose, is the width of one eye. The nose at the base is equivalent to the width of one eye. A vertical line can be drawn from either the left or right side of the bridge of the nose to intersect with the respective inner canthus. The mouth is equivalent to the width of two eyes. Vertical measurements can also be correlated to the width of the eye. The ear is two eye widths long. The face is six eye widths long or three ear lengths long.

100. C: The stomach is one of the four organs accessed using trocar guides during the aspiration process.

101. B: A vertical profile has the same amount of protrusion for the forehead, upper lip, and chin. If an imaginary vertical line was held in front of the face, all three of these points would touch it at the same distance. A concave face (least common) has a protrusion at the forehead and the chin, with a recessed upper lip. A convex (most common) profile has the most outward projection at the upper lip; both the forehead and the chin recede back from this projection. To account for a variance in facial profiles, there are 6 combinations of these forms: convex-concave, concave-convex, vertical-convex, vertical-concave, convex-vertical, concave-vertical. The first word designates the shape of the forehead from the eyebrows (recedes, protrudes, or is vertical) while the second designates how the lip and the chin relate in protrusion (the chin recedes, protrudes, or is vertical from the lip).

102. D: The canon of beauty is the standard of perfect proportions that is used to judge and compare the aesthetics of facial features. The canon of beauty depicts an oval face in which the face is two-thirds the length of the face at its widest point. If everyone met the standards set by the cannon of beauty, people would all have the same features. The classic proportions of a face are the divisions in which the face can be segmented into equal and comparable sections. These imaginary lines and measurements, based on the location, length, and/or width of other facial features, aid in reconstructing missing or traumatized features.

103. C: Extremely acidic conditions within the body cause an oxidation chemical reaction, triggering bilirubin (yellow coloration) to convert to biliverdin (green coloration). Formaldehyde used to be thought to cause the discoloration; however, it is the acidic environment that chemicals, including strong formaldehyde mixtures, can cause within the body as it acts as a reducing agent. The chemical reaction between proteins and aldehydes causes hydrogen ions to be released, which allows oxidation to occur. Most jaundice fluids include buffers and modifying agents that help balance the pH to prevent bilirubin from oxidizing into biliverdin. Formaldehyde or glutaraldehyde are used in these specialty fluids at low levels to provide preservation.

104. A: Anastomosis is when two blood vessels connect, either naturally or through a surgical procedure. Naturally occurring anastomoses allow for collateral circulation, providing a secondary source of blood flow to an area in case the primary one is compromised. They are commonly found around joints and in the intestines to ensure there are alternative methods of providing blood flow to areas with increased damage risk. Vasa vasora are the small blood vessels that supply blood and drainage to the layers of larger vessels. They are visibly apparent on larger arteries. Capillaries are the connection between small arteries (arterioles), the tissue of the body, and small veins (venules). An aneurysm is a compromised section of a vascular wall causing an enlarged, weak, and bulging area. Arterial aneurysms are more common, but they do occur in veins also.

105. C: The femoral artery is commonly used as a main injection site in embalming. Although the iliac, ulnar, and aortic arteries are sometimes used, this is uncommon.

106. B: A purse-string suture is a stitch that is used to close a rounded opening. It is made by stitching around the perimeter and pulling the stitches firmly to close the borders of the opening. The basket-weave suture (cross stitch) is a system of stitches that traverses the boundaries of an incision and is used to secure fillers and keep body tissues in place. The bridge stitch (simple interrupted suture) is a transitory suture consisting of independently cut and tied stitches that is used to maintain the location of tissues. The whip stitch is used to secure elongated incisions, such as those made during an autopsy.

107. B: The correct formula is to multiply 128 (the number of ounces per gallon) by the solution percentage (2) and divide that value by the index of the fluid.

108. C: A nasal tube aspirator is a 10" long and 3/16" diameter hollow bore instrument with a 90° curve used to remove fluid or purge from both the nasal and oral cavities. This aspiration instrument, like the trocar, is attached to 3/8-1/2" diameter plastic or rubber tubing, which is connected to the aspiration machine. Aspiration machines can be hydro aspirators or waterless aspirators. Autopsy or post aspirators are straight hollow-bore instruments with a large round, slotted head piece that allows liquid through but prevents fat and other materials from being sucked into the tubing when aspirating the cavity of autopsied bodies. Trocars are long, hollow-bore instruments with sharp points used to remove fluid and gas from the body during aspiration and used to inject cavity fluid into the torso.

109. B: A worm suture is used to close an incision after the embalming (arterial and cavity) is completed by pulling the margins of the incision under as they butt together, creating a hidden, flattened suture. This reduces the uneven edges of the incision or wound to create a smooth finish, eliminating jagged edges by pulling them under. The stitches are made outside of the incision and run parallel to the margins. The stitch enters and exits on the same side of the incision before crossing the incision to start a new stitch on the opposite side. When pulled, the tissue on the margin of the incision is inverted as it is pulled together. An intradermal suture is also a hidden suture, but the stitches run along the interior margin of the incision rather than along the external margin. The purse string suture can be used before or after embalming to close rounded holes or incisions. Once external stitches have been placed in a circular pattern following around the exterior margins of the rounded wound, both ends of the ligature can be pulled to close the hole. A baseball suture is a tight suture commonly used for large incisions like autopsy or donation incisions. The stitch starts on the inside of the incision and is pulled up through the exterior margin, then crosses to the opposite interior and out through the skin. It is pulled tight with each suture.

110. B: If the tissue is not firm and dry, there is no base on which to do the reconstructive work. When sutures will be done and any necessary wax or other restorative substances will be used, a firm and dry base allows these substances to be applied easily and also to retain their shape. This allows them to better perform their purpose.

111. C: A stipple brush, with its stiff and slightly separated tips, can be used to create an appearance similar to pores in the skin. A tapered, flat tip, or pointed brush will not create this effect.

112. C: The kidney is composed of portions that have hollow spaces along with other sections that are solid in nature. The lungs are also composed of both hollow and solid portions. The brain, pancreas, liver, and spleen are all solid organs. Other hollowed viscera include the heart, stomach, urinary bladder, gallbladder, small intestines, and large intestines. Aspiration removes fluid and gas accumulations from hollowed viscera.

113. B: If the body is not properly prepared for refrigeration, the cool, dry air begins to dehydrate the body. Surface dehydration is first seen in the eye lids, lips, and fingertips. Placing the body in plastic body bags or wrapping the body in plastic, rather than cotton sheets, prevents dehydration short-term. Initially, refrigeration is helpful in slowing rigor mortis and quickly cooling the body down. Decomposition is slowed and the blood remains liquified longer. This allows for the blood to more easily gravitate within the vascular system, which makes livor worse. However, this is not an issue immediately because livor mortis is intravascular, so the coloration can be cleared during arterial injection. Extended refrigeration causes significant embalming complications such as coagulated blood, gravitated fluid accumulations, accumulated gas, skin slip, and postmortem staining as the body begins to decompose. Refrigeration slows, but does not prevent, the process of decomposition.

114. B: A frontal view is observed by looking the decedent's face straight on. This allows the embalmer to analyze facial features directly. Bilateral curvatures and differences can be notated from this view. Pictures capturing a direct frontal view are helpful in cases of reconstruction to observe characteristics, facial features, and symmetries. A profile view observes the decedent or a picture from their side profile. A profile picture from both sides is helpful in reconstructions. Inverted views are when the decedent is observed from the head of the table, looking down their face. This change of view allows the embalmer to observe features and characteristics they may have missed using other views. This view can be achieved with a photograph by simply turning it upside down. A three-quarters view is observed when the head is turned at a 45° angle. This view helps establish the proper curvatures and proportions of the cheeks.

115. B: The chemical formula for formaldehyde is $\mathbf{HCHO}$ or $\mathbf{CH_2O}$. Formaldehyde molecules contain a carbon atom that is double-bonded to oxygen and has a single bond with each of the two hydrogens. This small aldehyde contains only one carbon. Formaldehyde is also called *methanal* or *methyl aldehyde*. Aldehydes have a general formula of $\mathbf{R - CHO}$. Dialdehydes have two aldehyde units, which makes their formula $\mathbf{OCH - R - CHO}$. Glutaraldehyde is an example of a dialdehyde with 5 carbons. Alcohols have the general formula of $\mathbf{R - OH}$. The simplest primary alcohol is methanol, or methyl alcohol, which has a formula of $\mathbf{CH_3OH}$. Carboxylic acids, also known as organic acids, have a general formula of $\mathbf{R - COOH}$. The smallest of these is formic acid, which has a formula of $\mathbf{HCOOH}$ or $\mathbf{CH_2O_2}$. Formic acid is created when formaldehyde undergoes oxidation.

116. C: The right and left iliac are exposed and easily accessible for embalming the lower extremities. As such, it is not necessary to use the femoral vessels. The ulnar arteries are usually not injected because they are in the wrist, and embalming of the arms is achieved through the axillary, brachial, or subclavian arteries. The jugular vessels are veins and are not injected; their arterial counterparts are the right and left carotids.

117. A: The zygomaticus major runs from the lateral portion of the zygomatic bone (origin), inferior to the corner of the mouth (insertion). When contracted, the muscle pulls at the corner of the mouth, pulling it superior and posterior (upwards and back). This movement helps create a smile. In structure, this muscle impacts the change of plane from the front to the side of the face. It also aids in creating the nasolabial fold and its projection. The depressor labii inferioris pulls the corner of the mouth inferior and lateral and the depressor anguli oris pulls the angle of the mouth inferiorly when contracted.

118. A: The first thing that needs to be done is to remove the cotton or other absorbent material left in the eye socket by the tissue bank enucleator. This is usually only temporarily absorbent, and has typically spilled out by the time the body is being prepared.

119. C: An aneurism needle is a small, blunt medical apparatus used in embalming. It is commonly used to make incisions into tissues, including the initial incision to raise the carotid artery and jugular vein for injection and drainage. A bistoury knife is a long, pointed medical utensil commonly used for removing excess body tissues. A hemostat or forceps is used to compress blood vessels and limit or prevent blood flow passage or drainage.

120. D: For a muscular suture, the needle enters the mouth between the lip and gums on the left side, enters the nasal cavity through the septum, and goes back into the mouth on the right side. Once the dentures, mouth former, or cotton are in place, the needle is then pushed through the tissue along the mandible where the lower lip meets the gums on the right side, exiting on the left side of the mouth where the lower lip meets the gums. The suture is then tied securely to close the mouth. Keeping the sutures close to the bone will limit puckering along the superior part of the chin. The mandibular suture starts by inserting the needle inside the mouth, at the base of the tongue, and pushing it down, out of the submandibular area of the chin. Using the same hole, the needle is reinserted and guided in front of the mandible, pushing it through inside the mouth where the lower lip meets the gums. This places the suture on each side of the mandible. Then, the dentures or mouth former are inserted. The upper portion of the suture is the same as the upper muscular suture. Entry is at the left side of the mouth, into the nasal cavity, through the septum, and back down into the mouth from the right nostril. The mouth is secured by tying the ends of the suture together. Needle injectors are used to tap in wire tacks, which are then twisted together to secure the mouth. A dental tie is when dental floss or thin ligature is secured to a tooth on the upper jaw and one on the bottom jaw. The two are then tied together to secure the mouth closed.

121. C: Drainage consists of blood, bodily fluids such as lymphatic and interstitial fluids, and arterial solution. Initially drainage consists of blood and its normal contents. As the arterial fluid is injected and distributed throughout the body, it begins to be incorporated into the drainage. Embalming fluid infiltrates the vascular system, entering interstitial space and tissues through the capillaries, pushing interstitial fluid out of the capillaries and back into the venous system where it is drained. Embalming fluid infiltrates the lymphatic system using lymph channels, which connect back to the subclavian veins. Postmortem arterial contractions cause most of the blood to enter the capillaries (85%) and veins (10%), while the rest remains in the arteries (5%). Gravity pulls blood to dependent capillaries, reducing blood in more elevated areas. If drainage becomes pure arterial fluid, the injection has short circuited, with something causing fluid to return at the drainage site rather than being pumped throughout the body.

122. C: Distribution is movement of arterial embalming solution through the body from the injection site to the capillaries where it enters the tissues. Distention is seen as the vascular system re-expands when arterial fluid is injected. These inflated vessels can be an indication of distribution to that area. Diffusion occurs when molecules in a solution of greater concentration move to an area with a lesser concentration until equilibrium is reached. Arterial diffusion in embalming occurs as arterial fluid leaves the capillaries (the intravascular area of higher concentration) and enters the interstitial space, mixing with the naturally present fluids of the body's tissues (the extravascular area of lower concentration). Dilution occurs as the arterial fluid enters the blood stream and interstitial spaces where it mixes with bodily fluids, reducing its concentration.

123. B: Ethically, funeral directors are obligated to provide quality, unjudging, respectful, fair, and dignified professional care to the decedent and their families while abiding by federal and state regulations and legislation. Various organizations involved in the funeral industry have published codes of ethics and standards that funeral homes, funeral directors, and funeral support staff should abide by. Organizations such as the Federal Trade Commission regulate pricing through the Funeral Rule to ensure consumers are being treated fairly and equally.

124. B: The blebs should be ruptured to drain the fluid. The tissue should be patted dry. Topical chemical preservatives should be applied to the areas that have blistered or show signs of blistering. This can be in the form of liquid chemicals or gels. These wraps and packs should stay in place to allow the chemicals to soak into and treat the problematic tissue. When the decedent is ready to be dressed and casketed, the packs should be inspected. Fresh swatches of cotton and plastic wrap should be applied to secure the area. The decedent should then be dressed in plastic garments. Absorptive, deodorizing, and preserving powders should be put inside the plastics to provide additional treatment and protection. Blebs always need to be treated. Bodies with blebs may need to be reaspirated to reduce the amount of fluid in the body. It can also reduce any built-up gas, reducing internal pressure which can lead to blebbing or purging. Reaspirating does not treat or drain blebs that have already formed.

125. B: When a family wants to see the deceased before there is time to do an extensive hair restoration, using a scarf on a woman or a head bandage on a man is an acceptable way to present the deceased. These familiar articles are items that cover injuries or abnormalities. People can relate to a scarf or a bandage more than an inadequate attempt at restoration.

126. B: The temporalis is one of the facial muscles. It is the strongest chewing muscle, and aids in the side-to-side and up-and-down movement of the mandible. The temporal is a bone, not a muscle, of the cranium. The levator labii superioris is the muscle that moves and lifts the upper lip. The corrugators are muscles that move the eyebrow inferiorly and medially. They can also form a frown when they are tightened.

127. D: Hydrolysis is a chemical change that occurs as a result of the introduction of water. Cell walls burst and their water is released. It is a very significant component of tissue decomposition. Vaporization is the term used to describe the transition of liquid matter to gaseous matter. Diffusion refers to the movement of molecules from a region of high measurable concentration to a region of low measurable concentration. Adsorption is the bonding of molecules from a gas or liquid. It is accomplished by passing the molecules over the outer layer of a surface and using filtration to capture the intended molecules.

128. C: All bodies received from another funeral home should be reaspirated, even if they arrived in a casket. They do not need to be completely undressed or removed from the casket unless problematic areas are discovered upon evaluating the body. Evaluations can be done by feel and by looking under clothing. The body can be aspirated while in the casket by pulling up the clothing and shrouding both the body and casket with protective cloths such as towels, thick absorbent sheets, or chuck pads. The nasal and oral cavities should be checked for fluid to ensure that they are clean and dry after traveling. If the body will be held for a few days, massage cream can be applied to the face and hands to prevent or limit dehydration. For extended delays, the body can be refrigerated. Wooden caskets can warp or be damaged in refrigeration. Metal caskets are more tolerant of refrigeration. Ideally, the body should be removed to a dressing table, stretcher, or refrigeration tray when refrigeration is needed.

129. A: Secondary dilution occurs when the arterial fluid enters the body. As the chemicals mix with blood in the vascular system and enter interstitial spaces, mixing with other bodily fluids, it is diluted. Secondary dilution must be factored into the selection of embalming fluid during the case analysis and during primary dilution. Primary dilution is when the embalming fluid is mixed with other coinjections and water in the embalming tank prior to injection. The embalmer mixes fluid anticipating secondary dilution and the needs of the body. An edematous body will require a stronger embalming concentration (less primary dilution) because there will be a greater amount of secondary dilution once the fluid enters the body. An emaciated body without signs of edema may have a greater primary dilution because secondary dilution will be assumed to be less than average.

130. D: In restoration, the cheeks are the focal point for establishing bilateral forms because their prominence and distance between one another varies from one person to another. The cheekbone is used as the transition point from the front of the face to the side of the face. Once the protrusion and distance are determined, all other features can be built. The forehead, chin, lips, nose, and eyes all have bilateral forms. The relationship and comparison between these features (curvatures, distance between each other, and projection) can be used to reconstruct the face and fill in missing or damaged features. The bilateral curvatures and differences can be viewed by looking at the face from a directly inferior or superior position (such as standing above the head and looking straight down at the face).

131. C: Long bone donation is the procurement of the hemipelvis, femur, fibula, and tibia through an incision made from the hip to the ankle. The procurement team will remove the bone and insert a ridged plastic pipe or rod to maintain some form to the legs. Veins, cartilage, tendons, and ligaments are also typically procured in addition to the bones. The vascular system is severely compromised which drastically impacts the embalming process. Some embalmers prefer to open the incision, clamp off disrupted vessels, and inject up the femoral artery or down the right carotid artery. If vasculars such as the popliteal artery are found intact, they can be used to inject the legs, followed by hypodermic treatment to achieve preservation. Other embalmers use a free flow method of injecting through the right common carotid artery. Arterial fluid will be distributed through intact vessels of the leg while free flowing out of disrupted vessels, saturating tissues. After injection is complete, sutures are removed, and the excess fluid is drained out. Hypodermic treatment is performed, embalming powders or gels are applied, and the incision is re-sutured. Additional bone procurements can involve the humerus, humeral head, proximal humerus, scapula, ribs, vertebra, and temporal bone.

132. A: Agonal hypostasis is a symptomatic progression by which blood pools and settles in the lowest parts of the body as a result of gravity. Hemolysis occurs when the walls of red blood cells are broken down and the hemoglobin they contain is released. Intermittent drainage (restricted drainage) is a method of drainage used during embalming that stops and starts the drainage at intervals while embalming fluid is being injected. Algor mortis is a condition that occurs after a person is deceased. There is a progression of temperature reduction as the temperature of the body decreases.

133. C: The left and right jugular are veins. They are not used for injection, but for drainage.

134. C: Prior to beginning an embalming, an evaluation of the body must be conducted to determine what methods and approaches will be used. Rigor mortis is noticeable upon observation of the body prior to beginning embalming. As the body is positioned and prepared for injection, it should be massaged and stretched out. Distention and drainage are observations made during the arterial injection that will determine if the embalming methods need to be readjusted to ensure proper distribution and preservation. Arteriosclerosis is not a preembalming consideration because it is discovered or observed once vessels are raised. It impacts distribution, leading the multipoint injections. Intrinsic factors considered during the preembalming analysis are internal influences such as the condition of the body (e.g., pathologies, microbial activity, moisture level, weight, gas, musculature), discolorations, chemicals/drugs (medical or illegal), and postmortem changes (e.g., algor mortis, hypostasis, rigor mortis, or postmortem staining). These are either determined from observation of the body or from information gathered from medical staff, family, and the death certificate. Extrinsic factors that influence the preembalming analysis are outside, environmental influences such as temperature, microbial activity from outside sources (not internal microbial activity), and time between death and embalming.

135. D: Potential pressure is the pressure level within the tubing connected to the embalming machine when it is turned on "inject" but the stopcock or rate of flow valve remains closed. Actual pressure is the force shown on the embalming machine pressure gauge when embalming fluid is being pumped through the body during arterial injection (the stopcock is open). The injection pressure is the level of pressure that counters vascular resistance; this is different throughout the body and not the same amount of pressure measured by the embalming machine gauge. Differential pressure is the calculation of rate of flow (potential pressure minus actual pressure).

136. D: The angulus oris eminence is a natural face marking that consists of a comparatively undersized, convex, raised area found lateral to the end of the line of closure of the mouth. The angulus oris sulcus is a natural facial marking groove found at each end of the line of closure of the mouth. The frontal process of the maxilla is the raised part of the upper jaw that protrudes slightly as it rises alongside the nasal bone to meet the frontal bone in the upper jaw. The frontal eminences are a pair of distinctive raised areas of the frontal bone found roughly one inch beneath the normal hairline.

137. B: The final stage of embalming analysis is the postinjection evaluations made based on the embalmer's observations. During this evaluation, the embalmer will determine what additional treatments are needed to ensure that the body is properly and sufficiently preserved and that the body looks pleasing. Treatments after observation can include hypodermic treatment to areas lacking sufficient preservation; resetting features if needed; purge prevention; hair and nail care; applying compresses to decubitus ulcers, skin slip, and wounds; and suturing and glueing areas as needed once leaking has been stopped. The three stages of embalming analysis are preembalming analysis (before embalming begins), injection analysis (during injection), and postinjection analysis (after arterial injection).

138. A: The equation used to determine primary dilution is:

$$\text{Index} \times \text{Volume of arterial fluid} = \text{Strength of solution} \times \text{Total solution volume}$$

When calculating how many ounces of arterial fluid are needed per gallon, the total solution volume is 128 oz (there are 128 oz in a gallon). In the scenario above, the calculation is: $20 \times Y = 2 \times 128$. In solving for the volume of arterial fluid, represented by Y, 128 oz is multiplied by 2 (2% solution), then divided by 20 (Index) to determine how many ounces of arterial fluid are needed per gallon of solution. Therefore, $Y = 12.8$ oz. If the embalming machine holds 3 gallons of fluid and a full tank is being mixed, the embalmer could calculate the number of ounces of arterial fluid required for the entire 3-gallon tank: 3 gallons equals 384 oz, multiplied by 2 to create a 2% solution is 768, which is then divided by 20, equaling 38.4 total ounces of arterial fluid.

139. A: It is recommended not to use a preinjection solution on decedents who have had an eye enucleation. The additional fluid can lead to swelling of the orbital cavity and tissue without adding any preservation qualities. Disrupted vasculature and traumatized tissues have an increased likelihood of swelling. Fluid follows the path of least resistance, so these traumatized areas receive more fluid than intact tissues, which have natural resistance and structure. Restricted cervical injections are recommended to allow more control over the fluid entering and draining from the head. They also provide the opportunity to inject the head and the body with different chemical mixtures. A slightly stronger solution is recommended to ensure that sufficient preservation reaches the damaged areas. Unnecessary movement should be avoided around the orbital cavity and tissue so not to further irritate the area. The rate of flow and injection pressure should be reduced to attempt to prevent swelling of the traumatized area.

140. D: Other embalmers who are in the room doing other work are allowed. Most states have laws that allow a medical doctor to observe the embalming process and even a member of the deceased's family. Any non-licensed people are prohibited, including the embalmer's husband or wife.

141. D: A hemothorax is when blood pools in the pleural cavity, typically as a result of an injury. Epistaxis is a bloody nose that occurs when blood pools in the nasal region. Hemopericardium is the condition in which blood pools in the pericardial sac of the heart muscle, and is often seen in an autopsy. Hemoperitoneum is the condition that occurs when blood collects in the peritoneal cavity.

142. B: Blood clots and coagulates can be removed from the heart and venous system. Arterial coagulants are not able to be pushed through the smaller arteries (arterioles) and capillaries.

Coinjection chemicals can aid in dissolving some of these coagulants so fluid can pass through the capillaries, but masses of clots and blood will not pass through them. Coagulants and clots move through veins more easily because veins increase in size as fluid is moved towards the heart. As arteries travel away from the heart, they decrease in size, which limits and restricts the movement of coagulants.

143. D: The most common nasal profile is the straight profile. It consists of a straight dorsum (anterior ridge) that can be classified as long, short, low tip or high tip. A convex or Roman nose has a bumped-up area along its dorsum length. The concave nasal form is when an area of the dorsum dips.

144. D: A funeral director can never refuse a viewing or identification viewing regardless of the disposition type selected by the family or condition of the body. Identification viewings for the next of kin should be encouraged and supported when disposition by cremation is selected. Identifying the deceased prior to cremation reduces the liability of the funeral home, ensuring that they have the proper person in their care. A funeral director can strongly suggest that the next of kin or other family members not see the body prior to disposition when there is extreme trauma or advanced decomposition. Identification in these cases is established by investigative parties such as police, coroners, or medical examiners. When a family member insists on a viewing or an identification viewing (with or without embalming) in these cases, the funeral director should do their best to restore features and stabilize the body to limit the duress a viewing may cause. Barriers such as stanchions can be used to keep the family at a distance; sheer or lace drapes can be used to conceal and partially shield the view of the decedent to hide and distort traumatic and restoration areas; a viewing window can be used to look at the deceased from another room; or partial viewings where only a portion of the body that has minimal trauma (a hand, a tattoo, etc.) can be used. A disclosure, indemnification, and waiver document should be signed by the family members who want to see the decedent to hold the funeral home and staff harmless for emotional duress and trauma that may be caused by viewing the body.

145. A: Phalanges are the numerous bones of the fingers and toes. The phalanges of the foot are the bones that make up the toes and the phalanges of the hand are the bones that constitute the fingers.

146. B: Intermittent drainage is when drainage is periodically closed while arterial fluid is being actively injected. Closing the drainage during injection can be a way to build pressure within the body to force fluid through areas subject to increased vascular resistance or when there are a lot of clots that need more pressure to push out. Concurrent drainage is continuous drainage throughout arterial injection. Alternate drainage is when drainage is opened when injection is turned off and then closed when the injection is restarted. Full body donation cases are typically embalmed by medical facilities without any drainage.

147. A: Cells are the basis of all living things. Cells are small life forms which function individually (single-celled organism) or as a group of cells in larger, more complex organisms. The human body is composed of trillions of cells, all of which vary in shape, size, structure, and function. The components of a cell consist of the plasma membrane, cytoplasm, nucleus, and organelles. Atoms are the smallest part of a chemical which cannot be broken down any smaller. Protons are positively charged particles in the nucleus of an atom. Molecules are one or more chemically bonded atoms.

148. C: Plastic garments that encase most of the body, covering the legs, arms, buttocks, back, and shoulders, and have a zipper closure along the chest are called unionalls. Coveralls are extended plastic pants, covering the body from midthigh to the midchest and midback. Capris are plastics that are a combination of stockings and pants, covering the feet, legs, and buttocks. Shirts are plastics that are used to contain the arms, shoulders, and trunk of the body. They have a front zipper just like unionalls. Shirts have an elastic band that rests on the body just above the waist.

149. B: Although the circle of Willis is exposed, it is the name of a formation of arteries and is not an opening. The foramen magnum is the large opening exposed at the base of the skull, where it meets the spinal cord.

150. B: Enzymes are chemical compounds that help to catalyze (speed up) chemical reactions in the body. They are also referred to as catalytic enzymes. Autolytic enzymes are produced by the body to break down cells and continue to function even after the body has died. Digestive enzymes help to break down food. Microbial enzymes are created by microorganisms such as bacteria and fungi.

151. A: Inactive dyes have no impact on the body's tissue coloration during embalming. The colors are just used so the embalmer can easily distinguish between the chemicals. Active dyes within the arterial fluid will deposit coloration to the tissues of the body. Active dyes can be in arterial fluid, or they can be a separate additive to the embalming mixture. Cosmetic dyes are active dyes in the form of active dyes in arterial fluid, supplementary active dye additives used in arterial injection, or active dyes within cosmetic products that will impact the color of the tissue through topical application (translucent tints and tinted creams).

152. C: The next of kin should be asked what they want to do with the flowers that are at the service. If there is an evening visitation, the family is typically asked after the visitation how they want the flowers handled. They may want specific flowers to be taken to the church, cemetery, family house, donated, or left at the funeral home to come back and get later. The family may also have flowers they would like to place inside the casket or remain in the casket following the viewing. Just like with personal belongings, jewelry, pictures, and memory items, the funeral director must ask the family what they would like done with them. Nothing can be assumed. For example, a casket spray typically stays at the graveside, however, a family may decide they want to take it home and use it as a center piece or break it into smaller arrangements for each of the children. Funeral homes often make a flower book for the family detailing the colors, flowers, and type of arrangements. Some flower books include the card and even a picture of the flower arrangement.

153. C: The standard insertion point of the trocar during aspiration is 2 inches superior and 2 inches to the anatomical left of the umbilicus. Using this location for insertion allows access to areas throughout the thoracic, abdominal, and pelvic cavities. The trocar can also be extended up into the neck from this point. If a point of entry 2 inches superior and 2 inches to the anatomical right of the umbilicus were used, the trocar would directly enter the solid tissue of the liver, making mobility more difficult. Aspirating someone who is morbidly obese may require an adjustment to the point of entry, or even need two points of entry, to sufficiently aspirate and treat all areas of the torso.

154. A: Postmortem clots have multicolored layers. The dark layer is composed of red blood cells and is dark in color. Gravity pulls the blood to the dependent areas of the vessel to form this layer. The top layer is composed of a jellied fibrin layer. Postmortem coagula consist of congealed blood cells stuck together to form a large, dark mass. Antemortem clots are repeating layers of platelets and fibrins that are formed during life. A thrombus or embolism are examples of antemortem clots.

155. B: An embalming case report should be completed for every decedent who enters the care of the funeral home whether they are embalmed or not. This form is used to document the condition of the body as it arrived to the funeral home; any treatments conducted, embalming or otherwise (e.g., aspirating or setting features for an identification viewing); postembalming treatments; and information about the funeral home, transfer team, embalmer, and decedent (name, date of death, cause of death, transfer information, possessions). Information should be documented in detail in all applicable sections and retained by the funeral home in the case file of the decedent. When transferred to another funeral home, a copy of the embalming case report should accompany the decedent. Embalming case reports have immense value for cases that end up going to court for any number of reasons (e.g., malpractice, alleged abuse, criminal trials, disinterments).

156. A: The right hypochondriac region of the nine abdominal regions is located on the upper right side of the grid. It contains a portion of the liver, kidney, greater omentum, small intestine, and the entire gallbladder. The nine regions divide the abdomen into nine sections by visualizing two vertical lines that extend up from the left and right midpoint of the iliac spine and the pubic symphysis and two horizontal lines; one that extends from the inferior margin of the 10th intercostal cartilage, and a lower line that extends from the iliac crest.

157. A: Infants, from birth to 18 months old, have delicate skin, more moisture within their tissues than older children and adults, small vasculature, and can present more accessibility challenges than older children and adults. Moisture within their tissues can increase with pathological conditions and treatments. As people age, moisture throughout the body continues to decrease. Infants have softer gum tissue, so needle injectors should not be used. As people age, they regress back to having soft gum tissue, especially in cases where teeth have been removed or lost. Although more difficult to access and smaller than adult cases, the common carotid and femoral arteries are usable primary injection sites in unautopsied infant cases. The abdominal aorta or ascending aorta can be used but accessibility is challenging, as this requires navigating the intestines or sternum.

158. B: Personal effects should be inventoried when the decedent arrives at the funeral home. Items should be documented on a personal possessions form in detail. Sheets and soiled clothing should be laundered prior to returning to the family. If the clothing is soiled beyond cleaning or was damaged in death or with the efforts of medical professionals, it should be documented and disposed of with biohazardous waste. Return of personal effects to the legal next of kin needs to be documented on this inventory record. Some funeral homes require the family to sign this form at the time they receive the possessions back. Always secure permission for transfer from the next of kin *prior* to transferring them into the care of the funeral home. Embalming or preparation for an identification viewing can be done once permission is received from the family.

159. B: Putrefaction is the decomposition of proteins. Proteins play an immense role in bodily structure and function, being primary components in skin, hair, nails, ligaments, tendons, cartilage, and connective tissue. Peptide bonds link two proteins together. Proteases are catalytic enzymes that break down these protein bonds during decomposition. Hydrolysis is a chemical reaction that triggers decomposition by breaking down a compound into smaller compounds or molecules when water is introduced. Deterioration of protein creates amino acids. Protein degradation significantly impacts embalming; the more amino acids, the more formaldehyde is required to achieve preservation because formaldehyde will bond with the amino acids. Fermentation is the decomposition of glucose (carbohydrates), resulting in organic acid. The breakdown of carbohydrates in the body does not produce enough organic acid to significantly impact embalming.

160. D: Kaposi's sarcoma is most often seen in those with AIDS. Though the reason for the correlation is unclear, it may be because of the breakdown of the immune system.

161. A: The four major types of preservatives used in embalming fluids are formaldehyde, aldehydes, alcohols, and phenols. Sterols are macrobiotic molecules that are present in plants and animals; they are not a preservative used in embalming fluid. Lipids (fats) are organic compounds present in plants and animals and are insoluble in water. They are an important part of cell membranes, but are not used as preservatives in embalming fluid.

162. A: When hemolysis of red blood cells occurs in a decedent and the result is post-mortem stain, the coloration made inside the body is referred to as *endogenous*. Fomites are non-living objects such as forks, countertops, door knobs, etc. They may have microorganisms on them left by a host that can be indirectly passed to another host. Atrophy is the condition that is characterized by a reduction in size or shrinking of a muscle or a part of the body. Exogenous pigments are those that originate from outside the location they infiltrate.

163. C: The head of a decedent should be kept in a straight position or angled 15° to the left. Funeral homes each have their own preference for which position they prefer. This positioning needs to occur when the body is positioned on the table prior to beginning the embalming process. The body will then fixate in the position the head is directed. The angle selected for the head will also factor in any trauma, swelling, or characteristics of the decedent that may need to be obscured. If there is trauma to the left side of the face, the head is kept straight or angled slightly to the left. Trauma on the viewing side may cause the angle to be increased slightly to the right. In cases with significant trauma to the right side of the face, the decedent may be reversed in the casket (full couch) or placed in a reversed-cap casket (half couch). Some caskets have tilting mechanisms for the interior bed to help position and angle decedents once they are casketed. Props and pillows can be used to angle or tilt the decedent in caskets that do not have a tiltable bed.

164. D: Leucopenia (also spelled leukopenia) is a condition in which a person has a diminished white blood cell count, so there is a decrease in the number of infection-fighting cells (leukocytes) in the blood. Hemophilia is a condition characterized by the failure of one's blood to clot appropriately. Leukemia is a form of cancer in which uncharacteristically high numbers of white blood cells are produced in undeveloped forms, meaning the blood and/or bone marrow are not functioning properly. Polycythemia is a condition characterized by an atypical amplification of the number of red blood cells or total red blood cell volume.

165. B: The external auditory meatus is the external opening into the ear canal. It is not seen from either the side profile or frontal view because it is posterior and medial to the tragus. The tragus is a small protrusion of cartilage originating off the cheek and extending over the external auditory meatus with a rounded edge. The external auditory meatus is the starting point in reconstructing the ear, aiding in proper placement. The opening is immediately inferior to the zygomatic arch, which is the midpoint for the length of the ear. The concha is the concave area directly superior to the external auditory meatus and inferior to the crus. The helix is the outer, external rim of the ear beginning at the crus, superior to the concha and external auditory meatus, and extending around and down the external ear to the lobe.

166. A: Somatic death occurs throughout the whole body when physiological and metabolic function is not able to be maintained. *Agonal*, which originates from the word *agony*, is used for the period of time prior to death or the process of dying. During the agonal period, the body increasingly loses the ability to support metabolic and physiological function. Somatic death can be broken down into three stages. Clinical death occurs first when respiration and the heart stop self-regulating; this is reversible with medical intervention. Brain death occurs following the cessation of respiration and heart function. Biological death is the death of smaller cells throughout the body tissues and organs. Some take more time to die than others, depending on their natural store of nutrients and oxygen. Brain and nerve cells take an average of five minutes, while muscle cells take 3 hours and cornea and blood cells take 6 hours.

167. D: Bacillus bacteria are typically shaped like cylindrical rods. Bacillus is one of the three general categories of bacteria based on their cellular shape. Vibrio bacteria have a curved shape. Vibrio is a sub-classification of the spiral group. Coccus bacteria typically have a spherical shape.

168. A: Organic chemistry focuses on analyzing carbon and carbon-based compounds and studying their properties, function, structures, and interactions. These compounds are found within living organisms. Inorganic chemistry focuses on the study of materials, gases, and elements that are not naturally occurring in living organisms. Biochemistry studies normal and pathological chemical qualities, functions, and interactions within living organisms. Physical chemistry studies chemicals at an atomic and molecular level.

169. B: Anatomical guides are when structures within the body are used to locate and identify other proximally located structures. When raising vessels, anatomical guides help the embalmer know if vessels are medial, deep, lateral, or superficial to the structure they have identified as their guide. Recognizing guides and surrounding structures to vessels will increase the proficiency of the embalmer. Linear guides are imaginary lines that the embalmer visualizes on the surface of the decedent to mark out internal anatomical structures, such as vessels. Anatomical limits are where a structure starts and ends, transitioning into or connecting to other structures.

170. A: Although syphilis can be contracted through kissing, placental transmission, and blood transfusions, approximately 95% of cases are due to sexual intercourse involving direct contact with the fluids or lesions of an infected individual.

Funeral Practice Tests #2 and #3

To take these additional practice tests, visit our online resources page:
mometrix.com/resources719/funeral

How to Overcome Test Anxiety

Just the thought of taking a test is enough to make most people a little nervous. A test is an important event that can have a long-term impact on your future, so it's important to take it seriously and it's natural to feel anxious about performing well. But just because anxiety is normal, that doesn't mean that it's helpful in test taking, or that you should simply accept it as part of your life. Anxiety can have a variety of effects. These effects can be mild, like making you feel slightly nervous, or severe, like blocking your ability to focus or remember even a simple detail.

If you experience test anxiety—whether severe or mild—it's important to know how to beat it. To discover this, first you need to understand what causes test anxiety.

Causes of Test Anxiety

While we often think of anxiety as an uncontrollable emotional state, it can actually be caused by simple, practical things. One of the most common causes of test anxiety is that a person does not feel adequately prepared for their test. This feeling can be the result of many different issues such as poor study habits or lack of organization, but the most common culprit is time management. Starting to study too late, failing to organize your study time to cover all of the material, or being distracted while you study will mean that you're not well prepared for the test. This may lead to cramming the night before, which will cause you to be physically and mentally exhausted for the test. Poor time management also contributes to feelings of stress, fear, and hopelessness as you realize you are not well prepared but don't know what to do about it.

Other times, test anxiety is not related to your preparation for the test but comes from unresolved fear. This may be a past failure on a test, or poor performance on tests in general. It may come from comparing yourself to others who seem to be performing better or from the stress of living up to expectations. Anxiety may be driven by fears of the future—how failure on this test would affect your educational and career goals. These fears are often completely irrational, but they can still negatively impact your test performance.

Elements of Test Anxiety

As mentioned earlier, test anxiety is considered to be an emotional state, but it has physical and mental components as well. Sometimes you may not even realize that you are suffering from test anxiety until you notice the physical symptoms. These can include trembling hands, rapid heartbeat, sweating, nausea, and tense muscles. Extreme anxiety may lead to fainting or vomiting. Obviously, any of these symptoms can have a negative impact on testing. It is important to recognize them as soon as they begin to occur so that you can address the problem before it damages your performance.

The mental components of test anxiety include trouble focusing and inability to remember learned information. During a test, your mind is on high alert, which can help you recall information and stay focused for an extended period of time. However, anxiety interferes with your mind's natural processes, causing you to blank out, even on the questions you know well. The strain of testing during anxiety makes it difficult to stay focused, especially on a test that may take several hours. Extreme anxiety can take a huge mental toll, making it difficult not only to recall test information but even to understand the test questions or pull your thoughts together.

Effects of Test Anxiety

Test anxiety is like a disease—if left untreated, it will get progressively worse. Anxiety leads to poor performance, and this reinforces the feelings of fear and failure, which in turn lead to poor performances on subsequent tests. It can grow from a mild nervousness to a crippling condition. If allowed to progress, test anxiety can have a big impact on your schooling, and consequently on your future.

Test anxiety can spread to other parts of your life. Anxiety on tests can become anxiety in any stressful situation, and blanking on a test can turn into panicking in a job situation. But fortunately, you don't have to let anxiety rule your testing and determine your grades. There are a number of relatively simple steps you can take to move past anxiety and function normally on a test and in the rest of life.

Physical Steps for Beating Test Anxiety

While test anxiety is a serious problem, the good news is that it can be overcome. It doesn't have to control your ability to think and remember information. While it may take time, you can begin taking steps today to beat anxiety.

Just as your first hint that you may be struggling with anxiety comes from the physical symptoms, the first step to treating it is also physical. Rest is crucial for having a clear, strong mind. If you are tired, it is much easier to give in to anxiety. But if you establish good sleep habits, your body and mind will be ready to perform optimally, without the strain of exhaustion. Additionally, sleeping well helps you to retain information better, so you're more likely to recall the answers when you see the test questions.

Getting good sleep means more than going to bed on time. It's important to allow your brain time to relax. Take study breaks from time to time so it doesn't get overworked, and don't study right before bed. Take time to rest your mind before trying to rest your body, or you may find it difficult to fall asleep.

Along with sleep, other aspects of physical health are important in preparing for a test. Good nutrition is vital for good brain function. Sugary foods and drinks may give a burst of energy but this burst is followed by a crash, both physically and emotionally. Instead, fuel your body with protein and vitamin-rich foods.

Also, drink plenty of water. Dehydration can lead to headaches and exhaustion, especially if your brain is already under stress from the rigors of the test. Particularly if your test is a long one, drink water during the breaks. And if possible, take an energy-boosting snack to eat between sections.

Along with sleep and diet, a third important part of physical health is exercise. Maintaining a steady workout schedule is helpful, but even taking 5-minute study breaks to walk can help get your blood pumping faster and clear your head. Exercise also releases endorphins, which contribute to a positive feeling and can help combat test anxiety.

When you nurture your physical health, you are also contributing to your mental health. If your body is healthy, your mind is much more likely to be healthy as well. So take time to rest, nourish your body with healthy food and water, and get moving as much as possible. Taking these physical steps will make you stronger and more able to take the mental steps necessary to overcome test anxiety.

Mental Steps for Beating Test Anxiety

Working on the mental side of test anxiety can be more challenging, but as with the physical side, there are clear steps you can take to overcome it. As mentioned earlier, test anxiety often stems from lack of preparation, so the obvious solution is to prepare for the test. Effective studying may be the most important weapon you have for beating test anxiety, but you can and should employ several other mental tools to combat fear.

First, boost your confidence by reminding yourself of past success—tests or projects that you aced. If you're putting as much effort into preparing for this test as you did for those, there's no reason you should expect to fail here. Work hard to prepare; then trust your preparation.

Second, surround yourself with encouraging people. It can be helpful to find a study group, but be sure that the people you're around will encourage a positive attitude. If you spend time with others who are anxious or cynical, this will only contribute to your own anxiety. Look for others who are motivated to study hard from a desire to succeed, not from a fear of failure.

Third, reward yourself. A test is physically and mentally tiring, even without anxiety, and it can be helpful to have something to look forward to. Plan an activity following the test, regardless of the outcome, such as going to a movie or getting ice cream.

When you are taking the test, if you find yourself beginning to feel anxious, remind yourself that you know the material. Visualize successfully completing the test. Then take a few deep, relaxing breaths and return to it. Work through the questions carefully but with confidence, knowing that you are capable of succeeding.

Developing a healthy mental approach to test taking will also aid in other areas of life. Test anxiety affects more than just the actual test—it can be damaging to your mental health and even contribute to depression. It's important to beat test anxiety before it becomes a problem for more than testing.

Study Strategy

Being prepared for the test is necessary to combat anxiety, but what does being prepared look like? You may study for hours on end and still not feel prepared. What you need is a strategy for test prep. The next few pages outline our recommended steps to help you plan out and conquer the challenge of preparation.

Step 1: Scope Out the Test

Learn everything you can about the format (multiple choice, essay, etc.) and what will be on the test. Gather any study materials, course outlines, or sample exams that may be available. Not only will this help you to prepare, but knowing what to expect can help to alleviate test anxiety.

Step 2: Map Out the Material

Look through the textbook or study guide and make note of how many chapters or sections it has. Then divide these over the time you have. For example, if a book has 15 chapters and you have five days to study, you need to cover three chapters each day. Even better, if you have the time, leave an extra day at the end for overall review after you have gone through the material in depth.

If time is limited, you may need to prioritize the material. Look through it and make note of which sections you think you already have a good grasp on, and which need review. While you are studying, skim quickly through the familiar sections and take more time on the challenging parts.

Write out your plan so you don't get lost as you go. Having a written plan also helps you feel more in control of the study, so anxiety is less likely to arise from feeling overwhelmed at the amount to cover.

Step 3: Gather Your Tools

Decide what study method works best for you. Do you prefer to highlight in the book as you study and then go back over the highlighted portions? Or do you type out notes of the important information? Or is it helpful to make flashcards that you can carry with you? Assemble the pens, index cards, highlighters, post-it notes, and any other materials you may need so you won't be distracted by getting up to find things while you study.

If you're having a hard time retaining the information or organizing your notes, experiment with different methods. For example, try color-coding by subject with colored pens, highlighters, or post-it notes. If you learn better by hearing, try recording yourself reading your notes so you can listen while in the car, working out, or simply sitting at your desk. Ask a friend to quiz you from your flashcards, or try teaching someone the material to solidify it in your mind.

Step 4: Create Your Environment

It's important to avoid distractions while you study. This includes both the obvious distractions like visitors and the subtle distractions like an uncomfortable chair (or a too-comfortable couch that makes you want to fall asleep). Set up the best study environment possible: good lighting and a comfortable work area. If background music helps you focus, you may want to turn it on, but otherwise keep the room quiet. If you are using a computer to take notes, be sure you don't have any other windows open, especially applications like social media, games, or anything else that could distract you. Silence your phone and turn off notifications. Be sure to keep water close by so you stay hydrated while you study (but avoid unhealthy drinks and snacks).

Also, take into account the best time of day to study. Are you freshest first thing in the morning? Try to set aside some time then to work through the material. Is your mind clearer in the afternoon or evening? Schedule your study session then. Another method is to study at the same time of day that you will take the test, so that your brain gets used to working on the material at that time and will be ready to focus at test time.

Step 5: Study!

Once you have done all the study preparation, it's time to settle into the actual studying. Sit down, take a few moments to settle your mind so you can focus, and begin to follow your study plan. Don't give in to distractions or let yourself procrastinate. This is your time to prepare so you'll be ready to fearlessly approach the test. Make the most of the time and stay focused.

Of course, you don't want to burn out. If you study too long you may find that you're not retaining the information very well. Take regular study breaks. For example, taking five minutes out of every hour to walk briskly, breathing deeply and swinging your arms, can help your mind stay fresh.

As you get to the end of each chapter or section, it's a good idea to do a quick review. Remind yourself of what you learned and work on any difficult parts. When you feel that you've mastered the material, move on to the next part. At the end of your study session, briefly skim through your notes again.

But while review is helpful, cramming last minute is NOT. If at all possible, work ahead so that you won't need to fit all your study into the last day. Cramming overloads your brain with more information than it can process and retain, and your tired mind may struggle to recall even previously learned information when it is overwhelmed with last-minute study. Also, the urgent nature of cramming and the stress placed on your brain contribute to anxiety. You'll be more likely to go to the test feeling unprepared and having trouble thinking clearly.

So don't cram, and don't stay up late before the test, even just to review your notes at a leisurely pace. Your brain needs rest more than it needs to go over the information again. In fact, plan to finish your studies by noon or early afternoon the day before the test. Give your brain the rest of the day to relax or focus on other things, and get a good night's sleep. Then you will be fresh for the test and better able to recall what you've studied.

STEP 6: TAKE A PRACTICE TEST

Many courses offer sample tests, either online or in the study materials. This is an excellent resource to check whether you have mastered the material, as well as to prepare for the test format and environment.

Check the test format ahead of time: the number of questions, the type (multiple choice, free response, etc.), and the time limit. Then create a plan for working through them. For example, if you have 30 minutes to take a 60-question test, your limit is 30 seconds per question. Spend less time on the questions you know well so that you can take more time on the difficult ones.

If you have time to take several practice tests, take the first one open book, with no time limit. Work through the questions at your own pace and make sure you fully understand them. Gradually work up to taking a test under test conditions: sit at a desk with all study materials put away and set a timer. Pace yourself to make sure you finish the test with time to spare and go back to check your answers if you have time.

After each test, check your answers. On the questions you missed, be sure you understand why you missed them. Did you misread the question (tests can use tricky wording)? Did you forget the information? Or was it something you hadn't learned? Go back and study any shaky areas that the practice tests reveal.

Taking these tests not only helps with your grade, but also aids in combating test anxiety. If you're already used to the test conditions, you're less likely to worry about it, and working through tests until you're scoring well gives you a confidence boost. Go through the practice tests until you feel comfortable, and then you can go into the test knowing that you're ready for it.

Test Tips

On test day, you should be confident, knowing that you've prepared well and are ready to answer the questions. But aside from preparation, there are several test day strategies you can employ to maximize your performance.

First, as stated before, get a good night's sleep the night before the test (and for several nights before that, if possible). Go into the test with a fresh, alert mind rather than staying up late to study.

Try not to change too much about your normal routine on the day of the test. It's important to eat a nutritious breakfast, but if you normally don't eat breakfast at all, consider eating just a protein bar. If you're a coffee drinker, go ahead and have your normal coffee. Just make sure you time it so that the caffeine doesn't wear off right in the middle of your test. Avoid sugary beverages, and drink enough water to stay hydrated but not so much that you need a restroom break 10 minutes into the test. If your test isn't first thing in the morning, consider going for a walk or doing a light workout before the test to get your blood flowing.

Allow yourself enough time to get ready, and leave for the test with plenty of time to spare so you won't have the anxiety of scrambling to arrive in time. Another reason to be early is to select a good seat. It's helpful to sit away from doors and windows, which can be distracting. Find a good seat, get out your supplies, and settle your mind before the test begins.

When the test begins, start by going over the instructions carefully, even if you already know what to expect. Make sure you avoid any careless mistakes by following the directions.

Then begin working through the questions, pacing yourself as you've practiced. If you're not sure on an answer, don't spend too much time on it, and don't let it shake your confidence. Either skip it and come back later, or eliminate as many wrong answers as possible and guess among the remaining ones. Don't dwell on these questions as you continue—put them out of your mind and focus on what lies ahead.

Be sure to read all of the answer choices, even if you're sure the first one is the right answer. Sometimes you'll find a better one if you keep reading. But don't second-guess yourself if you do immediately know the answer. Your gut instinct is usually right. Don't let test anxiety rob you of the information you know.

If you have time at the end of the test (and if the test format allows), go back and review your answers. Be cautious about changing any, since your first instinct tends to be correct, but make sure you didn't misread any of the questions or accidentally mark the wrong answer choice. Look over any you skipped and make an educated guess.

At the end, leave the test feeling confident. You've done your best, so don't waste time worrying about your performance or wishing you could change anything. Instead, celebrate the successful completion of this test. And finally, use this test to learn how to deal with anxiety even better next time.

Review Video: Test Anxiety
Visit mometrix.com/academy and enter code: 100340

Important Qualification

Not all anxiety is created equal. If your test anxiety is causing major issues in your life beyond the classroom or testing center, or if you are experiencing troubling physical symptoms related to your anxiety, it may be a sign of a serious physiological or psychological condition. If this sounds like your situation, we strongly encourage you to seek professional help.

Online Resources

Due to our efforts to try to keep this book to a manageable length, we've created a link that will give you access to all of your online resources:

mometrix.com/resources719/funeral

It's Your Moment, Let's Celebrate It!

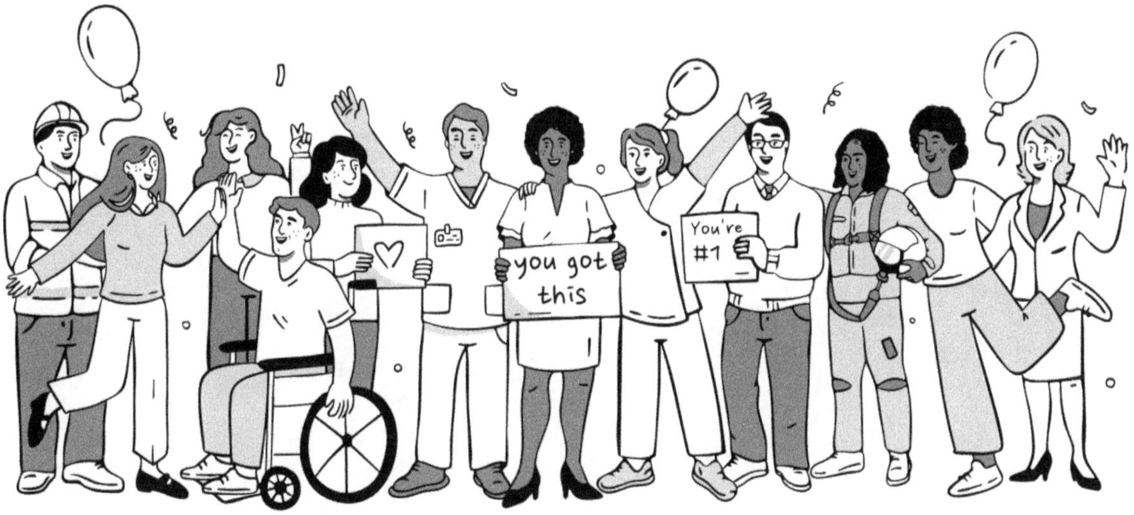

Share your story @mometrixtestpreparation

www.ingramcontent.com/pod-product-compliance
Lightning Source LLC
LaVergne TN
LVHW062147200926
848484LV00007B/1877